Trauma and Resilience in Contemporary Australian Policing

Andrew Paterson

Trauma and Resilience in Contemporary Australian Policing

Is PTS Inevitable for First Responders?

Springer

Andrew Paterson
Chandlers Hill, SA, Australia

ISBN 978-981-16-4415-3 ISBN 978-981-16-4416-0 (eBook)
https://doi.org/10.1007/978-981-16-4416-0

This Springer imprint is published by the registered company Springer Nature Singapore Pte Ltd.
The registered company address is: 152 Beach Road, #21-01/04 Gateway East, Singapore 189721, Singapore

Prologue

My Experience of Trauma

I began my first postgraduate degree in social work at the end of 1973. I took 12 months to complete the Postgraduate Bachelor of Social Administration degree and during that time was offered part-time work by the then Department for Community Welfare.[1] The Department was interested in me supervising a group of young offenders who lived in the Adelaide City square mile who were also known to be using illicit drugs. I accepted the position half time to begin with and later went full time as time permitted. The young men were challenging and as I was at the beginning of my social work career, I focused on engaging with them and their families in order to offer them opportunities for rehabilitation at an early stage in their criminal careers.

Crisis Care Unit and SAPOL

After 12 months in that role, I learnt about the possibility of the establishment of Crisis Care Unit. Crisis Care was a bold and unique innovation on the part of the Department for Community Welfare and South Australian Police. The objective was to establish a 24-hour, 7 days a week Crisis Intervention Program staffed by psychology and social work graduates who worked predominately with the police in responding to domestic violence. The unit—once established—was intended to offer on-the-spot services to police patrols who had attended domestic violence incidents and requested the attendance of Crisis Care staff. These were the early days of a focus on domestic violence from an operational policing perspectiven 'interest in domestic violence and SAPOL were predominately motivated by their desire to save time attending and re-attending such incidents. At this point in SAPOL's operational history, the department had a policy of non-intervention in family matters. This

[1] DCW was the South Australian Government's Welfare agency with responsibility for child welfare, youth justice and emergency financial assistance.

meant that police patrols would attend domestic violence incidents, restore the peace and at least temporarily stop the violence, usually without laying charges against perpetrators. They would then take some details of what was occurring and resume their patrol duties. Crisis Care marked a new era in SAPOL in that it was the first time that the organisation had become operationally involved with professionals other than their own sworn staff. It was decided after my appointment that before I recruited staff for the unit, I should spend 3 months in police patrol cars observing what police officers were doing in the field and also promoting the unit through my contact with officers. I was at that stage working closely with a senior police Superintendent named Ray Killmeir who at that time was responsible for police training and who later became Deputy Commissioner of South Australia Police. He was a thoughtful, highly intelligent and pragmatic individual, and together we worked through what we foresaw as significant difficulties in terms of blending the SAPOL para-military culture and that of the proposed Crisis Care Unit. My presence in the patrol cars gave me an opportunity to observe what police officers did and also it gave police officers an opportunity to ask questions about the proposed Crisis Care operation so that they could begin to prepare to work with it should they be so inclined.

I began my patrol activities in late 1975, and this was less than 12 months after police women in South Australia had come into uniform and began to undertake the same duties as their male colleagues. This was a time of significant change as many male police officers had reservations about working with female police in the field. Many told me quietly that they were concerned that they now had an extra responsibility, that of protecting their female partners from violence when it became a possibility. Police officers who attended domestic violence situations in 1975 were usually part of what were called "mixed patrols". Mixed patrols consisted of a male and a female officer; the latter were considered by virtue of their gender and history in policing to be more interpersonally competent when tasked to domestic violence incidents.

Crisis Care became operational in early 1976 and after a reasonably slow start gained the confidence of operational police. This was clearly indicated by the frequent requests from police for assistance in their family-related duties. We noted that the majority of such requests came from younger patrol officers.

A few years after the unit's establishment, I was asked to negotiate a siege where somewhat surprisingly the officer in charge announced on a loud hailer to the person within the building that I was coming in to talk to him in order that we might "sort something out" adding that "he is not a copper". I entered the premises knowing that the person inside was armed with a shotgun and after 3½ hours of intense conversation and negotiation, I was able to leave the building in his company. He was subsequently charged with offences, but after a short time the charges were dropped. This was a particularly stressful event for all concerned. But it was a profoundly vertical learning experience for me in terms of dealing with that kind of situation and its emotional aftermath.

The process of learning to manage and support a Crisis Intervention agency at that time was complex, and I was determined to replicate the best qualities of my previous managers in terms of the way in which I managed the Crisis Care Unit itself. There was a very intense level of collegiality and camaraderie within the unit. We were initially a staff of only eight professional people, plus one clerical officer. We covered the metropolitan area of Adelaide 7 days a week, 24 hours a day and the process was very much one of learning on the job and sharing our insights and expertise with each other as we became more competent and experienced. The only literature to which we could refer at that point was based on psychiatric insights after critical incidents, largely in the United States of America (Parad and Caplan 1969; Caplan, 1964; Smith, 1977). This was Crisis Intervention theory in its earliest form.

One of the major concerns was the need to be accepted as competent and useful by operational police. This happened slowly. Police in those days were particularly strategic and practically minded. They had little time for what they perceived as "touchy, feely" aspects of social work, and so we were motivated very strongly to make practical decisions that lead to outcomes which enabled police officers to hand over the responsibility for particular families to us rather than to continually attend their disputes without achieving useful, long-term outcomes.

My other profound learning experience was around police culture and the culture of the justice system. I learnt quite quickly how closely knit police officers were and how they relied upon each other to remain healthy in the context of what was often a stressful and demanding job. I enjoyed the adrenalin around police operations, and I appreciated strategic thinking as applied by police officers and gradually realised that the police we worked with were intelligent, thoughtful and dedicated to "the job". These were smart people. My principal police colleague, Chief Superintendent Ray Killmeir, would frequently send a police cadet around to the secret location of Crisis Care bearing an envelope which contained an article from a journal such as *Psychology Today* with a note attached saying "read this and ring me. Regards Ray". A tutorial would usually follow where we discussed the implications of the research for our work. We developed a close working relationship with a majority of police officers on patrol and the unit over the years and developed significant expertise in this area. Similar Crisis Units were introduced around Australia in the early 1980s.

This was the beginning of my close professional working relationship with SAPOL. This was also the period in which DSM 3 first defined Post-Traumatic Stress Disorder. I became acquainted with the concept through a working relationship with some psychologists who were establishing the then Vietnam Veterans Counselling Service. At Crisis Care, we had become aware that a disproportionate number of Vietnam Veterans were amongst perpetrators of domestic violence during our attendances through police referrals. My discussions with the psychologists establishing the Vietnam Veterans Counselling Service covered a whole range of issues but included the expression of my view about sending young men to a conflict like Vietnam, knowing that they would be exposed to significant risk, many of them being conscripts. Upon their return from Vietnam in 1977/78, the same young men were shunned by some sectors of South Australian society. I could not understand why having sent young men to that conflict where they had seen what they saw and had done what they did and then upon their return society either ignored their psychological trauma or referred to it as a disorder. My view was that we were probably unjust in defining their response to Vietnam as a disorder. I felt more inclined to see it as a natural response to a profoundly significant set of unnatural circumstances. My view has not changed significantly over the ensuing years.

I also became aware that strategic and practical thinking was critically important in terms of the crisis intervention context. We needed to work with SAPOL, usually with individual police officers, to establish ways in which we could best deliver our services to police and also to other members of the community through our after-hours responsibility for the Department for Community Welfare. At this point, I was working shifts when I could, as well as being on call 7 days a week after hours. The on-call responsibilities often involved being woken in order to give my approval to such activities as taking young people into the temporary care and control (Guardianship) of the Minister for Community Welfare. During this period, I learned the implications of being on shift, I learned about the impact of sleep deprivation and a great deal about the immediate aftermath of being involved in critical incidents laced with high levels of adrenaline.

When I left Crisis Care in 1982, I was weary. One evening in 1980, while sitting at home I suddenly began trembling violently although I knew that I was not ill and certainly was not cold. Our general practitioner attended and considered that I was probably undergoing some kind of stress reaction which he temporarily medicated. I then began a process of defining what was happening to me as well as trying to work through the experience. This was not PTSD. It was something else. Over the following months, I recovered slowly but realised that what had befallen me was some kind of anxiety state that related directly to the stress and pressure I had been under over the 6 years during which the Crisis Care Unit established itself. I took some leave against the advice of senior colleagues within the Department for Community Welfare because they considered that taking leave on the grounds of stress may well disadvantage my future career.

The Ash Wednesday Bushfires

On February 16, 1983, disastrous bushfires swept across South Australia and Western Victoria killing 75 people. I clearly remember the morning of the day, as it was unusually dark, windy and suffocatingly hot. I was then District Manager of a suburban Community Welfare Centre in Adelaide's inner South East, recovering from the exhaustion following my Crisis Care tenure. That evening, I sat with my family watching television reports of the devastation, with a sense of frustration that I was no longer part of the Crisis Care Unit and therefore unlikely to be involved in meaningful crisis intervention relief activities. I need not have worried about that as our home telephone rang the following evening directing me to prepare to travel to Mt Gambier the next day to organise and support a local social work team to work with families of those who had been killed in the fires. I flew south in a small twin-engined aircraft and was told by the pilot who had been airborne above the south east on Ash Wednesday that he had witnessed nothing like the fires during his long career. He told of solid sheets of flame 2,000 feet above the pine forests that covered much of the region and of mature forests flattened like sticks by the backdraft of the flames. I looked down in awe as we came in to land.

That afternoon, I met with six local social workers employed by the state welfare department (my organisation), the Education Department and local health agencies. All were young, inexperienced and desperately trying to recall what their lecturers had taught them about supporting victims of extreme trauma. We spent the first day covering those issues and then allocated families to each worker to contact and offer support and counselling. These were the very early days of disaster relief strategies and services. We responded by utilising the theory and practice of crisis intervention, drawing on my time with the Crisis Care Unit. It was demanding work. I met a farmer in the middle of his paddock as he stood twisting rusting wires together to form a fence no longer needed as no animals on his property had survived the fires. His pregnant wife and three children had died trying to escape the fire after he had directed them to do so. He was left with the clothes he was wearing. After a conversation during which we outlined resources he might wish to access, he turned to me and said, "This must be very difficult for you, dealing with all this tragedy". I was speechless.

Two weeks into the experience, it was announced at one of our regular planning meetings that a professor of psychiatry from the University of Queensland would be joining us and would be working with me for the next week. I was less than delighted, expressing the view that the last thing I needed was an academic psychiatrist peering over my shoulder. My respect for that profession had been negatively impacted by the Crisis Care experience. I was directed to fly home that evening to spend some time with my family whom I had not seen for a fortnight and to meet Prof. Beverly Raphael at the Adelaide Airport the next morning to fly back to the south east and to brief her during the journey. I met the Professor as arranged and she introduced me to a young Psychiatrist, Dr Sandy (Alexander) McFarlane who took notes of our in-flight conversation on the back of several aircraft sick bags, having forgotten to bring a note pad for that purpose (McFarlane, 1986). I became aware very quickly that the Professor was vastly experienced in disaster responses and was enormously impressed by her insights and ability to engage with the community in which we were working. Some 30 years later, she introduced me to Post-Traumatic Growth Theory which formed the basis of my present research (Raphael, 2014). Both she and the now Prof. Sandy McFarlane became world authorities in dealing with post-disaster trauma as well as making significant contributions to trauma theory generally in military and first responder contexts. Both contributed to my decision to translate experiences such as the Ash Wednesday response into my subsequent career with victims of trauma.

I returned to my duties as District Manager and 12 months later flew to the national Disaster College at Mt Macedon, Victoria, to meet with others who had been involved in the aftermath of Ash Wednesday fires in similar roles to mine. We gathered for what we thought was an operational debrief and were ushered into a theatre and shown uncut footage of the fires for some 15 minutes. When the lights came up almost everyone in the room was in tears and showing signs of distress. The organisers were shocked. These were the very early days of critical incident debriefing and before the realisation that helpers were often significantly impacted by the events surrounding their intervention. I was unable for many years to talk of my Ash Wednesday experiences, both in private and during presentations without becoming emotional.

Victims of Crime Service

After a period of 7 years working as a District Manager for the Department for Community Welfare, I was offered the opportunity of a secondment into the fledgling Victims of Crime Service in Adelaide. Previously when engaged in a state tour promoting the recent establishment of the Rape Crisis Centre at Adelaide's Queen Elizabeth Hospital, I encountered a retired Commissioner of Police from Queensland named Ray Whitrod. Ray had left Queensland in the early 1980s, having disagreed with the then Premier Joh Bielke Petersen about the government's inaction with regard to corruption within Queensland police. Ray upon his arrival in Adelaide, settled into retirement but after some years, was approached by the parents of some of the young women who had been murdered by Christopher Worrell as a part of a series of homicides that became known as the Truro murders. The bodies of several of the young women Worrell murdered were dumped in paddocks outside Truro in the Barossa Valley of South Australia. Victims of Crime Service was in the very early stages of its development as Whitrod responded to the request for help from the parents of some of the young women who were murdered and began establishing what became a voluntary organisation largely staffed by family members of those who had been murdered.

Ray was enthusiastic about the new organisation and contacted me to see if I could assist with setting up some processes for VOCS around the retention of information and the establishment of records that would enable the service to prosper. In 1989, I applied for the position of Executive Director of Victims of Crime Service. Ray was delighted to receive my application, and he and then VOCs Board Chair John Halsey interviewed me at the somewhat primitive VOCS offices and quickly informed me that I had been successful in gaining the position.

I saw my responsibilities as enabling the professionalisation of the organisation as well as being clinically involved utilising my skills as a social worker. Over the first 2 years of my appointment, I was able to add several professional staff to those who were already present when I arrived and to engage volunteer staff in ways that were more suitable to their skill and commitment levels. It was also clear that a significant proportion of my responsibilities would involve raising the profile of crime victims within the justice system as well as publicising the services that the organisation made available to individuals and families affected by crime and violence. I developed a caseload that largely consisted of family members of those who had been murdered and also did a great deal of work debriefing cash handlers after armed robberies which were prolific at that time. It was clear that advocacy would be particularly important as SAPOL at that stage was the most sympathetic section of the justice system as far as victims of crime were concerned. This was largely because they were present immediately after the victimisation occurred and were therefore sympathetic to the victim's experience as well as focused on instituting processes that would lead to charges, trials and justice being dispensed to those who had caused the victimisation in the first place. The court system largely ignored victims of crime in the late 1980s and early 1990s, valuing them only in so far as they offered themselves as witnesses for the prosecution. Our role at VOCS therefore was to offer support and counselling to victims of crime as well as trying to change aspects of the justice system that were presently not offering them recognition or status as victims of crime.

My work with families of homicide victims was confronting, as I would usually make contact with the family shortly after the homicide had taken place. The families were always in states of disengagement, shock and acute grief. I realised quite early in the process that my role at that point in their experience was simply to engage with them and then stay engaged as they worked through the early stages of their grief that frequently turned to anger and sometimes focused on the inadequacies of the justice system they were experiencing.

As the years passed, I realised that no one that I worked with in the situation I have just described could have been diagnosed with PTSD in terms of my observations of them. They were possessed by grief, they were often depressed, they expressed high levels of anger and a sense of injustice about what had happened particularly when they encountered the intricacies and complications of the justice system that left them feeling confused and isolated. My role as an advocate was critically important in that as well as supporting them through their grief I was also able to represent them within the system and seek to explain its processes. At this time, I was also involved heavily in critical incident stress debriefing. I travelled to the United States of America as I had developed a close working relationship with the National Organization of Victim Assistance which was based in Washington DC. I undertook a 3-week training programme in the United States with National Organisation of Victim Assistance and the Federal Bureau of Investigation implementing what I later realised was the Mitchell model of critical incident stress debriefing. This I practiced regularly and realised its effectiveness both with victims of armed robbery and secondary and tertiary victims of homicide that had occurred in institutions, public places and private homes. I recall being summoned to a university college in Adelaide after a young student had been murdered by a fellow student. The students themselves were shattered by what had occurred as were their teachers and those who administered the college. We had one debriefing session and at one point in that session, I realised that I was the only person in the room who was not in tears. Debriefing clearly was intended to allow people to express their emotions and to begin the process of dealing with what had occurred. Many expressed the view that they found my presence and demeanour encouraging, and particularly cash handlers were prepared at that point for a normal recovery as well as the possibility that they may be involved in future armed robberies. One of my achievements at Victims of Crime Service was to create and present a training programme for cash handlers that prepared them for armed robbery and gave them advanced information about possible reactions and responses to it. We talked with victimised cash handlers about possible reactions, described such responses as normal and encouraged people to stay in touch with us as they worked through their trauma. That was the beginning of my focus on the concept of resilience. I was profoundly interested in what contributed to the capacity of those who were able to deal with such life-threatening experiences adequately and in a short period of time and equally with those who could not.

During this period, I spent a great deal of time in the company of operational police. SAPOL was at that stage developing its Victims of Crime branch, and I worked with mainly female police officers as that process began and continued. Later, I was also heavily involved in the training process when a small group of female Sergeants decided that domestic violence training was critically important to middle managers (Sergeants) and devised a series of training modules with which I became involved as a presenter. I spent time with police officers at national conferences as I had done when the Crisis Care Unit was developing. At such times, I developed close relationships with police that enabled them to unload their concerns about some of the duty-related experiences they had had. They often became emotional at such times. At this point, I began to realise the cost for some individuals of a long career in policing.

Mobilong Prison

I developed a working relationship with the Department for Correctional Services in an endeavour involving improved communication between that Department and Victims of Crime. During one such meeting with the then CEO Sue Vardon, she asked me whether I would be interested in a career with Correctional Services. She informed me that the General Manager's position at Mobilong Prison[2] was about to be advertised and she suggested that I should give serious thought to applying for that position. Her motivation was to change her Department's culture by injecting "outsiders" into middle management positions. I applied, and after 6 years at Victims of Crime Service was appointed General Manager of Mobilong Prison at the end of 1995. This was a significant change of role as I transferred from Victims of Crime Service where I had small staff and a relatively small budget to Mobilong Prison where I was responsible for 70 staff, 200 prisoners and a budget of approximately $6 million in 1995/96.

When I began my time at Mobilong as General Manager, there was much consternation among the prison staff who considered that having a social worker in charge of the institution might be a problem. They consoled themselves with the view that as a result of my experience with victims, I would probably not be "soft" on prisoners. Over the ensuing months and years, I was able to convince them that all could be well if we were able to consider our duties, our responsibilities and our legal obligations in open-minded and innovative ways. My basic strategy at Mobilong was to spend a great deal of time in the prison itself, walking around by myself, talking to prisoners

[2] Mobilong is a medium security, State run prison at Murray Bridge, seventy kilometres from Adelaide. In 1995, it housed 200 prisoners.

and staff about the operation of the prison and their individual circumstances. This was an effective strategy in terms of me becoming aware of potential crisis situations before they turned into crises and also it reassured the staff and some prisoners that I was interested in their well-being. I also made a point of encouraging innovation as staff members were encouraged to make suggestions with regard to changes in the way we approached running the prison and its rehabilitation programmes. During this time, I also gained an understanding of criminal behaviour from the perspective of the offenders and developed a broader knowledge of what contributed to initial and continuing criminal activity.

I was comfortable with the para-military culture of Mobilong Prison and Correctional Services and valued it greatly. As part of my responsibilities, I spoke often and at length with unit managers in the prison and with those who staffed the various facilities and sections within it. I reinforced my view that management and leadership involved listening, supporting and encouraging staff to participate in the process of change within institutions. The Correctional Services experience also reinforced my view of the "us and them" syndrome where people on the ground in prisons referred to Correctional Services headquarters as "bullshit castle". I became acutely aware during my Correctional Services experience of the danger of organisations not being open to change and the absolute imperative that strategic thinking in terms of such change should be unhurried and comprehensive. After 2 years in Corrections, my contract was terminated and I established Empower Justice Services, a consultancy that focused on crime prevention, restorative justice, critical incident debriefing and training. I ran the consultancy for the next 13 years.

Empower Justice Services P/L

Once more, I found myself working closely with police officers, this time in crime prevention working with police intelligence Sergeants around criminal activities and their location as well as working with many colleagues that I had previously engaged with in my other roles within the justice system. My activities around critical incident debriefing continued, again in the context of armed robbery as a result of referrals from SAPOL officers, petrol station franchisees and other cash handling organisations. Our younger daughter became a police officer during this period and subsequently married a fellow police officer so I was given another view of the police organisation, as it were from within the family. I watched with great interest the changes that occurred in our daughter's life and how she adapted from having been a professional social worker to a professional police officer. She embraced her new culture, becoming a competent patrol and family violence operative over the 19 years she has served.

The Empower Justice Services experience enabled me to engage with the justice system from a different perspective. This time in the context of innovation and also from the perspective of a person who was now independent of allegiances to the "silos" and departments within the justice system.

Teaching At University

In 2010, I was approached by Flinders University to apply for a role as a Field Education Coordinator within the social work programme. For the following 6 years I supervised students on placement often within the justice system and again observed their engagement from the perspective of that systems impact on individuals. A significant part of my innovative activity in this role at Flinders was the establishment of police placements within family violence investigation units at SAPOL.

I was also encouraged by academic colleagues to consider undertaking postgraduate study. My initial negative response to the suggestion was that of a practical hands-on practitioner, but later I began considering the opportunities that postgraduate study might offer for me to put my career in some perspective and consider my experience within the systems in the context of academic research. My early intention was to continue my interest in trauma by studying police, ambulance, fire and correctional services officers but after being encouraged to "focus"; this was refined down to the point where I decided to study resilience among police officers only. I approached this from a social work perspective. I was encouraged by the development of the positive psychology movement who in my opinion were adapting their practice to that of one close to social work, in terms of their new objective of looking for strengths and positives in people's experiences rather than only negatives and pathology.

In a 2013 conversation with Prof. Beverley Raphael whom I had first met during my engagement during the 1983 Ash Wednesday bushfires, I was introduced to "Post-Traumatic Growth" theory. Tedeschi and Calhoun were referenced by Prof. Raphael who encouraged my immediate attention to their research. Before I began the research, I engaged with a psychologist over a 2-month period to ensure that I had a good platform from which to launch myself into the study. The psychological debrief that I undertook reviewed and reflected my career as the particular psychologist I consulted had worked with me in the 1970s establishing the Vietnam Veterans Counselling Service. This was a good way of clearing the slate and preparing me to engage in the research with an open mind.

Contents

Chapter 1
Introduction

They call it 'The job' because it's not a job. That's the joke.
SAPOL Senior Sergeant, 28 years' service
What disturbs men's minds is not events, but their judgements on events
Epictetus 55–135 AD
Any abnormal reaction to an abnormal situation is normal behaviour
Victor Frankl

Abstract This chapter introduces the research question: "How resilient are South Australian Police Officers" and summarises the themes that arose from the 50 interviews as well as the research design and method. The themes included power, organisational executive culture, the feminisation of policing since the 1970s and the impact on police culture, death and bodies, the constant companion of operational police, keeping well, coping in the operational context, asking for help when traumatised, a risky action for operational police, sleep, its critical importance to well-being and resilience, resilience, its meaning and importance to policing, PTSD and policing, the media, and the contemporary expectation that trauma exposure will inevitably cause injury and post-traumatic growth theory. How it applies to policing and resilience. This chapter also examines traditional and more contemporary theories of policing and the impact, if any, they have on the way police organisations see their role in the "good order" of society. A brief history of South Australia Police, a summary of the research methodology and a description of the cohort of police officers interviewed conclude the chapter.

1.1 How Resilient Are South Australia Police Members?

My 35 years of experience in the South Australian justice system has been characterised by trauma experienced by others and at times by myself. Police officers have populated my professional career as I worked with them in several roles. In the 1970s, an early domestic violence support programme allowed me to engage with operational police colleagues on patrol. In providing support to crime victims

A. Paterson, *Trauma and Resilience in Contemporary Australian Policing*,
https://doi.org/10.1007/978-981-16-4416-0_1

in a non-government agency, I worked with officers whose taskings [1] involved their contact with the same group. As a consultant, I worked in intelligence-led crime prevention activities and as a prison manager I enlisted the support of police officers when inmates broke the law while incarcerated or when my staff needed assistance to maintain the good order of the prison. I have had significant experience working with police officers as a colleague whilst being "unsworn". At times, I have acted as a confidant to officers in conversations that they may not have had with sworn colleagues. Often they talked of duty-related challenges such as injuries sustained by them and their capacity to inflict harm (sometimes terminal) on others. At such times, they often became emotional, expressing a vulnerability not expressible elsewhere in their organisation. I have been consistently impressed by their resilience and sometimes wondered how it was maintained. This study explores those issues, changes in police culture, how women fare in "the job" and how management strategies impact their well-being. My experience, my age and my understanding of the language of policing, all contributed to the rich data that came out of the long interviews and that informed the thematic structure of this research. Contemporary ethnographic research into policing and its culture has not achieved this level of detail and insight (Faull, 2017; Henry, 2004; Loftus, 2009). The topic-specific literature around trauma, resilience and growth through traumatic exposure is embedded in the themes from the interviews which form the chapters of the book.

1.2 Aims of This Study

This research project sets out to explore mechanisms that police officers use to "normalise" their experiences to preserve the delicate professional balance between "coping" that Henry (2004) calls "psychic numbing" and being responsive to victims and survivors in their everyday work environment. Recent advances in post-traumatic growth theory will be considered, which set out to re-interpret exposure in a positive context, as well as preventative experience in Australia and internationally.

There are five aims directing this research:

1. To research current literature, both academic research and that generated from within police organisations, and to frame and understand trauma theory. This analysis spans from military service and "shell shock" in World War One, through "battle fatigue" in World War Two and PTSD responses after the Vietnam War and subsequent conflicts (Jones & Wessely, 2005). Such theory is now applied to non-military contexts quite broadly (Seligman, 2011).
2. To compare current PTSD theory with post-traumatic growth theory in terms of the tendency of current PTSD models to predict the "inevitability" of some traumatic responses and to medicalise the treatment of the condition once diagnosed. Systems theory, also known as "Field Theory" (Lewin, 1951) is a typical

[1] A "tasking" is a direction to a police patrol to attend an incident that warrants police attention. They are "tasked" to attend.

social work approach that looks beyond the individual and his/her internal predicament, to the factors such as personal, familial, organisational, social and structural that may influence recovery and re-engagement. It will too form a theoretical framework for this thesis as the interviewer seeks to address the complex issues around individual relationships within families, police organisations and the community in which policing takes place. Saleebey summarises these relationships thus, "As we discover the desires, talents and interest of each person…we hone our skills in recognising, appreciating, valuing and utilising that which is already there. In a sense, we co-create with individuals and various social settings a mutually enriching partnership and exchange" (Saleebey, 1996:54).

3. To obtain qualitative data into policing, trauma and resilience through interviews with serving and retired police officers. Such interviews will be based on biographical research approaches (Roberts, 2002; Zinn, 2004) which encompass the use of life stories; in this case, police careers from the perspective of the officer. This approach has been suggested by the growing availability of autobiographical accounts of police careers so far encountered by the researcher (Horner, 2011; Rogers, 1999; Sparkes, 2013). Interviews were conducted with the intent of exploring with officers how they have maintained resilience over their careers and what factors, in their view, contributed to a long and healthy experience, or otherwise, of policing.
4. To identify and define the influence of command structures and police culture on the development of resilience or susceptibility to post-traumatic reactions as part of police activities and to examine the importance of exposure to death and injury in the line of duty to the development of healthy trauma responses and to examine the place of "dark humour" in the development of resilience in police officers.
5. To examine the effectiveness of contemporary critical incident debriefing approaches when offered to police after exposure to serious critical incidents.

The literature referenced for this research is embedded in the thematic chapters and covers the history and development of trauma theory and its recent application to the experience of "first responders" including police officers. Post-traumatic growth theory offers a more positive view of the impact of trauma, defining opportunities for individuals, whilst being impacted by trauma exposure to also experience personal (and professional) growth. A qualitative approach, unusual in this scope in most policing research due to access problems not experienced here, was chosen to make the voices of these officers and clinicians clearly heard, as they tell their own stories of resilience, service and challenge. Police management literature rarely addresses managing the mental well-being of officers. This research focussed on the impact of SAPOL management and leadership on the resilience of those officers interviewed. The final research aim seeks to clarify from an operational police perspective the value of critical incident debriefs in the context of a vigorous, largely academic debate about the value of offering such opportunities to first responders.

1.3 My Conversation with the Data

I considered myself a practitioner, and gained undergraduate and postgraduate qualifications to enter my profession and relied on an ongoing study, both structured and informal to develop and maintain my skills. Often, I invited academics to observe my activities, shifts at Crisis Care, training sessions in the victim support agency that I led and visits to the prison. That was a kind of pay-back for all they had developed in me and an attempt to inform their academic activities with practical experience. When I began this research, the topic was never in doubt, as I had formed views about trauma, PTSD, debriefing, psychology, psychiatry and the justice system that were based on my experience at a personal and professional level. Policing fascinated me. I liked working with coppers. I appreciated the way they thought and how we tackled systemic change as well as operational challenges. I enjoyed being part of the culture and recognised how privileged I was to be accepted into it. The no-nonsense approach to problem-solving we shared was important to me and that impacted my management style and the way I thought about priorities.

I knew that policing was stressful as I observed what lay behind the culture and competencies of the police I worked with and got to know. I recognised that police developed skills and strategies that worked for highly unusual situations, including humour, the ability to "numb" their responses to other's trauma and deep camaraderie. Often, when attending national conferences with police officers as we did particularly in the 1970s and 1980s, my police colleagues would open up, with the help of a few beers. They talked of the responsibilities of the job and the tasks that had challenged them. They became emotional while doing so without apparent embarrassment.

The interviews were arranged with little difficulty after the invitation letter was published in the Police Association magazine. Emails and phone calls followed. Some policemen who knew me were the first to make contact, including a cohort of Sergeants from South Coast to whom I had presented some months earlier about my research. As I completed my presentation, I was surrounded by Sergeants, holding out business cards, telling me to contact them when I commenced interviewing. I knew that we had struck a significant research topic among present and past officers and that they recognised that the project could have the potential to change SAPOL's approach to trauma through their career stories.[2]

My first interview was with a veteran officer, a woman with 40 years of experience, who was a Victim Contact Officer when I was at the Victims of Crime Service. That was a strong start, followed by a STAR group sergeant who had been shot on duty, then the oldest serving SAPOL member, and a Vietnam Vet who was very clear about why he was "well". I was aware that I spoke and understood the language of policing, and I did not need to ask questions about those issues. I often waited quietly while

---

[2] Interviews were conducted in public places such as coffee shops, at Flinders University, police stations, Police Association offices and in the officer's homes. Only two officers were interviewed in public where there was no problem with confidentiality as we were able to find quiet corners to talk.

the officers sat in silence gathering their thoughts during the interviews. As many of them acknowledged, these were not conversations they had experienced previously.

I began each interview by asking: "when did you join?" and "why did you join?" That led naturally into their career trajectories and into the confronting aspects of their career experiences. I always only needed to ask clarifying questions to keep the conversation flowing. I asked about sleep patterns, whether they "had ever been close to the edge", what strategies they used to "keep well" and what career highlights and achievements they experienced. At the end of each interview I asked, "on a scale of 1–10, one being I have wasted my career in a hopeless, un-appreciative organisation, dealing with society's dregs with few positive outcomes, and ten being I would do it all again, I have achieved a great deal, worked with great colleagues with many fantastic outcomes". Most of them responded immediately with a score. The scores were surprising, thirteen 10s, ten 9s, thirteen 8s, seven 7s and two 6s. I either did not ask or did not record the other three responses.

The interviews were fascinating, exhausting and, according to those interviewed, unique. I took handwritten notes which proved easier than I had envisaged. I was aware that my social work communication and listening skills were important to the way the interviews developed as was my age and experience. Most of the policemen I had not met knew of my professional history. When handed information and consent sheets, all the interviewees read them carefully and when finished looked up and said "right" or something similar. None held back, telling of their experiences and challenges with care and relish. Some of their detailed accounts of incidents were challenging for both of us. During the interview with a senior sergeant recently retired from major crime, who reckoned he had investigated over 200 homicides and suspicious deaths, "towards the end I had had enough of grief, dickheads and dead bodies". I was writing notes, head down when he said "sorry mate!" I looked up and saw that he was crying. We were in a coffee shop. He quickly regained control and later asked if such a response was normal. I replied in the affirmative.

Some interviews were conducted over several sessions where long-serving officers felt that more than one meeting was necessary. One was a very recently retired detective senior sergeant, a real "old school copper" who joined in 1974 and who had very high standards of care for his team members and a palpable sense of duty and achievement. He said, "you need a very high degree of intelligence to be a good cop". And, "integrity in policing is very important; you're either a copper or a crook". I also interviewed an elderly retired Deputy Commissioner. We met three times at his home. I had worked closely with him when establishing Crisis Care in the mid-1970s. We kept in touch over the years through his daughter, now an Assistant Commissioner in SAPOL. I attended her graduation with her father in the late 1980s. Before our daughter commenced her academy course in 2001, we visited him and I watched with great pride as the two talked about policing. She addressed him as "Sir" throughout the conversation, apologising when he suggested she use his first name, saying that out of respect, she could not. I sent six pages of notes to him after our final research meeting and he responded by sending a 30-page typed document, which is an autobiography covering his enlistment in 1941 at the age of 15 to his retirement in the late 1980s. It is profoundly insightful, particularly describing how he became a competent and caring manager.

I interviewed 15 women as a part of the cohort. Some I had worked with in Victim Support, some worked in family violence, some were in child abuse investigation, some on patrols, some were detectives, and the highest rank among them was that of sergeant. Those who enlisted in the 1970s and 1980s told of extraordinary levels of discrimination and harassment that included sexual assault on the job. That, they said was the most confronting aspect of policing, their operational duties were a breeze in comparison. Part-time work and parenting was always difficult in the culture of those days and has changed little since. Female police married to male police are only too aware of the barriers imposed by parenting and police male/female roles as they watch their husbands and co-parents of their children climb promotional ladders not available to them. I was astonished by the strength of these women and very aware of the contribution they had made to their organisation despite formidable barriers.

The present sophistication of SAPOL domestic violence services available to victims in South Australia is the result of the determination of a group of female Sergeants in the 1990s who recognised that the then state welfare agency, obsessed with child protection had taken its eye off the DV ball. They realised that Sergeants were the key and organised DV awareness training for them in which I participated as a presenter. It was a major turning point for SAPOL and a potent indicator of the "feminisation" of the force. I interviewed one of those female Sergeants for this research who joined in 1968, 6 years before women came into SAPOL uniformed service. She was trained for a mere six weeks and on graduation had no powers of arrest, and entered into a social work role within the organisation. She married a fellow officer, who was discriminated against as a result. She saw her career as unremarkable, I disagreed. A younger, female detective was really clear about her work in the Family Violence section, "I like doing something I feel strongly about, working with other agencies, making the process less distressing for victims". She was aware of the changes in SAPOL due to the promotion of women into top jobs and could see the potential for significant change through them.

Thirteen Sergeants were interviewed. It became clear that those among them who had patrol teams were under most organisational stress with a strong sense of responsibility for the well-being of their charges who were mostly younger officers. They were constantly under a great deal of pressure from higher commissioned officers who were risk-averse and less than supportive of their middle managers "Everything that goes wrong is blamed on the shift manager". They perceive this as a lack of trust in their judgement and professionalism. They offer debriefs "after difficult jobs", notice changes in the demeanour of individuals within their teams and offer feedback after good and negative job outcomes. All of this without SAPOL training in these areas, "we don't get any training but use a common-sense approach" said one. Another, deeply frustrated with SAPOL (the organisation) said, "My team time my 'for fuck's sake' outburst when I come back on shift after time off. It's now down to twenty minutes". I am convinced that Sergeants are crucially important to the well-being of the organisation. With appropriate (basic) training in early intervention, debriefing and support they could become the foundation of very effective strategies that would be of enormous benefit to them and their troops. This, in the context of "command and control" approaches to executive management, tend to show no concern for the well-being of front-line officers. One Sergeant said, deeply dissatisfied with SAPOL, "I get my satisfaction from looking after my troops", and "if you show weakness, you're out, there's no loyalty (from SAPOL) you're just a number!".

I interviewed eight Commissioned Officers, one Deputy Commissioner, (retired) three Chief Superintendents (two retired, one recently), two Detective Chief Inspectors (both retired) and two Inspectors (both operational). Many non-commissioned officers complained that their higher-ranked colleagues lacked understanding of the stresses and strains of operational policing. Said one, "Commissioned Officers forget where they have come from". Those senior officers I interviewed clearly had not as they recounted their early career experiences with precision. Many talked of how they worked on "becoming a good boss" and how they had tried with varying success to bring change to SAPOL where they felt it was most needed. Some criticised "piss poor management" they had experienced on the way up the SAPOL ladder. One created a leadership programme for Sergeants, which although successful and well-received was discontinued. Some contemporary Sergeants interviewed for my research would have relished the opportunity to participate. The same Chief Superintendent, aware of the gap between commissioned ranks and those below said, "Many cops think,' the jobs fucked', I invite them to come and sit on my side of the desk. There have been three police shootings in my career. The bosses were there, looking after the troops".

A retired Detective Chief Inspector was similarly thoughtful when recounting his career experiences, including "feedback from victims" and his capacity to compartmentalise traumatic experiences as critically important to his well-being. Another retired Detective Chief Inspector recounted that at gruesome crime scenes he had no problems, they came afterwards, "I used to go into my kids bedrooms while they were asleep to touch them to make sure they were warm". And referring to the issues around the transition after promotion, "It was a barrier being commissioned although the feedback was positive about my involvement".

A recently promoted Inspector after a 15-year operational career, including in the STAR group, was very clear about changes in SAPOL that were needed to increase the levels of well-being. Recommending a new emphasis on pro-active monitoring of staff well-being, an emphasis on exercise and fitness, and a more rigorous recruiting process he said, "There are too many broken cops. We need more support for the people on the road who are getting flogged!".

These senior officers had clear memories of their operational service and similarly focussed insights and suggestions into organisational change. How those beneath them organisationally had developed the perception of distance between "them and us" was not easy to discern. It may well be a distance that the executive group in SAPOL seek to create and maintain.

Many of the interviews resulted from other interviews as (for example) child exploitation investigators, major crash and major crime officers and Special Task and Rescue Group officers recommended the research and interviews to colleagues.

One sergeant, after his interview, recommended to a colleague who had been shot on duty that he contact me. A STAR[3] group Sergeant in an email sent after I had interviewed him and his wife in their home said, "I have passed your details on to other members at my work and they may be in touch with you".

Only two officers interviewed were motivated by very high levels of frustration and negativity about SAPOL, the others participated to tell their story and to outline the strategies they used to stay well. Another significant factor for them was justifiable pride in their career and what they had accomplished.

The STAR group officers interviewed (five) were different from the others. Aware of their elite status in the organisation, they were carefully recruited and bonded very tightly. One explained that when off-duty he became aware of his colleague's involvement in murder-suicide involving children while it was unfolding. He was relieved he said not to be on shift but sent supportive texts to those who were. These were officers who are acutely aware of the fact that they were at the pointy end of policing and their coping strategies reflected that: "I'm affected, I'm saddened, I feel for those involved, I have had tears, it doesn't affect me, I don't let it affect my life. It's like watching a movie!" said one, after over 20 years in the STAR group. A younger colleague, after recovering the body of a person who had drowned received texts from his STAR group colleagues: "Afterwards I got two or three texts from other team members saying 'good job', you are now a proper diver!".

Two of the officers interviewed had been diagnosed with PTSD. Both when making contact with me, asked if I wanted to interview them as they had been diagnosed and therefore might be seen to lack resilience. I assured them that I did. The younger of the two, recently diagnosed, while serving in the country, had attended three fatal motor vehicle accidents (MVAs) in a 10-day period. He received a phone call from SAPOL's Employee Assistance Programme asking, "Are you OK?" This Officer had been offered one psychological review in 8 years, and had formed the view that "debriefs are usually operational, not about you…". After finding a person who was reported missing and then died in 40°C heat several days after, the Senior Constable while "bagging" the deceased was reminded of his 5-year-old son's head. While driving to his station with the decomposed body at the back of his ute, he pulled over "and just broke". In treatment and doing well he added, "Resilience training/building is important. I've kept it a secret for too long".

The other officer was back on the job after his diagnosis, and was philosophical about his lot, "My PTSD has gone up and down. From hyper to laconic. There is a solid group who I trust, people know me!" adding, "I have seen a lot of death and violence, countless suicides, vulnerable and innocent people. It could have been me!" He was, however, less than enthusiastic about SAPOL's response to his trauma-related issues, "In terms of the SAPOL rehab and injury management people, I wouldn't cross the road to piss on those pricks!".

---

[3] Special Task and Rescue group are elite officers carefully selected and trained as first responders to critical incidents involving armed offenders. They also conduct underwater body recovery taskings and rescues.

Several officers interviewed had had episodes of depression and anxiety, one being diagnosed with a "dissociative disorder". They were able to make contact with psychological assistance through SAPOL, as the direct result of an understanding senior officer. Some also saw the writing on the wall and transferred it to other SAPOL sections as they recognised their levels of exhaustion. The importance of psychological education to understand what was happening to them was crucial to these officers. Most did it for themselves with the help of the Internet. One officer, who described himself as a "high functioning alcoholic", got help through SAPOL after his new wife insisted to do so. He is now in control of his drinking. Policing, he said "is a self-medicating culture camouflaged by a social culture. We have quiet beers now in people's houses". Alcohol was a constant theme in the interviews conducted with longer-serving officers.[4] Until the arrival of drink driving legislation in the 1980s, it clearly had an important debriefing function. A younger officer, when interviewed, was clear that "there is no positive relationship between alcohol and coping".

Suicide within SAPOL was regularly mentioned by the officers interviewed. They were all concerned that colleagues should decide to take that option and fearful of the implications for themselves and the organisation. All reported a lack of response from higher command when suicides occurred within SAPOL. An example cited was a complete lack of internal response after a suicide in a Southern police station. No commissioned officers contacted those closest to the deceased officer and all had to apply for special leave to attend his funeral. All those who mentioned colleagues committing suicide also assumed that rates among police were high, an assumption not supported by much research. Attending civilian suicides taxes the resilience of officers. Many mentioned such tasks as confronting. When "their own" do the same, they are shaken.

I interviewed an officer who had been shot on duty. He was well supported by SAPOL, given time to recover and open access to peers in the job who had also been shot. He received psychological support from within and outside SAPOL. This was a visible injury as well as a traumatic one. SAPOL coped well with that.

The interviews were very draining for me. Not because of the graphic detail, but more to do with the levels of concentration required of me to note what was said accurately. I was invited to visit the Police Historical Society one Thursday morning by its Chair, a retired Detective Chief Inspector. I interviewed four retired officers in total, before and after lunch. I was exhausted and elated by the process. I am acutely aware of the value of the data collected. The need to do it justice and my awareness of its uniqueness has been challenging. The process has been a privilege. As Christine Nixon, retired Chief Commissioner of Victoria Police said of her troops, "These were people who cared deeply about their duty and their capacity to perform it".

The six psychologists and psychiatrists interviewed were with one exception highly critical of the way SAPOL executives manage their member's mental health. One described SAPOL as a toxic psychiatric environment. Several described how officers who "they wanted out" were bullied by management and subjected to multiple

[4] See more detail in Chap. 5 "Coping, keeping well.".

unnecessary reviews and tests to hasten their departure. All agreed that PTSD rates in SAPOL were low and that most officers so diagnosed were "exhausted by what they have seen". All were critical of the lack of a discernible mental health policy in SAPOL and most were clear in their view that most trauma-related problems they encountered in SAPOL members were related to "command and control" management not operational experiences. These interviews were valuable in that they confirmed the themes that emerged from the 50 officer interviews.

1.4 The Interview Themes

The qualitative interviews conducted for this research form a unique contribution to the literature of policing, resilience and trauma studies. The themes that emerged from the 50 conversations with officers and the six with psychiatrists and psychologists who treat and assess some of their colleagues became the basic structure of this thesis. They are in the following sections.

1.4.1 Power, Organisational and Police Culture, "the Job"

This chapter offers SAPOL officers, past and present, an opportunity to give voice to their experiences of management and leadership. In line with much of the policing literature, albeit giving more detail to essential change, they have expressed clearly what must happen to ensure that present and future generations of SAPOL members and police in other jurisdictions are lead and managed by middle and executive leaders in ways that build on their well-being and mental health in "the job".

1.4.2 Feminisation of Policing

In this chapter, the voices of women police in South Australia are researched in the context of significant detailed interviews for the first time. Echoing recent reviews, these women have described careers in policing not primarily challenged by everyday crime and mayhem, but rather by systemic discrimination, bullying and harassment. These are the voices of women who are insistent on change that will allow future generations of their female colleagues to focus on their duties without the extra challenge of surviving bullying, harassment and discrimination so that they can continue in "the job". The level of resilience they have developed to do so is almost unimaginable.

1.4.3 Death and Bodies

This chapter featured clearly the voices of the police officers interviewed describing how they have coped with many forms of death encounters as they have carried out their duties. It reveals the role of police culture, the passing down of wisdom from older to younger officers and the pride experienced officers express in the importance of the skills they develop in this area.

1.4.4 Keeping Well, Coping

Police officers interviewed for this research were not vulnerable individuals whose duty-related experiences sentenced them to a PTSD diagnosis. They clearly coped with the challenges of their chosen profession in a variety of ways that indicated their awareness of the need to take responsibility for their own mental health.

1.4.5 Asking for Help

This research is unique in that it confirms through interviews with officers and clinicians the depth of the need for change within SAPOL. Asking for help should be natural and encouraged, not a career-ending risk. Recent developments in this area (Carroll, 2015) show promise of much-needed change.

1.4.6 Sleep

Sustaining sleep is a skill that those interviewed either acquired through experience or genetic inheritance. Those who lacked such an advantage accepted troubled sleep as a price they paid for being in "the job" devising strategies such as sleeping on rostered days off or simply putting up with their lot. The majority had learned to sleep well, again in the absence of input from SAPOL, this being a significant indicator of their resilience.

1.4.7 Resilience

The police officers interviewed in this study were well aware of the need for them to take the initiative to develop and maintain their own resilience. In volunteering to be interviewed they were acknowledging their view that SAPOL does little for its members in this area, leaving responsibility for their well-being up to them.

1.4.8 PTSD and Policing

This study has enabled the voices of the SAPOL officers interviewed to be heard, revealing their optimism and pride in their identity and career achievements despite their awareness of the hazards of their profession. Their knowledge of PTSD is significant, they are aware of colleagues who have been "broken" and they have taken steps to remain well in the knowledge that their organisation ('SAPOL") will do little to assist them.

1.4.9 Post-traumatic Growth in Policing

I argue that police officers are not the hapless, slow-moving ignorant targets of inevitable PTSD diagnosis (McFarlane, 2011) but rather thoughtful, well-researched individuals whose sense of duty encourages them to adopt measures that contribute to their long-term well-being, personal and professional growth. The 50 interviewees show clearly that such a diagnosis is not inevitable as McFarlane suggests, even in the absence of significant support from SAPOL.

In recognizing these themes in the interviews, they became the structure for this research. To ensure clarity of analysis, an embedded literature review structure was configured. Instead of a single chapter which may result in a reification of complex issues and a disconnection from my original evidence, I decided to separate the literature reviews into each designated chapter. The resultant structure ensures a tight alignment of data, theory and interpretation.

1.5 Research Design and Methodology

A qualitative research approach was adopted, using biographical research methods (Apitzsch & Siouti, 2007; Gardner, 2001; Roberts, 2002; Zinn, 2004), which "aim[s] toward treating social actors as knowledgeable, intentional agents, active and reflective in the constitution of their own identity (ies) and social worlds" (Gardner, 2001:187). Gardner warns against the researcher accepting one person's view or definition of a situation, suggesting that "triangulation" of accounts will lead to a clearer version of what actually happened, which was a feature of the proposed research where 50 police officers were interviewed. Gardner also argues (2001:194) that biographical knowledge is "practical" or "pragmatic" in that it is a "contingent way of interpreting the world, constructed and reconstructed through multiple and ongoing time–space specific encounters with other (single and collective) actors and bodies of knowledge". This is supported by the autobiographies written by police officers who have been diagnosed with PTSD. There are clear commonalities of experience and process that reinforced and "triangulated" through the interview process.

Biographical knowledge can be utilised in two ways as research:

1. As a mode of access to "the lived experience of the actor" (Gardner, 2001:196) and
2. As an account that "partially informs and is informed by its positioning in multiple networks of agents and wider, fuller frames of reference" (Gardner, 2001:196).

Apitzsch and Siouti (2007:9) build on this approach asserting that "the main idea of biographical-narrative interview is to generate a spontaneous auto-biographical narration which is not structured by questions posed by the interviewer, but by the narrator's structures of relevance". Zinn (2004:7) sees biographical research as "analysing the development of the individual personality in the life course", assuming that individuals during their life experiences form a "coherent" description of the meaning of, in the case of this research, their police career. Winlow (2001:536/2001b) although researching populations at more than arm's length from policing is very clear that ethnographers such as himself need to adopt observational (and interactive) techniques to "tease out the essential essences grounded in visceral action". Much of policing is well described as "visceral" and Winlow's research has much in common with the way I approached officers interviewed in my cohort.

A process of thematic analysis was applied to the research (Cresswell, 1998; Guest et al., 2011) in order to analyse the data obtained from the interviews to appropriately analyse themes that emerge. Themes are defined as "patterns across data sets that are important to the description of the phenomenon and are associated with a specific research question" (Daly et al., 1997:162). The themes then become the categories for analysis as the research unfolds (Fereday & Muir-Cochrane, 2006).

There were two sources of primary data: Interviewees, who are serving and retired police officers, were invited to outline their police careers, with reference to when they first joined the service, memorable incidents, achievements and frustrations. I occasionally asked clarifying questions, based on the PTSD checklist (Weathers, 2013) and the post-traumatic growth inventory (Tedeschi & Calhoun, 1996). This inventory has also been widely used under controlled and verified clinical conditions (Shakespeare-Finch, 2013). Emphasis was placed on how resilience has been maintained, including departmental assistance or otherwise, family and relationships, recreation and self-care. Three psychiatrists and three psychologists who had all either treated or assessed officers were also interviewed. This "triangulation" clarified accounts of lived experiences obtained during the narrative approaches used.

1.5.1 The Sample

A total of 50 sworn police officers were interviewed who were operational or retired. Three psychologists and three psychiatrists who treat or assess SAPOL members were also interviewed. As a condition of obtaining approval to conduct the research from the Flinders University Faculty of Social and Behavioural Sciences research ethics committee, I agreed to also make an application to the SAPOL Research and Survey Coordinating Committee (RSCC). The Executive Officer of the committee made it clear that if approval was given it would require that SAPOL exercise editorial rights over the final study report. This was of considerable concern to both myself and the Social and Behavioural Sciences Ethics Committee at Flinders University. Scraton and Chadwick (1987) record a similar problem around research into the Prison Department in the United Kingdom in the 1970s where the Home Office's view of "proper research" (p. 11) conflicted with that of the researchers whose interest was seen as a threat. It was, therefore, no surprise that after the application was made, the SAPOL Research and Survey Committee responded as follows:

> After careful consideration of your proposal, I regret to inform you that the RSCC is unable to approve your application. The proposed field of work has already being considered (SIC) internally to be undertaken within the organisation (Hoff, 2015).[5]

After consultation with the Chair and Deputy Chair of the Social and Behavioural Sciences Ethics Committee, I was asked to provide the answers to two questions:

1. Did the proposed research require the input and collection of SAPOL data? The answer was "no" as this was a qualitative approach.
2. Would the police officers interviewed be officially representing SAPOL? Again the answer was "no" as the interviews were to be focused on the experiences of the officers in confronting traumatic situations and their strategies around the preservation of their health and well-being.

The ethics committee also asked for a letter of support from the Police Association (Union) which was forthcoming (Carroll, 2015. See Appendix B). I was given final ethics approval to commence interviews within a week of those requirements being met. All police officers interviewed, volunteered to participate in the study as a result of a letter written to the Police Association Journal. The response from police officers was immediate with a wide cross-section of members making contact with me by email, text or telephone. In addition, a group of operational Sergeants had previously expressed their willingness to be interviewed after I had presented to a training day for South Coast Local Service Area Sergeants some six months earlier. Word of mouth recommendations from officers already interviewed also resulted in further expressions of interest and contacts as the interviews proceeded.

The Police Association made its offices available for me to meet participants and conduct interviews, others were conducted in police stations including headquarters

[5] See full text of the letter in Appendix C.

and on-campus at Flinders University as well as in the private homes of participants. Two early interviews were conducted in public at coffee shops. Although no privacy issues arose, the practice was discontinued as the process developed. Some interviews (three in total) required more than one meeting. Most took one to two hours to complete.

All participants were informed prior to the interviews of the lack of approval for this research from SAPOL Research and Survey Coordination Committee. None withdrew as a result. Twelve female officers were interviewed and 38 were male officers. Five of the female officers were retired at the time of their interview, and eight male officers were retired. A broad range of rank was represented with 20 Senior Constables, 22 Sergeants, four Inspectors, one Superintendent, two Chief Superintendents and one (Retired) Deputy Commissioner. Years of service varied from 5 years of operational experience to several officers who had served 40 years or more. Four Special Task and Rescue group Officers were interviewed. Two of the 50 interviewed had been diagnosed with PTSD.

Information sheets were either emailed to officers before the interview or provided at the beginning of the interview process.[6] Consent forms were filled out and signed by participants at the commencement of each interview after the purpose of the project was explained and any questions answered. Handwritten notes were taken by me during the interviews, these were typed up and sent to the participants for feedback after the interviews were completed, to ensure accuracy. All those interviewed participated with a high level of relaxation and enthusiasm, many commenting that they found the interviews "helpful" and some even called the process "therapeutic". It was clear from comments made that most participants had not engaged in such a conversation before. Some became emotional during the interviews. None required or requested professional referrals to counsellors after the interviews had been completed.

1.6 Sapol History and Structure

In order to effectively engage with South Australian police officers in the context of a qualitative open-ended interview format, a comprehensive context for the study is necessary. Part of that context comprises an understanding of SAPOL culture and how that influences the well-being and resilience of the police officers the organisation employs. A significant factor in this is the history of the organisation from which its culture and traditions have developed. SAPOL has its own Historical Society, a group of mostly retired police officers who spend one day each week at its offices located at the Thebarton Police Barracks attending to the police museum located on-site, developing a record of the history of the organisation and assisting researchers to locate documents and other items of historical interest. The Historical Society was of immense value to me in writing this section.

---

[6] See Appendix A.

The South Australia Police, constituted in 1838, 2 years after the colony of South Australia was proclaimed. Unlike the other states, South Australia was never a penal colony. The need for a police force was not foreseen by those planning the colony in the 1830s as it was assumed that only upstanding, law-abiding citizens would be admitted to the new colony whose settlers did not include transported felons as in Victoria, New South Wales and Queensland (Hopkins, 2003). However, it soon became clear that persons entering South Australia from the eastern states and those absconding from locally docked shipping constituted a law and order problem that had to be addressed. The resulting police force was modelled on that established by Robert Peel in London in 1829 and comprised 20 constables commanded by Inspector Henry Inman. The vast distance was an early problem as settlements were established in Port Adelaide, Port Lincoln and Kangaroo Island, the latter two necessitating several days of travel to be reached.

General orders issued in 1861, included the directive that "the mounted police force in South Australia is a Service specially adapted to smart active unencumbered unmarried men" (General order No. 18). This requirement expresses the need for members to focus on their duties. Further regulations required "each man to devote his whole time to the police service" (Hopkins, 2005:12) and "no man in the police force shall marry without permission". Days off were rare, working days commenced at 08:30 h and concluded around 22:30 h.

The period 1850–1890 saw significant increases in emigration into the developing colony and by the end of that period the whole of South Australia had been explored and outlying police stations established. During this period and up to 1911, the Northern Territory was administered by South Australia and the Overland telegraph line between Adelaide and Darwin was constructed necessitating a police presence to protect the line from "uncivilised aboriginal tribes" (Hopkins, 2005:26). Therefore, policing was—and is—implicated in colonization. During the period from the 1850s to the turn of the twentieth century, police stations were established throughout the state as the rail and road networks were developed. Many police "troopers" lived under challenging conditions, both in terms of rudimentary accommodation, extremes of climate and the vast distances that separated them from "backup" when it was required (Killmeir, 2016).

Changes in methods of transport had a significant effect on policing, particularly after privately-owned motor vehicles appeared on South Australian roads in 1915 (Hopkins, 2003). The first recorded road fatality involving a car and a pedestrian occurred in 1915. By 1956, the road toll had risen exponentially, and that year 12,530 road accidents were recorded with 167 fatalities. Random breath testing was introduced in 1986, thus having a direct impact on police alcohol culture as will be analysed later in the thesis.[7]

In lieu of a more structured training approach for new recruits, a "catechism" for police cadets was introduced in 1870 (Hopkins, 2005) in the absence of formal training, which outlined the duties, responsibilities and basic legal issues surrounding police duties. Forty years later, little had changed with regard to the preparation of

[7] See "Coping", Chap. 5.

adult recruits for their careers in policing. Most trainings took place "on the job" as recent recruits were exposed to their duties under the supervision of more experienced senior colleagues. Police Academy training was military in nature involving high levels of regimentation and little academic or legal input. Those trained during this period often joined at the age of 16 or younger and were schooled in etiquette, public speaking and typing as well as basic legal matters over a 4-year period interspersed with frequent periods of practical exposure to police work (Killmeir, 2016).

In the 1960s, all training was transferred to the Police Academy at Fort Largs where it now included, "physical fitness, ceremonial drill, equitation, police procedures and law in that order of priority" (Hopkins, 2003:100). In the 1970s, the police Studies certificate was introduced in co-operation with TAFE (Training and Further Education) colleges which broadened the training syllabus significantly, allowing police officers access to relevant tertiary studies relevant to forensic science and social sciences more generally. In 2003, Commissioned Officers aspiring to the rank of Superintendent were required to complete a Graduate Certificate in Management at the University of South Australia (Hopkins, 2003). In the twenty-first century, police training embraces those who join with tertiary qualifications and encourages aspirational Commissioned Officers to pursue further academic qualifications in the areas such as law, management and criminology.

SAPOL has a 180-year history of British Peelian style policing, which began in the context of an Australian settlement that was different from the penal colonies to the East, West and North of the country in that it was free and democratic, a social experiment "down under". In my next chapter, I define the context of this study in the twenty-first century understanding of how such democratic police organisations have changed in response to the challenges now faced, including that of recognising the need to acknowledge that policing has its problems and the psychological and physical well-being of those in "the job".

1.7 Theories of Policing

SAPOL functions amongst what Manning (2010) describes as "Anglo American Democratic Policing" nations. These include the United Kingdom, the United States of America, Canada, Australia and New Zealand. Manning identifies such approaches as "democratic policing-focussed on deterrence and prevention, reactive and responsive to public concerns, uniformed, visible and order maintaining at best" (p. 47). Scratona and Chadwick (1987:19) also make reference to the "liberal democratic model" of police work which assumes "the maintenance of order and the enforcement of the law within a democratic framework". Such policing is "benign" in the sense that it has a clear focus on reactive responses to crime and disorder, crime prevention and remaining politically neutral as it resolves societal conflict with a minimum of force. In this sense, argues Manning, "police affect democracy and democracy affects them" (p. 4). Such policing sits comfortably with SAPOL whose police cars proudly claim by way of signage that they are "Leading the way to keeping

South Australians safe". Scraton (1985: 8) is very clear that "police are no more than citizens in uniform" engaged in "policing by consent" in his rebuke of police and policing during Margaret Thatcher's Prime Ministership. Scraton's (1999/2009) accounts of the aftermath of the 1989 Hillsborough soccer stadium disaster where 96 people died, and the subsequent perversions of justice and truth that followed, portray a police organisation that is by any definition far from democratic, rather oppressive, excessively violent and driven by its political masters. SAPOL during the turbulent years of protest in South Australia against the Vietnam War and the later South African sporting tours showed itself to be far more constrained, less violent and more ready to negotiate with protestors before, after and during such protests. The right to protest was respected although senior officers at the time admitted that they felt conflicted when policing protests while sharing the political views of the protestors. Bruggeman (2016:2) defines policing in this context as "intentional action involving the conscious exercise of power or authority that is directed towards rule enforcement, the promotion of order or assurance of safety". He argues that "the police should symbolise objectivity, transparency and decency, act as a protector, not for certain groups only, but for all citizens. Be present, wherever and whenever necessary, twenty four hours a day, seven days a week for the benefit of societies at large" (p. 1). Bruggeman concludes that policing based on common values, such as freedom, liberty, justice and fundamental rights, is truly democratic. I would further argue that due in part to its history and genesis, SAPOL is particularly so.

If I am to constructively engage in a critical study of South Australia police and their levels of resilience, I need to seek the answer to a basic question posed by many researchers, "Is there a theory of policing, and if there is, how are such theories constructed and who constructs them?" Manning (2010: 132) is clear that "there is no theory of policing, nor even a systematic failed attempt". Sparrow (2016) theorises police work in terms of what they do, using examples such as an at best, lukewarm commitment to community policing and intelligence lead policing, soft and hard policing, minimum and maximum policing, zero-tolerance policing and "broken windows" community policing, as well as order maintenance policing as evidenced in NYPD initiatives of the 1980s and 1990s. Harcourt (1998:298) refers to the "The fine art of policing" as a "quality of life initiative" including approaches referred to above as well as hot spots policing. Reiner (2010) suggests that for policing theorists consider no less than ten questions before they commence their research. These include the nature of policing activities, the identity of those who become police officers, their motivation for doing so, what powers and discretion they possess and exercise, what social functions they fulfil, who polices the police and how can "the developing purposes and practices of policing be understood?" (p. 16).

Police in South Australia attend to a wide variety of tasks, not confined to law enforcement or social service (SAPOL, 2016). They offer sophisticated responses to social problems including domestic violence and child abuse in cooperative relationships with other professional groups, including legal practitioners, social workers, psychiatrists and psychologists, medical practitioners and many others. Much of what they do is "social work" and in the period of my professional career, SAPOL has moved from a policy (and practice) of non-intervention in family matters such as domestic violence to a very interventionist approach responding to perpetrators with restraining orders and (when breached) incarceration. Victims are now treated with respect and referred on to often overwhelmed support agencies outside of SAPOL in many cases.

However, democratic policing such as that practised in South Australia has many internal challenges, as described by Manning (2005:29), thus "management and managerialism are shaping the practices of the top command and officers above the sergeant level" and in terms of policing in the United Kingdom, "There is also a tension in the UK, albeit centred at Bramshill Police College, between crime control and analysis and police management and leadership concerns more generally" (p. 35). Berkley and Berkley (1969), in his consideration of the identity of, "The democratic police officer" asks, "How is it possible (for police) to treat citizens equally when the police organisation is capricious?" He urges democratic police organisations to be less punitive, more egalitarian and fair, both within society and their own managerial cultures. The democratic police officer, argues Berkely, should have a high standard of professionalism, based on sound education, training and supervision. In discussing David Sklansky's (2007) contribution to the democratic policing discussion, he adds, "The issue of democracy within police organisations, as noted above, has rarely been of concern" (p. 15). SAPOL might increase its concern in this area by heeding Peter Cotton's (2016) suggestion in the recommendations of his mental health review of Victoria (Australia) police by adopting a person focussed management style rather than its present "command and control" approach. This, argues Cotton, would make a significant contribution to the well-being and resilience of its members.

This management approach is a theme that was often referred to by my interview cohort as representing a major stressor, far more challenging than the everyday mayhem, violence and death that is a central factor of their duties. Sergeants, in particular, refer to the ascendance of managerialist risk aversion as a major stressor and source of frustration for them. This is supported by much trauma-focussed research into policing and related first responder organisations (Chae & Boyle, 2013; Gilmartin, 2002; Marin, 2012; McFarlane, 2011; Peters, 2009; Stinchcomb, 2004; Toch, 2002; Violanti, 2014) that clearly portrays "command and control" management approaches in organisations such as SAPOL, coupled with an obsession with risk, contributing directly to high levels of stress among officers. Manning (2010:188) argues with regard to police management in the UK that "given the first principle of fair hiring and evaluation, police should seek to be fair in hiring, internal evaluation, promotion and demotion, transfers and disciplinary treatment of employees, whether sworn officers or civilians". Further, Greene (2014:38) asks, "who now comes to the police profession, with what expectations and abilities and what does this mean for the social and occupational organisation of the police" and "how are police organisations now managed, and with what changes and implications?" (p. 39). He goes on to opine that "Simply put, in a large number of studies, the question is not what works, (in policing) but what forces are shaping policing and how do people react to these forces and to the police?" It is therefore increasingly clear that democratic policing has a stress and trauma problem, not directly acknowledged in the discussions of policing theory referred to above but clearly evident in the trauma literature which has a different focus, the well-being of those who police democracies.

This chapter has explored the context of contemporary "democratic" policing, both at an international and more local level. It is argued here that there has been little thought given by police organisations to the impact of their management approaches and lack of psychological support for officers after "out of the ordinary" (by policing standards) incidents, and that as a result, there exists a crisis in contemporary policing that must be addressed. It is no longer acceptable at a personal, professional and organisational level that officers are left to take care of their own well-being in the context of an expectation by many in the media and helping professions that unwanted traumatic responses to operational duties and the way they are managed are almost inevitable.[8] Such issues form the basis of my study in the embedded literature reviews within the thematic chapters that follow.

References

Apitzsch, U., & Siouti, I. (2007). Biographical analysis as an interdisciplinary research perspective in the field of migration studies. *Research Integration.*

Bruggeman, W. (2016). Pearls in policing: Exploring the boundaries of policing. *Pearls in Policing.* Hong-Kong.

Berkley, G. E., & Berkley, G. E. (1969). *The democratic policeman.* Beacon Press.

Chae, M. H., & Boyle, D. J. (2013). Police suicide: Prevalence, risk, and protective factors. *Policing: An International Journal of Police Strategies & Management, 36*(1), 91–118.

Cotton, P. (2016). Victoria Police Mental Health Review. An independent review into the mental health and well-being of Victoria Police employees. Australia.

Carroll, M. (2015). Support letter. A. Paterson. Adelaide, South Australia: Police Association of South Australia.

Cresswell, J. W. (1998). *Qualitative inquiry and research design: Choosing among five traditions.* Sage Publications.

A Faull 2017 Police work and identity: A South African ethnography Routledge

J Fereday E Muir-Cochrane 2006 Demonstrating rigor using thematic analysis: A hybrid approach of inductive and deductive coding and theme development International Journal of Qualitative Methods 5 1 80 92

G Gardner 2001 Unreliable memories and other contingencies: Problems with biographical knowledge Qualitative Research 1 2 185 204

KM Gilmartin 2002 Emotional survival for law enforcement ES Press, PMB 233 2968

Guest, G., et al. (2011). *Applied thematic analysis.* Sage.

Harcourt, B. E. (1998). Reflecting on the subject: A critique of the social influence conception of deterrence, the broken windows theory, and order-maintenance policing New York style. *Mich. L. Rev, 291*(293), 309–329.

VE Henry 2004 Death work: Police, trauma, and the psychology of survival Oxford University Press

Hopkins, C. (2003). South Australia Police 1838–2003 A history of the development and operations of the force from its establishment. South Australian Police Historical Society Inc.

Horner, P. (2011). *Jack knife: The crashing of a policeman—NSW police and PTSD.* New South.

[8] See Chap. 2 "Power, organisational and police culture, 'the job".

E Jones S Wessely 2005 Shell shock to PTSD: Military psychiatry from 1900 to the Gulf War Psychology Press
Loftus, B. (2009). *Police Culture in a changing world.* Clarendon Studies in Criminology.
Lewin, K. (1951). Field theory in social science. Selected theoretical papers edited by Dorian Cartwright.
Raphael, B. (2014). Telephone conversation. A. Paterson. Adelaide, South Australia.
PK Manning 2005 The study of policing Police Quarterly 8 1 23 43
McFarlane, A. C. (2011). *Many paths, one purpose. Expert forum.* Australian Centre for posttraumatic mental health.
Peters, R. F. (2009). *Police under pressure (A donkey on the edge).* HEAS Publications.
Roberts, B. (2002). *Biographical research.* Open University Press.
LK Rogers 1999 Posttraumatic stress disorder: A police officer's report Proctor Publications
D Saleebey 1996 The strengths perspective in social work practice: Extensions and cautions Social Work 41 3 296 305
SAPOL. (2016). SAPOL Annual Report. S. A. Police. Adelaide South Australia, Government of South Australia.
Scraton, P., & Chadwick, K. (1987). *Law, order and the authoritarian state: readings in critical criminology,* Open University Press.
Sparkes, A. (2013). *The cost of bravery.* Australia: Penguin Group, Australia.
Sparrow, M. (2016). *Handcuffed: What holds policing back, and the keys to reform*, Brookings Institution Press.
JB Stinchcomb 2004 Searching for stress in all the wrong places: Combating chronic organizational stressors in policing Police Practice and Research 5 3 259 277
RG Tedeschi LG Calhoun 1996 The posttraumatic growth inventory: Measuring the positive legacy of trauma Journal of Traumatic Stress 9 3 455 471
Toch, H. (2002). Stress in policing. *American Psychological Association Journal.*
Violanti, J. M. (2014). *Dying for the job: Police work exposure and health.* Charles C Thomas Publisher.
Weathers, F., et al. (2013). *The PTSD checklist for DSM 5 (PCL-5).* National Centre for PTSD.
Zinn, J. O. (2004). Social contexts and responses to risk network (SCARR).

Chapter 2
Power, Organisational and Police Culture: "The Job"

Abstract The focus here is on police culture in Australia and across the globe. What does the international literature say about how police are organised and managed, what is effective leadership in the context of policing and how, if at all, do police organisations change? The interview data around this theme is examined and discussed in terms of how executive police management impacts the resilience of police members lower in the pecking order and what officers themselves consider effective leadership and management to be. The use of the phrase "the job" is examined, how it describes the nature of their task for many officers and how such a cultural descriptor impacts coping with the rigours of policing.

2.1 "The Job"

Police officers worldwide refer to their profession as "the job". As confirmed by a retired Detective Senior Sergeant, "in the seventies when we were young, we were married to the job". A Detective Senior Constable told me, "I love the job, it's about the ability to help someone and make a difference". The use of the word resonates and the connotation was revealed in a comment from a Sergeant referring to his early career when stationed on the West Coast of South Australia, "I loved the job at Ceduna. They call the job the job because it isn't a job, that's the joke". What this means is that policing isn't a "job", it's a calling, a family and much more. In response to my question, "How has the job been for you?" one officer answered, "In general good, it's a great job, it's more than a job it can become people's whole lives". This chapter will examine data from the officer interviews and literature addressing police culture, leadership and management in terms of their impact on the health, resilience and well-being of contemporary police in "the Job". Institutional and political power is also a real issue in this context. The exercise of power within SAPOL, often in the context of paramilitary "command and control" approaches (Cotton, 2016), has a profound impact on the well-being of operational officers. Chapter 3 demonstrates clearly how this impacts women in the form of bullying and harassment. Cotton's "people centred management" is an important key to a significant change in this area.

A. Paterson, *Trauma and Resilience in Contemporary Australian Policing*,
https://doi.org/10.1007/978-981-16-4416-0_2

2.2 Police Culture. What Is It?

The importance of policing culture and its impact both positive and negative on the health and well-being of police officers is central to this research (Gilmartin, 2002; Higgs & Bettess, 1987; Loftus, 2009; Marin, 2012; Peters, 2009; Prenzler, 1994). Organisational history is also an important factor in understanding how culture develops (Crank & Crank, 2014).

Volkman (2007) describes typical police cultural characteristics that include pride and perfectionism, rigidity, bonding between officers against a common foe ("them"), the development and use of language unique to the profession as well as a professional focus on safety and security. Police are process and action-oriented, loyal to other members of the police "family" and deeply suspicious of outsiders (Henry, 2004; Horner, 2011; Mckay, 2005). Police culture has been traditionally masculine and resistant to organisational and operational change. Loftus (2010) defines police culture as "an adaptation to the realities of police work" (p.4) and this is supported by a plethora of literature written usually by experienced veterans of policing outlining how many years of service impacted on them at the level of personality, social interaction and family life, as well as their attitudes and values towards acceptable societal behaviour and those in society (the "them") who don't conform (Baker & Das, 2013; Bushey, 2015; Horner, 2011; June, 2013; Littles, 2011).

Crank and Crank (2014: 4) warn against studies of police culture "stripping cops of their humanity" and counsel the avoidance of the oversimplification of their organisational structures, policies and behaviours. They also point out that language is critically important to policing and that its values, beliefs, rituals and habits "are full of historical prescriptions and common sense that guide actions" (p. 66). Culture, argue Crank and Crank, is little more than "collective sense making".

Silverii (2014) explores how police officers change from recruitment to retirement outlining five "liminal" phases of the police personality. The Academy teaches the "us and them" of policing, the initial field exposure encourages recent graduates to "forget the academy" as they move toward the states of independence and autonomy critical to the effective exercise of their professional discretion in the field. The next phase described as "don't rock the boat" occurs as older officers move towards retirement. The final phase returns the officers to the "us versus them" mentality, but more gently with the benefit of years of field experience. The central themes of police culture according to Silverii include operational activity ("crime fighting and making a difference") shared values, shared experiences, shared behaviours and shared efforts in the field. Such sharing is partly responsible for the close bonds that develop between officers, often described by them as "camaraderie".[1]

Crank and Crank (2014) and Loftus (2009) emphasise group cohesion, often an issue when police corruption and injustice is alleged (Scraton, 1985; Scraton & Chadwick, 1987). This includes a shared image of strength and authority intrinsic to the police role and territorial control as both are seen as central to police culture. An argument that will emerge later in this research refers to the emphasis on strength

[1] This will be examined in detail in Chap. 8 "Resilience".

and toughness which can often impede the timely seeking of help and support for individual officers as trauma-related problems develop. Kirby (2013:109) argues further that culture encompasses "values, norms, perspectives and craft rules which inform police conduct" and agrees that issues such as suspicion, cynicism, isolation and solidarity with colleagues, conservatism, male machismo, racism and "can do leadership" characterise police organisation in cultural terms. Flannery (2015:62) in the context of treating psychological trauma further describes police officers as "action oriented, self-contained deferential men and women where complaining is not acceptable behaviour". The latter reference is again to the "strength and toughness" that often inhibits individual police officers from seeking support at vulnerable moments in their careers as well as police organisational policies that ignore or underplay stress factors inherent to policing.

Smith describes police culture in terms of defensive attitudes, a general lack of emotional response and firm resistance to change both organisational and cultural. Continuing the theme of psychological self-sufficiency, Smith goes on to describe police attitudes to help-seeking, thus "those services are there for wimps, those who can't cope with the job, not for real men" (p.277). Loftus (2010:4) describes a culture of "serving others, making a difference, contributing to the greater good" and sees police officers as "continually suspicious, leading socially isolated lives and displaying defensive solidarity with colleagues". She continues, "Police culture encompasses the images officers have of their role along with their assumptions which underpins and informs their conduct" (p. 5).

Police culture can also be seen as a "protective factor" in terms of work-related stress in policing. According to Pole et al. (2006: 208) "resilience is a function not only of the individual but also of the circumstances of the environment in which he or she finds himself/herself". Chae and Boyle (2013) support such a view naming "social support" a significant component of police culture, in preventing unwelcome trauma-related responses to the more challenging and confronting aspects of police work.[2]

2.3 The "Police Family"

Police officers at the beginning of their career are assured that police organisations have similar values to a functional family. The message imparted to young police officers is that you support and back up your colleagues and that the police organisation takes care of its own in a variety of ways. For the five police officers whose autobiographies are referenced in detail in my PTSD and policing chapter, this was not a reality. Allan Sparks, after being diagnosed with career-related PTSD began a long period of sustained litigation against New South Wales Police and describes his feeling of being "discarded like a piece of shit". His recovery left no option to return to his former duties, as far as New South Wales Police were concerned, and

[2] This will be discussed further in Chap. 5: "Keeping well, coping".

he was damaged beyond repair (Sparkes, 2013:160). Esther Mckay (2005) similarly accuses the organisation of making her feel inadequate, having been offered little training by NSW Police in terms of stress management and no psychological support or debriefs as she spent 17 years as a crime scene examiner, her duties filled with carnage, grotesque injury and death. She was diagnosed with PTSD and discharged in 2001 being deemed medically unfit for duty. Horner (2011; 234) alludes to his disillusionment in very clear terms as "police family bullshit". His career challenges were met with no input from his organisation, so he increasingly relied on alcohol to survive, a strategy that resulted in his dismissal from police service. US officer Ken Rogers (1999) was accused of being a malingerer by his organisation who disputed his PTSD diagnosis and denied in court that his police experience and duties had contributed to it. His account clearly indicates how such an organisational response contributed to his mental deterioration. Belinda Neil (2014) was similarly forced to undertake 4 years of duty of care legal action against New South Wales Police before she received a financial settlement after her "hurt on duty" PTSD diagnosis. Geoff Bernasconi (Mckay, 2010:209) after diagnosis had "no call to say that he was valued" from the Department and describes his "feelings of abandonment" (p. 249). All of the police officers whose careers are referenced here were given no choice and left their police careers "hurt on duty" once a PTSD diagnosis had been made. Alan Sparkes (2013: 153) says "and the police seem no better able to handle a mentally ill son. As far as the department was concerned if you wanted to be treated like a leper, just leave work with a mental illness".

Police culture is complex and multi-faceted and is the "glue" that holds police organisations together as a "family" which has a unique role and extraordinary powers and discretion in society. The paramilitary, top-down command structures, where orders and authority are not openly questioned, and the clear divisions created by the rank structures, as well as the stressors that inevitably accompany policing, all contribute to the well-being or otherwise of police officers. Most researchers in this area agree that police culture is a product of what officers do, how they view the world and how they perceive each other as part of a family that has in common experiences of society that "normal" citizens don't share. They share an "us and them" perception of the world and when resilience is required they bond to that end. Culture is, therefore, a central component of this study.

2.4 Police Organisational Culture

Some of the more recent research literature focussing on policing and trauma seeks to change the focus from the everyday stressful experiences of officers in the field to the way in which they are managed and how their organisations function (Cotton, 2016; Dollard et al., 2003; Garner, 2008; Hanson & McKenna, 2011; McFarlane, 2017; Shane, 2010; Sparrow, 2016; Stinchcomb, 2004). "Command and control" approaches to management, typical of most police organisations, are usually justified by the need for clear, decisive action in the context of critical incidents (Burke,

2016) but often result in a lack of consultation, unjustified interference by senior officers in operational decision-making, a lack of feedback around positive operational outcomes and frustration relating to higher-level decision-making that avoids consultation with lower ranks. These issues are well summed up by former New York City Police Commissioner Lee P. Brown:

> The command-and-control culture of the police department doesn't treat officers as intelligent, creative and trustworthy people. It allows them very little discretion. It is designed to make sure they don't get into trouble, don't embarrass the department, and don't get their supervisors into trouble (Cited in Webber, 1990:113).

Stinchcomb (2004:266) also makes the same point that "rigid policies, reluctant decision makers, anger between male and females, demanding supervisors and micro-managing administration" as well as "treating workers (police officers) like children, rigidly hierarchical and overly bureaucratic" structures are inherently stressful. She goes on to point out that the absence of communication and consultation, little or no feedback around performance and a lack of opportunity for lower ranks to contribute to departmental policy, all add to the malaise that stems from issues other than operational challenges of everyday policing. Violanti (2014:8) in an article addressing suicide in police organisations makes a similar point, "hopelessness emerges from the social, milieu and structure of the police organisation and not from the danger of policing".

Much of the contemporary police management literature considered in this research shows little sign of awareness among police educators and leaders of these issues. Boon (2015:8), however, breaks that constraint, "there is little doubt that to be successful, a leader has to gain the support of followers by being visible, approachable, honest, fair and competent". Baker and Das (2013) interviewing police chiefs from across the globe express the view that "the best way of finding out about people is by talking with them" although most of those high-ranking police interviewed by Baker and Dass expressed little interest in extending their management focus to that of stress factors that may impact on their profession. Cook and Tattersall (2010:12) in a handbook for Senior Investigating Officers opine that "leaders (compared with managers) inspire and motivate", but remain silent about the management of trauma and stress among their colleagues.

2.5 Police Management and Leadership

Many of the 50 officers interviewed for my research expressed clear views about what they saw as effective management and leadership in policing. Most of them identified management as an aspect of the department that addresses organisational, administrative and bureaucratic factors and "leadership" at a more operational level, which was more concerned with achieving organisational and professional goals and valuing and taking care of officers in that context. Leaders are seen as "hands on", inspirational, consultative and trusting, having the ability to give feedback, positive and negative, in effective ways that encourage skill and professional development, and constituting a positive role model for younger and more inexperienced officers. The interview data below in its sheer volume alone expresses the concerns of those interviewed effectively. The greatest challenge to their resilience, according to those officers interviewed, is the way they are led.

Police management literature clearly distinguishes between management and leadership. Stinchcomb (2004:261) sees "autocratic management practices whose key ingredient is control" as a major contributor to work-related trauma responses, identifying micro-management, rigid policy structures and reluctant decision-making as symptoms of typically poor management practices in policing. Shane (2010) agrees observing that "individual coping mechanisms"[3] are developed by officers to cope with operational stressors, but those emanating from "job context" are more difficult to create and maintain. Such issues, often referenced by SAPOL officers at interview, include being second-guessed in the field when, for example, a senior officer overrules an order given by a Sergeant to his/her team, when the punishment for minor offences is too severe and when there is a lack of recognition and positive feedback for jobs well done.

Parsons et al. (2011) in a study involving senior police officers in South Australia identified "command and control" approaches to management in SAPOL, concluding that as most police are not trained to be managers, their focus is usually on compliance rather than facilitating communication and consultative leadership. Evidence of such a lack was frequently referred to by SAPOL officers including some of the significant ranks who saw themselves as self-taught in management practices, usually relying on "common sense". Many officers during my interviews commented on SAPOL's typical approach to seemingly regular organisational restructures, where genuine, open communication with those on the ground is, in their view, always lacking. Cotton (2016) in his report into Victoria police focussing on the mental health of the organisation calls for "an overarching leadership framework" and a new emphasis on "people oriented leadership" (Cotton, 2016:40). This, in Cotton's view, includes the development of team-based "structures and processes" that foster support, open communication and consultation in decision-making, as well as clarity around expectations characterised by feedback, discussion, debate and learning, between management and officers under their command. With reference to leadership, Cotton envisages an organisation where leaders are role models in such areas, stating that "excessively directive leadership, (command and control) causes disgruntlement and reduces morale and engagement" (p. 41). People-oriented leadership, says Cotton, has profound positive implications for the mental health and well-being of employees, particularly in police organisations where at present such leadership is a rarity.

Boon (2104:8) describes an effective police leader as "being visible, approachable, honest fair and competent", and goes on to distinguish such leadership from management, thus "leadership is strategic, whereas management is tactical", but refrains from including in the "tactical" any reference to strategies addressing health

[3] See Chap. 5: "Keeping well, coping".

and well-being. One officer interviewed for my research commented that SAPOL senior management was noted for their lack of visibility to the lower echelons saying, "I have never been in my ten year career in the city, in the same physical space as the Commissioner". An officer who served in the London Metropolitan police before joining SAPOL compared his experience in the United Kingdom to South Australia, "Management in the UK would regularly go out in a patrol car just to keep in touch. It should happen here!" Cook and Tattersall (2010:12) also argue that "leaders (compared to managers) inspire and motivate". One way of doing so, according to many officers interviewed, involved senior officers showing an interest in the most difficult areas of policing such as family violence investigation. A Sergeant working in that area was resigned to that reality, "There's no time for SAPOL to care about its people. We are never asked, is everyone going OK. That is the way policing is". Fleming and Lafferty (2003) confirms this in an interview with Sir Peter Fahey, Chief Constable of Manchester Police in the United Kingdom, quoting him as saying, "Future leaders must see each member of staff as an individual whose skills and experience must be drawn out and utilised". Sir Peter, perhaps heralding a new era of police organisational research goes on, "We can benefit from the advice of academics, providing they take time to write for practitioners and not just for themselves" (p. x. Forward).

Garner (2008), himself an experienced American senior officer, argues that "the police leader as counsellor should avoid being aloof, uninterested and seemingly uncaring". Garner goes on to point out that if seen that way such a leader will be unlikely to receive from his "troops" requests for help or advice that might support their careers and relationships. This is often reflected in the interviews conducted with SAPOL members, who rarely express their readiness to seek help from their leaders particularly those above the rank of Sergeant, without a high level of confidence born of a similar perception. Garner (2016:7) from an American perspective agrees stating that "the Sergeant in today's law enforcement organisation has the best job in America, they have more fun and more influence on the success of a police organisation than anyone else". Orrick (2008:159) comments that officers seeking good leadership look for trust, hope and positivity, as well as evidence that they are valued as individuals. Poor supervision, argues Orrick, indicates that many officers are "over managed and under led" which inevitably leads to negativity and disillusionment on their part. A significant, contemporary organisational focus on risk management was seen by some of those interviewed as a problem in terms of creating an environment of trust and positive communication. "Risk management now influences everything we do and say", said one, adding "There are quotas, not targets, the message is don't achieve their quotas, next year they will want more".

2.6 Management and Leadership: The Data from the Interviews

This, as indicated above, was a central theme of the interviews. Officers frequently referred to the importance of effective management, their experience of managers in the organisation and the impact of para-military structures on the way they are led. Leadership was clearly distinguished from management, often those interviewed expressing the view that support and feedback are lacking and that once commissioned, senior officers accept and repeat management styles that cause widespread discomfort throughout SAPOL. This is well represented in the following from a Detective Sergeant, "We were hammered in the media, and at no time did management come in and say "how are you guys going?" This comment refers to an investigation into a long-running child abuse matter. Workloads, particularly in domestic violence and child abuse investigations, are another issue frequently raised, "if we point out our ridiculously high workloads to management, if we raise the issue…the response is always "do you need to come out of the area?" This frustration feeds much discomfort among specialised investigators, who are highly committed to more recently introduced policing activities such as family violence investigation and child protection that draw some criticism from more traditional colleagues who see policing as "catching crooks". One such specialist said that

> The workload and the frustration born out of SAPOL's attitude. No extra staff despite doubling of workload. No acknowledgement of the importance of what we do compared to traditional Policing, child protection and DV don't get enough resources…there's still a lot more work to do in these areas. There is still a strong view in SAPOL that we are glorified Social Workers!

There is clear evidence here of SAPOL's readiness to accept new operational responsibilities such as domestic violence interventions, a far cry from traditional policing, without the extra commitment needed to resource such services appropriately. Since the 1970s, SAPOL has moved from a "no intervention in family matters" (Paterson, 1984) policy where, for example, a domestic violence perpetrator would be advised not to do it again, to a twenty-first-century regime where intervention orders, arrests and direct cross-departmental interventions are the order of the day. The major stressor for this officer is not the confronting aspects of policing domestic violence, but rather the lack of resources to police it adequately and the lack of practical, operational recognition by senior officers of its importance.

Issues around organisational trust and communication are real for many officers, "I first started to worry about the organization when rules meant everything … you have to trust people in the organization". Officers referred to the Commissioned Officer (Inspector and above) at the management level of their organisation as "SAPOL" clearly portrays an "us and them" perspective. "SAPOL don't trust us to make a decision, they don't believe us or trust us" and in line with much of the more recent stress-related police literature, "What stresses us most is the organization", and "The biggest stressor in the job is management. It's a case of the troops V SAPOL. The bosses are only interested in SAPOL, you don't start out in the job that way!", and more negatively, "I was diagnosed with PTSD and mild depression. Was refused WorkCover. SAPOL disagreed with the diagnosis. I took sick leave and PASA (the police union) sued SAPOL. Management don't care. We are cannon fodder!" This view of "SAPOL" was regularly expressed by many of those interviewed. There is evidence of a major separation between "the troops" (ranks up to and including Sergeant) and the "bosses" (Inspector and above). The latter are regularly accused of forgetting what operational policing is like, as represented in "they don't start out in the job that way!" Said another in the same vein, "Commissioned Officers forget where they have come from". And further, "Patrols need the greatest skills. Bosses and Criminal Investigations Branch (detectives) should be required to go back on patrols to keep up their skills and awareness".

For this reason, operational leadership at Sergeants level is clearly of crucial importance, with many officers recalling positive and negative experiences of SAPOL middle management, "Bad supervisors, with bad management skills put a lot of stress on you", and more positively, "I had two old school Sergeants who were very good, you kept away from arse–hole Sergeants". Another Senior Constable said, "A team is only as good as it's Sergeant, it's not an easy role. I have a fantastic Sergeant". She went on, "Sergeants are very important but a lot of them are old school and not aware of options as far as stress issues are concerned". The awareness of "stress issues", and the capacity to intervene in a timely way before such issues become serious and debilitating is a skill set often referred to by the Sergeants themselves. Team leaders often have to deal with and handle problems that team members have outside of SAPOL "you would notice if team members were withdrawn or argumentative" said one Sergeant, adding, "every shift you were aware of physical or mental issues. If I saw changes, I would call them in for a chat". "Other team members would tell me if they thought colleagues were in trouble". A retired Senior Sergeant, referring to "outside" impacts on officer's well-being added, "Sergeants are critical to the health of their teams. 40% of the time the problems team members have are personal relationship issues".

Training in team leadership and management was seen by many Sergeants as an important issue. Many of those interviewed were sure that from an organisational perspective, leaders are of necessity, born and not made. They disagreed, one very clear in his belief in the value of training in this area, "To achieve Sergeant's rank, I undertook twenty subjects in an Advanced Diploma of Justice Administration. There was no SAPOL training in team management", said one interviewee reinforcing what much of police management literature argues around police management styles and a lack of organisational input into such areas (Burke, 2016; Parsons et al., 2011; Webber, 1990). It is assumed, at least in SAPOL and probably in other police jurisdictions, that the elevation to a Sergeant or Commissioned rank endows the recipient with leadership and management skills. Those interviewed for this research clearly thought otherwise. This was reinforced when I asked a competent and respected Sergeant, "Where did your management approach come from. Were you trained as a team leader?" She answered, "We don't get any training, but use a common-sense approach with things like hot debriefs after an incident". She added after some thought, "experience in handling people over the years led to my management style. I learnt by trial and error. Diplomacy and negotiation were central and important". It is not hard to imagine the benefits that SAPOL and other police organisations might accrue when even minimal training and education, preferably sourced from outside of the organisation, was offered departmentally to Sergeants and Commissioned officers alike. Cotton (2016) could not be clearer in his recommendations to Victoria police around such possibilities.

A retired, high-ranking officer was also clear about the most desirable qualities of effective leaders and managers: "I didn't have to deal with bosses as much due to my early promotion but had to learn how to be a good one". When asked what that entailed, he responded in answer to the question, "What's a good boss? Credibility". And further, "I had some Sergeants you would walk over hot coals for, bad Sergeants had closed minds, made rash decisions and were not approachable".

A Senior SAPOL Officer earlier in his career created a leadership programme for Sergeants:

> The Leadership Enhancement Programme was a real innovation. "******** suggested we include Darlington (southern Adelaide suburb) Sergeants as well. Twelve Patrol Sergeants were involved. We started with a morning tea. We set up a learning environment. They were going ahead in leaps and bounds. We challenged them to have their teams humming along. They developed confidence in themselves that enhanced and elevated their skills. We found the right balance between quantitative and qualitative input. There's little difference in leadership between us and General Motors Holden or the Submarine Corporation. The Leadership Enhancement Programme was about developing skills in leadership.

This programme, devised by a now-retired Chief Superintendent, was very short-lived. Little value, it seems, is placed on such innovations by SAPOL executive management. Preparation for leadership at Sergeant's level is often limited to the observation of others in the role and one's own experience of their approach to management and leadership. This is well expressed by the officer who set up the ill-fated programme described above, "We load everything onto Sergeants, we don't give them in-service training", The number of Sergeants who volunteered to be interviewed for my research and their levels of organisational frustration supports his view. Another retired high-ranking officer explained his perspective of the same issue, "I had three hopeless beat Sergeants! I learnt not how to do things". Referring to another senior officer at an early stage in his career, he went on, "The Sergeant was nuts. I learned how not to handle people". Another Sergeant describing his own leadership style expressed this expectation of his team, "The performance I expect from my team. I expect from myself. I like to lead by example".

Another high-ranking officer commented linking effective person-centred leadership with the central focus of this research, "Leadership training is also of critical importance" and "we need to support leadership at all levels. Leadership has a lot to do with resilience, well led troops are more likely to bounce back". This again demonstrates a central theme of this research, in that there is clear evidence that some high-ranking SAPOL officers have given this issue deep thought, evidenced by the use of terms such as "well lead" and "resilience".

Sergeants themselves were very conscious of their responsibilities, "I was never an arsehole, when things went wrong I pointed out that things don't work out all the time, you don't win all the time" and continued "people will follow you because they want to". The distinction between leadership and management approaches was clearly made by this Sergeant, "We need leaders not managers. We need to work out of loyalty not fear! We don't have many leaders in this job. SAPOL has many managers but very few leaders". Again, this long-serving, vastly experienced officer, shortly after his retirement, shows a significant level of insight into the basic ingredients of leadership. Obviously, such skills were developed from experience, from the often-mentioned "common sense" without specific leadership training input from SAPOL.

A Senior Sergeant expressed his awareness of the responsibilities of management at this level clearly during his interview, "Every day I sent my team out they could have been killed". This is a clear indication of the close bonds between police leaders at this level and those they lead. These bonds are cultural, effective and sustaining. It would appear, however, that those who lead at this level find their own resilience difficult to maintain. They are the focus of much risk-averse management and would greatly benefit from "people centred management" (Cotton, 2016) to underpin their own resilience.[4]

"Unsurprisingly, many officers of lower rank referred to the lack of management skills above them in the organisation due to a lack of training and a promotional process that was usually based on factors other than competence and management qualifications". The Department often has poor upper management skills. Some "Commissioned Officers" are there for the kudos and were made up "promoted" because of sponsors "within the organisation". This Senior Sergeant, who had no intention of seeking further promotion, went on, "We come to work to have fun. I've worked earlier in my career with some fantastic Sergeants. They say this is how I want it done. You don't want to disappoint this kind of leader. We are basically serving the community". This comment extends the perception of the need for a high quality of leadership beyond its impact on those led to the effectiveness of what they do in terms of impact on the community served.

Many interviewees were very clear that the leadership qualities of managers had a great deal to do with high morale and satisfaction among lower ranks. "There is a big correlation between positive management and the well-being of the team" said one, and another Senior Officer speaking of leadership and its impact on organisational well-being commented bluntly, "I'm not sure it's the gruesome experiences that get to you, you get through that with black humour. Support from colleagues and a few beers after work. The real problem is piss poor management practices and a lack of leadership! The internal working environment of any organization impacts on staff". This is yet another clear example of a long-serving, high ranking officer who is keenly aware of his organisation's deficits in this area and frustrated by the failure of his attempts to change it over a long career.

A significant factor in terms of leadership in policing is the capacity to give positive feedback when it is due (Cotton, 2016; Garner, 2008, 2016; Hanson & McKenna,

[4] See my recommendations section.

2011). Many who were interviewed saw this as far superior to a "command and control" approach where senior officers expect competence and compliance and rarely comment when a task is done well. This was well summed up by a Senior Constable thus, "You are never going to get praise. If you get it, enjoy it, you shouldn't expect it!".

A young Senior Constable summed up the importance of such a response very clearly, "Positive feedback is important. When your Sergeant says you did a good job! The first body I recovered in Water Ops off Granite Island. We were at Mt Gambier training when we were called in and arrived at Victor Harbor at three am. We spotted the body quite quickly. Afterwards I got two or three texts from other team members saying "good job, you are now a proper diver! My Sergeant congratulated me. When I got home, I and my partner had a drink as celebration".

Said a colleague referring to the same, apparently rare experience in the context of cultural support, "Team bonding is important, the blues family is very much alive, there are many different areas you can work in SAPOL, you can be as motivated as you like. It's really good when you get positive feedback from a Sergeant or a boss". The distinction made here between a Sergeant and a "boss" is also significant paralleling another commonly made between "SAPOL" and operational officers.

Another Senior Sergeant summed this up by saying, "Recognition is important as well. One Boss said after a big event, you blokes have gone through a shit day….thanks". His wife showed me after our interview concluded, a letter from the Coroner to SAPOL management praising the STAR group after a particularly challenging murder/suicide case. Her husband said, "I could frame this". A Chief Superintendent showed an apparently rare awareness for a person of his rank of the same issue, "It's important to recognise good work both individual and the team". A younger female Senior Constable added, "There is a lack of positive feedback. I am really proud of much of what I've done. I've had some really bad managers, one resulted in a PASA[5] complaint when a manager tried to drive me out because I was part-time. I've had some very good managers, my current boss is amazing, and I would like to be like him". Some Sergeants were, however, somewhat reticent about positive feedback, and cautioned against too much of a good thing, "Don't give too much praise, I had to be careful about not using praise too often, only when they handled a difficult job well" adding, "we dealt with bad outcomes behind closed doors, I never belittled individuals in front of their peers".

The present emphasis on risk management in SAPOL is seen by many of those interviewed as a problem that has a profound impact on the way SAPOL managers lead: "Risk management now influences everything we do and say. The required standards for our work is above and beyond what humans can do. There are quotas not targets, the message is don't achieve the set targets, or next year they will want more". Such disincentives are also clearly stated in much of the policing literature (Denhardt & Denhardt, 2010; Garner, 2008, 2016; Gilmartin, 2002; Granter et al., 2015; Padhy et al., 2015; Paton, 2009; Pearson-Goff & Herrington, 2013; Sparrow, 2016) where officers feel that the majority of their career-related stressors are located

[5] Police Association of South Australia. The police union.

not in their operational activities but in the way such duties are impacted upon by management practices such as those described here.

Delving more deeply into what constitutes more positive and effective leadership, a retired senior constable gave an example from her career experience, "“***** was a great Sergeant, she was intelligent and had an easy going nature. I had a Sergeant in the country who was kind and did the job as it was meant to be done. He was a leader not a manager. That kind of flexibility was only evident in the country". Kindness, in this context seems a far cry from the more usual "command and control".

Another Senior Constable, commenting on a positive example of leadership commented:

> I was involved in a pursuit, kids driving the car, they tried to ram our fleet,[6] they hit a stobie pole[7] at 100 km per hour, I kept driver's airway open till medics arrived. The car caught fire. I was pretty rattled!" A Chief Inspector arrived and said, there's nothing wrong here, we'll back you 100%. This was unusual, that Chief Inspector had a lot of respect from the troops, most bosses are worried about themselves.

This refers to the high levels of risk aversion experienced by many in the lower ranks. This Chief Inspector stood out because he was prepared to take the risk of reassuring his "rattled" colleagues that he would support them in the inquiry that would inevitably follow such an incident. Most of the similar ranks would offer no such support.

Leadership at the executive level is also seen as critically important, "Scipionne (Chief Commissioner) in Victoria is a good example of a leader who supports his people. We need leadership, not management". I asked one officer, "What have you enjoyed about policing?" "Being on a good team that is stable with good senior people who give free reign but back up when necessary. I had two years in that posting working with ******* who was a Senior Constable instructor who worked shifts, he was inspiring, his whole attitude was around a team effort, leadership and positive support".

A Chief Superintendent who, early in his career was promoted to Senior Constable First Class with supervisory responsibilities, recounted how out of concern for junior officers confronted by death and injury said, "I'd go down to the Morgue if I knew there was an inexperienced team there". That, he opined, was "leadership and good management". Most of the officers I interviewed, agreed. It is very clear from this comment that such approaches operate far beyond the "command and control" practices described elsewhere by other more junior officers. There is an often expressed hope from those interviewed that this might become the management norm, rather than the exception.

Some senior officers are well aware of the issues canvassed above by those interviewed. One responded to those concerns thus, "Many cops think 'the jobs fucked' I invite them to come and sit on my side of the desk. There have been three police

---

[6] Patrol car.

[7] "Stobie" poles are power poles made of concrete and steel in South Australia and named after their inventor.

shootings in my career, the bosses were there, looking after the troops". Significant here is the insight from this high ranking officer after more than fifty years in "the job" that there is a significant distance between "SAPOL" (him) and those who see disengaged managers as the reason why "the job's fucked", rather than their inevitable and constant exposure to trauma and dysfunction.

Looking towards an organisational future of cooperation and creative leadership, a recently promoted Inspector suggested that "You have to work with people in the job, not against them". And further, with regard to his perception of the changes required to create and maintain resilience, "In terms of well-being, I have plans in my head around changes in SAPOL in this area. A footy club monitors its player's welfare. I am sure work performance in affected by levels of well-being. We need pro-active monitoring of staff, offer gym memberships, catch them before they break. We've got a whole lot of broken coppers we can't put anywhere. People should be rotated rigorously". At some point, the overwhelming consensus from the lower ranks about the need for change in management style, coupled with similar views from those now rising towards higher command, might create a tipping point for change. The benefits in terms of the well-being of "the troops" and their resilience would be positive beyond estimation.

2.7 The Organisation and Change: The Literature

Each interview inevitably lead to a conversation about "the organisation", SAPOL. Officers develop relationships with their employer that vary from the expected "pissed off' minority, through those who tolerate the organisation and those who become a part of the management structure through promotion. As indicated in my discussion of leadership and management, when an officer referred to "SAPOL" he or she meant the organisation, and strangely seemed in the process to distance herself/himself from it as in "From SAPOL's perspective police do a job and the consequences are not an issue" and "SAPOL needs to acknowledge that everyone in the job has an exposure to trauma". A senior officer commented further, "The internal working environment of any organisation impacts on staff, the trauma comes from the work stuff, not the {operational} dramas!".

Interestingly, some of those interviewed made a clear distinction between what they do professionally (policing), and the organisation as in an Inspector's comment about his career "I wouldn't change a thing! That's more about policing than it is about SAPOL. I don't trust the organisation". Such a distinction is featured in some of the qualitative international research literature around policing. Henry (2004) refers to the SAPOL equivalent in New York City, the NYPD, as "the Department" with the same emphasis as expressed by the South Australian officers above. This describes "the structures, policies and procedures and to some extent the people that comprise the police agency at any given time" (Henry, 2004: 107) and is in the same sense as that described by the South Australian officers, a distinction or separation between operational and managerial realities that has profound implications among other things for the wellness and resilience of officers. Said one, "The biggest stressor is identifying our enemy inside the job. The enemy is within".

Gilmartin (2002) in his advice to operational and retired officers emphasises his view that "emotional survival" depends on the ability not to allow "the Department" to incite levels of frustration and anger that impact on the individual's health. "Control what you can control" is the message, "and let the rest go!" This is reflected in the anger shown at interview by one officer, "SAPOL is a big fucking machine. I say to coppers, they don't hate you mate, they don't know you exist!".

Several officers interviewed were clearly able to see the difference between "the job" and the department. Said one, whose life partner, also a police officer had been in his view, badly treated by SAPOL "I don't like the organisation, but I try not to let it affect my work, I still enjoy the job". Such disenchantment is confirmed by Paton (2009) who relies on the life-course model to chart police careers, arguing that "organisational systems and procedures sustain bureaucratic and political imperatives". These he argues, fuel much of the disenchantment that is expressed above. Within police organisations, as in many others, there are two worlds, that of the operational constable and their immediate supervisors and the department, in this case, "SAPOL". Violanti and Paton (2006:90) also focus on the impact on health by the organisation in policing, reaching the conclusion that "organisational factors may be more important in predicting PTSD than exposure to (operational) events". Peters (2009:18) concurs in discussing why the New South Wales Police Department has had difficulty responding to the emotional (job-stress-related) needs of its officers, "You are expecting loyalty from an organisation, which by definition is unable to show this emotional trait". Most officers interviewed had few expectations of SAPOL in this area. Said one, "I have the usual frustration with the organisation, no hierarchy can deal with the trauma for me…we hate welfare and all that stuff, the reviews each year are just crap!".

In terms of organisational change in policing, the literature is clear about the need for continual change in response to changes in society and its expectations of police officers (Baker & Das, 2013; Kirby, 2013; Sparrow, 2016) and surprisingly in terms of the conservatism often attributed to them, many officers interviewed agreed, "We need a cultural change…change must start from the top down" and another more positively, "It's a good job, with great potential to be better. SAPOL is not progressive enough!".

2.8 The Organisation: Data from the Interviews

Officers interviewed all had a view of the organisation and its positive and negative qualities. The "us and them" distinction is not unusual in large organisations, and SAPOL is no exception. There is among the lower ranks a view that once an officer is commissioned and no longer operational her or his credibility decreases having joined the "them" of policing. This is well expressed by the comment of a long-serving Senior Constable, "The biggest stressor is identifying our enemy inside the job. The enemy is within. Micro managing and bullying is the central issue".

A Senior Constable expressed his view of another issue, "The organisation is still extremely risk averse, which is more about risk to the organisation. Is there anything that is going to make the organisation look bad?" This was said in the context of a conversation about a domestic violence related murder that took place in public space and elicited criticism of SAPOL's processes around victim protection.

A retired Detective Senior Sergeant in his criticism from a somewhat jaundiced and angry perspective said, "We didn't trust our bosses". Criticising stress management within the organisation, he went on, "There is no mechanism in SAPOL to save people, the psych unit is useless". Giving an example of a 25-year-old psychologist who, in his view, "knew nothing", he went on, "cops are discarded by the organization. We don't circle the wagons any more, dogging[8] is rampant. We now have a culture of lagging. Does this extend to someone who is stressed?" As well referring to "command and control" approaches to management in SAPOL, went on, "It's always about discipline not about development". A retired Senior Constable made a similar albeit briefer comment referring to the organisation's interest in the impact of trauma on officers, "From SAPOL's perspective police do a job and the consequences are not an issue".

A Senior Constable, opined, "SAPOL needs to acknowledge that everyone in the job has some sort of exposure {to trauma}". It needs to change the focus from "who's to blame". Again, this being a reference to seemingly unsympathetic "command and control" approaches that have failed to quench this individual's enthusiasm for "the job". A Senior Constable made the same point commenting, "SAPOL needs to teach people how to be good at their job. We are a controlling organisation".

A Sergeant, accepting that a level of frustration about such issues was inevitable, acknowledged, "I have the usual frustration with the organisation, no hierarchy can deal with trauma for me, it's nice to know they are thinking {about trauma and its impact} but I believe it is just 'ticking the managerial boxes' we hate welfare and all that stuff, the psych reviews every year are just crap!".

Another Sergeant, seriously injured on duty and returning to work was disappointed, "The organisational response to my later injuries hit me hard. I was not sleeping, eating or wanting to train. I lost interest in the job. I had mild depression. I said to myself, this can't affect me! What can I do? I got treatment for the depression. I saw a psychiatrist once!".

A Sergeant saw the growing involvement of women in SAPOL at high ranks as a positive "Policing has changed as women in management become more involved in SAPOL politics, women are now less likely to be seen and not heard. The lower ranks are more inclined to question things".

A Detective Senior Constable in response to the question, "Has the organisation been supportive of your career" was unequivocal in his answer, "No! In 2009, my teenage son got into some trouble. I went to {police} Welfare for support, they

[8] Informing on colleagues.

informed me of disclosure requirements, I walked out". "I couldn't afford to let any defence lawyer get a sniff. I paid for a private counsellor. I'm having some family issues. I wouldn't go to Employee Assistance". Another officer, although clearly happy with her career and its outcomes, echoed a similar level of distrust and caution, "I wouldn't change a thing! That's more about policing than it is about SAPOL. I don't carry my warrant card when I'm off duty. You do that early in your career. I don't trust the organisation. If I saw something off duty I would not intervene, I would phone for a patrol!".

Others saw a clear need for organisational change, "We need a cultural change, for example, what if the CEO of a police department was not a copper? Change must start from the top down". And, in terms of his readiness to criticise the status quo a retired Senior Constable offered addressing his ex-bosses, "You see me as a problem but I'm your greatest ally because I'm prepared to tell you the truth!" Another added, "It's a shared responsibility. It's not just up to management. The job is what you make it. Some coppers organisational expectations are unrealistic. SAPOL needs to provide these opportunities, remove psycho-social hazards. Get rid of non-supportive management and bullying and harassment". In similar terms, referring to effective leadership advocated for by Cotton (2016) and others, a psychologist added, "I could go out and do a debrief, but if their Superintendent said 'how are you guys doing?' The power of that was immense!" He went on, "The tone of any school is set by the Principal. SAPOL is no different! The top needs to respond to the new order". He concluded, "If they did so upper management would be impressed with the reduction in Work Cover costs".

Sergeants, those who lead their teams on the operational front line, were acutely aware of their responsibility for the safety and well-being of each member, and were caught in the middle of the gap between those doing "the job" and "SAPOL". They were also at ease with expressing their frustration around management and leadership issues, especially their lack of training to identify early signs of trauma or exhaustion among their teams and to respond effectively in their best interests. The high number of Sergeants who were interviewed (22) was a clear indicator of their concerns and their hope that independent research such as this might contribute to much needed (in their view) change.

2.9 Where Next?

SAPOL along with many police organisations world-wide is under significant pressure to re-think its approach to management and leadership in the light of criticism through reports such as Cotton's (2016) that focus on the impact that traditional "command and control" strategies have on the mental health and well-being of its officers. Those interviewed for this research were as one in enjoying "the job" despite, not because of the way they are managed. A lack of interest in management training at all relevant levels in SAPOL reveals an executive view that the organisation has little to learn from the literature or civilian understandings of what constitutes such activities in terms of the health of the organisation. Sworn officers would welcome a change that incorporates the possibility of positive feedback when it is due, less micro-management and risk aversion and access to training and development opportunities, particularly for Sergeants that would make them more comfortable with their leadership responsibilities.

This chapter has given SAPOL officers, past and present, an opportunity to give voice to their experiences of management and leadership. In line with much of the policing literature, albeit giving more detail to essential change, they have expressed clearly what must happen to ensure that present and future generations of SAPOL members and police elsewhere are lead and managed by middle and executive leaders in ways that encourage their well-being and mental health in "the job". The data above is comprehensive, the message is from the front line and issues a challenge to SAPOL and the Police Association of South Australia (the Union) to embark on meaningful and comprehensive changes in management and leadership culture.

References

Baker, B. F., & Das, D. K. (2013). *Trends in policing: Interviews with police leaders across the globe,* vol. 4. CRC Press.

Boon, B. (2015). *Blackstone's leadership for sergeants and inspectors.*

Burke R. J. (2016). *Stress in policing: Sources routledge consequences and interventions.*

Bushey K. (2015). *My LAPD journey: From street cop to commander.* USA: Graphic publishers.

Chae, M. H., & Boyle, D. J. (2013). Police suicide: Prevalence, risk, and protective factors. *Policing: An International Journal of Police Strategies & Management, 36*(1), 91–118.

Cook, T., & Tattersall, A. (2010). *Blackstone's senior investigating officers' handbook.* Oxford University Press.

Cotton, P. (2016). Victoria police mental health review. An independent review into the mental health and well-being of Victoria Police employees. Australia.

Crank, J., & Crank, J. P. (2014). *Understanding police culture.* Routledge.

Denhardt, J., & Denhardt, R. (2010). Building organizational resilience and adaptive management. In *Handbook of adult resilience* (pp. 333–349).

Dollard, M., et al. (2003). *Occupational stress in the service professions,* CRC Press.

Flannery, R. B. (2015). Treating psychological trauma in first responders: A multi-modal paradigm. *Psychiatric Quarterly, 86*(2), 261–267.

Fleming, J. & Lafferty G. (2003). Equity confounded? Women in Australian police organisations. *Labour & Industry: A journal of the social and economic relations of work, 13*(3): 37–49.

Garner, G. W. (2008). *Common sense police supervision: Practical tips for the first-line leader.* Charles C Thomas Publisher.

Garner, G. W. (2016). *Leading cops: Decision making for the law enforcement leader.* USA: Charles C Thomas.

Gilmartin, K. M. (2002). Emotional survival for law enforcement. *ES Press, PMB, 233,* 2968.

Granter, E. et al. (2015). Normalizing extreme work in the Police Service? Austerity and the inspecting ranks. *Organization, 22*(4): 512–529.

Hanson, R., &McKenna, P. F. (2011). Respectful leadership: The emergence of upward nobility as a way of life in policing. *Policing, 5*(4), 287–299.

Henry, V. E. (2004). *Death work: Police, trauma, and the psychology of survival.* Oxford University Press

Horner, P. (2011). *Jack Knife: The crashing of a policeman- NSW police and PTSD.* New South Wales: Australia, Zeus Publications.
June, D. L. (2013). *What they didn't teach at the academy: Topics, stories, and reality beyond the classroom.* CRC Press.
Kirby, S. (2013). *Effective policing? Implementation in theory and practice.* Springer.
Littles, M. (2011). *The police wife: Bullets in the washing machine.* Self.
Loftus, B. (2009). *Police culture in a changing world.* Clarendon Studies in Criminology.
Marin, A. (2012). *In the line of Duty.* Ombudsman's report. Ontario, Canada.
McFarlane, A. C. (2017). Improving internal practices to support emergency services. *Mental Health strategy for first responders: Tackle stigma &enhance prevention strategies.* Melbourne Australia: Criterion Conferences.
Mckay, E. (2005). *Crime scene-true stories from the life of a crime scene investigator.* Viking (Penguin) Australia.
Mckay, E. (2010). *Forensic investigator.* Viking (Penguin) Australia.
Orrick, D. W. (2008). *Recruitment, retention, and turnover of police personnel: Reliable, practical, and effective solutions.* Charles C Thomas Publisher.
Padhy, M, et al. (2015). Optimism and Psychological Well-Being of Police Officers with Different Work Experiences. *Sage Open, 5*(2): 2158244015580852.
Parsons, A., et al. (2011). Effective policing: Management influence and the commitment of senior police personnel. *Policing & Society, 21*(1), 1–26.
Paterson, A. (1984). *Women Police in South Australia in 1974: The beginnings of a chequered career.* Unpublished mini thesis.
Paton, D. (2009). *Traumatic stress in police officers: A career-length assessment from recruitment to retirement.* Charles C Thomas Publisher.
Pearson-Goff, M. & Herrington, V. (2013). Police leadership: A systematic review of the literature. *Policing* pat027.
Peters, R. F. (2009). *Police under pressure (A donkey on the edge).* HEAS Publications.
Pole, N., et al. (2006). Resilience in retired police officers. *Traumatology, 12*(3), 207–216.
Prenzler, T. (1994). Women in Australian policing: An historical overview. *Journal of Australian Studies, 18*(42), 78–88.
Scraton, P. (1985). *The State of the police.* Pluto Pr.
Scraton, P., & Chadwick, K. (1987). *Law, order and the authoritarian state: readings in critical criminology.* Open University Press.
Shane, J. M. (2010). Organizational stressors and police performance. *Journal of Criminal Justice, 38*(4), 807–818.
Silverii, L. S. (2014). *Cop culture: Why good cops go bad.* CRC Press.
Sparkes, A. (2013). *The Cost of Bravery.* New South Wales, Australia, Penguin Group, Australia.
Sparrow, M. (2016). *Handcuffed: What holds policing back, and the keys to reform.* Brookings Institution Press.
Stinchcomb, J. B. (2004). Searching for stress in all the wrong places: Combating chronic organizational stressors in policing. *Police Practice and Research, 5*(3), 259–277.
Violanti, J. M., & Paton, D. (2006). *Who gets PTSD?: Issues of posttraumatic stress vulnerability.* Charles C Thomas.
Violanti, J. M. (2014). *Dying for the job: Police work exposure and health.* Charles C Thomas Publisher.
Volkman, V. R. E. (2007). *Traumatic incident reduction and critical incident stress management.* USA: Loving, Healing press.
Webber, A. (1990). Crime and management: An interview with New York City police commissioner Lee P. Brown. *Harvard Business Review,* 111–126.

Chapter 3
The Feminisation of Policing

Abstract SAPOL women came into uniform with the same job and person specification as their male police colleagues in 1974, largely as a result of emerging equal opportunity legislation. This chapter outlines from their perspective, the struggle, including bullying, harassment and prolific gender-based discrimination, for them and their capacity to thrive in a very challenging environment. Recent inquiries by Commissioners of Equal Opportunity in several Australian states are referenced, indicating that contemporary female officers are not immune to the 1970s experiences of their predecessors but that much progress in terms of their cultural contribution to policing has been achieved. The interview data is rich in evidence of female resilience in policing and of the nature and effectiveness of their coping mechanisms and interpersonal skills. Their impact on a male-dominated policing culture is well described as are the changes they have wrought and the future they face.

I first began working with SAPOL in 1975, just 12 months after women had entered SAPOL uniformed service. I was at that time setting up the Crisis Care programme to assist officers with domestic violence taskings. Before the service commenced I spent three months in police cars on patrol, usually assigned to "mixed patrols" consisting of male and female officers as they were often tasked to "domestics" as they were then called. As my brief history of women in SAPOL (below) reveals these early female pioneers were seen by their male colleagues as an extra responsibility and a potential problem "when things got tough". In the intervening 43 years, a great deal has changed with regard to the role of sworn female officers in SAPOL and a great deal has remained the same. Recent reviews examining sexual harassment and bullying in SAPOL and Victoria police (Jenkins, 2015; Vincent, 2016) highlighted a continuing problem, which was confirmed by many of the female officers I interviewed for this research, particularly those whose service commenced in the 1970s and 1980s. But there has been great progress in the way in which male officers (apart from those described by my interviewees as "dinosaurs") now work with their female colleagues with very few such concerns. Women have risen through the ranks to join executive SAPOL management and my interviews reveal that their colleagues at the patrol officer level and above have brought significant change to the way in which police cope with the traumatic challenges of their operational duties. The women

A. Paterson, *Trauma and Resilience in Contemporary Australian Policing*,
https://doi.org/10.1007/978-981-16-4416-0_3

interviewed are more open to expressing emotional responses in positive ways, more likely to seek support when stressed from colleagues within and professionals and family members outside of the organisation. The data from my interviews show they have ushered in a significant change to the "macho" culture of policing. Traditionally based on a military model, most police organisations have been characterised by a masculine culture (Brough, 2016; Burke & Mikkelsen, 2005; Charlesworth & Robertson, 2012; Paterson, 2014; Winlow, 2001) which contributes significantly to the lack of organisational attention to issues around duty-related trauma and its impact (McKay, 2005).

In 1995 policewomen constituted 13.5% of the total of 42,517 sworn officers employed in Australia. By 2005/2006, this figure had risen to 23% of a total of 45,986 officers employed in this country (Paterson, 2014). This chapter will explore the possibility that the presence of significant numbers of operational policewomen has softened the masculine culture to the extent that some emotional reactions to operational out of the ordinary traumatic events (e.g. the death of a child) may now be more acceptable as stress relief and protective measure than previously.

3.1 Women in SAPOL: A Short History

South Australia's first policewoman was appointed in 1915. Fanny Kate Boadicea Cocks had been appointed as the first full-time Juvenile Court Probation Officer in 1906. As a former school teacher, she offered advice to parents after conducting investigations into young offender's home lives, sought and found work for them and reduced re-offending rates of probationers down to a mere 3% (Higgs & Bettess, 1987). In 1909, amendments to the State Children's Act (Higgs & Bettess, 1987) empowered police constables to arrest children in crisis or moral danger, who were judged to have unfit parents or who were destitute. The stigma attached to male police officers taking such actions led to the appointment of Kate Cocks and colleague Annie Ross. The State Children's Council in 1914 suggested that "the advisability of appointing a small number of police women whose duties shall be the protection of the morals of young girls" (Higgs & Bettess, 1987:11). Despite resistance from the then Commissioner of Police, and with the support of a raft of community organisations, the two women were sworn in as police constables, commencing their duties on December 1, 1915. Some expressed the view that their appointment would raise the standards of the police, "for what body of public servants is more ridiculed for their inefficiency, for their obsolete methods, for their clumsy tactics, than the present day police" (Higgs & Bettess, 1987:12). This was the beginning of a journey for female officers that would lead to their present equal duties and pay as well as the opportunity to contribute to the culture of contemporary policing and all its challenges (Loftus, 2009; McKay, 2005; Neil, 2014; Nixon, 2012; Prenzler, 1994; Prenzler & Heyes, 2000; Paterson, 2014).

Both Cocks and Ross were committed members of the Methodist Church, Annie Ross having worked as a "licenced lying in homes Inspectress" before her appointment as a police officer. Such homes cared for single pregnant young women for up to six months after the birth of their child. The two women were appointed with pay and conditions equal to those of their male colleagues, apparently a first in the British Empire (Higgs & Bettess, 1987). This equality laid the foundation for the contribution future generations of female officers would make to the culture of SAPOL, including positive aspects of dealing with the stresses of the job (Nixon, 2012). Duties for the pioneering duo included child protection, the policing of prostitution, patrolling streets and beaches to ensure propriety among courting couples, meeting trains and steamships at Port Adelaide to escort arrivals to safe accommodation, conducting enquiries for state government departments, rescuing young women from "immoral surroundings", placing women in institutions and conducting arrests including absconders from state homes. As well, with an increase in staffing for the women police branch after one year of operation, enquiries were conducted into "white slave traffic, ill treatment and neglect of wives by husbands, mentally deficient persons and aged, destitute and drunken women" (Higgs & Bettess, 1987: 38).

Sub-Inspector Fraser, an officer in charge of the Pt. Adelaide police station where two women police were later stationed, described the value of their work in these terms, "That a great deal of their work is social work, and by some is not regarded as "police work" there is no denying that it is "good work" and I maintain that it is police work for by this work a great deal of crime is prevented" (cited in Higgs & Bettess: 40). Social work in Australia at this time was in its infancy, with church organisations (including the Methodist congregations) tending to the needs of the poor and disadvantaged, particularly women and children (Mendes, 2005). This "good work" continued through the 1920s and 1930s, with women police playing a prominent role in the allocation and distribution of welfare support during the great depression. When Kate Cocks retired from police service in 1934 she was succeeded by Mary Wilcher, who now commanded 15 policewomen. Their duties remained firmly in the area of social work activities dealing with family issues, prostitution, abortion, gambling and the protection of young people whose amorous activities placed them under the firm moral gaze of the law. Women police, however, during this period also assisted their male colleagues in the investigation of a wide range of criminal offences, including rape, carnal knowledge, incest, bigamy, assault and drunkenness.

During World War Two the work of the women police "leaned even more toward social work and the protection of morals" due in no small part to the influx of servicemen into South Australia during this period (Higgs & Bettess, 1987). In 1953, a trio of young women recruits undertook for the first time the same training as male cadets at the Thebarton police barracks. 1955 saw the introduction of night and evening shifts for women police officers, enabling them to attend and investigate domestic disputes and sexual offences including rape.

The challenges to policing of the 1960s and 1970s were met with ever-increasing involvement and reliance on women police officers. The "bodgie and widgie"[1] teenage phenomenon of the 1960s (Moore, 2004), the increasing incidence of illicit drug use, the sexual revolution stemming in part from the availability of the contraceptive pill from 1961, as well as protests against the involvement of Australia in the Vietnam War all featured women police in investigations, arrests, crowd control and other critically important aspects of policing at that time (Higgs & Bettess, 1987).

In 1968, a major review of SAPOL including policies, practice and organisational structure was undertaken with the view to decentralising services from headquarters in the Adelaide City centre to surrounding and outlying suburbs and regions. Part of the review focussed on women police members. After months of uncertainty, the Women's Police Branch was closed and women police entered uniformed service. Initially "mixed patrols" were tasked with domestic disputes and matters involving women and children (Paterson, 1984) but the women later assumed equal duties and responsibilities and continued with equal pay.

3.2 Women in Policing: The Informing Literature

Women police in South Australia celebrated 100 years in "the job" in 2016. A brief history of their movement into the occupation was introduced in this chapter. Female officers were given the same job and person specification as their male colleagues in 1974 and began uniformed duties that year. This was due to a re-organisation in the force at that time and prefigured anti-discrimination and equal opportunity legislation introduced in the 1970s and 1980s in Australian jurisdictions (Prenzler, 1994). The operational arrival of female officers was greeted with scepticism and concern by many of their male colleagues (Wilkinson & Froyland, 1996). A retired Detective Senior Sergeant explained when interviewed for my research, "When women came into uniform in 1974 we hoped they would be resilient, none of this cry baby stuff, tears were at home or with your (shift) partner". What this officer meant by "cry baby stuff" is not clear, but he does portray the sense of uncertainty that this innovation caused among male officers at that time.

"Mixed patrols" consisting of one male and one female officer began only after the female officers were interviewed by the spouses of the male officers to ensure propriety with a view to the long patrol hours the new crews would spend together. These mixed patrols were routinely tasked to "domestics" as they were then called as the presence of a female officer was considered to be an advantage in terms of allowing female victims to talk with an officer of the same gender (Higgs & Bettess, 1987).

---

[1] "Bodgies and widgies" were young people who dressed in tight jeans and sported unusual haircuts, congregating in public places as a challenge to the conservative culture of the time. See (Moore, 2004).

Progress since this period in terms of the empowerment of female officers has been slow but sure and largely due to their promotion through to the executive management of the organisation. The more recent reviews by Jenkins (2015) and Vincent (2016), although confronting are a very clear indicator of how the resilience of women "in the job" is still severely tested day to day.

The literature around the resilience of women in policing is scarce. Often the focus is on the vulnerability to the stress of women officers who are seen as a besieged minority in a male-dominated occupation (Blok & Brown, 2005; Fleming & Lafferty, 2003). Policewomen often still face a unique range of duty-related stressors by virtue of their gender, including sexism, disapproval by colleagues, a lack of role models and a significant career disadvantage if they decide to have children as well as a lack of appropriate mentoring in the context of their acceptance into the macho, male-dominated policing culture (Ménard & Arter, 2014; Paterson, 2014; Jenkins, 2015; Vincent, 2016). Women police officers in my interview cohort, especially those who served in the 1970s and 1980s all referred to the stress-related challenges of their career choice in terms of discrimination rather than those relating to operational experiences. In her "Advice to women beginning a career in policing" (2003) United States Police Chief Penny Harrington goes no further than her first paragraph to warn young female officers that they "need to be aware of the discrimination issues still remaining so that they will recognise them when they arise" (p. 1). She goes on to outline the perils of "becoming one of the boys" aligning with "cowboys" in the job, as well as "malcontents" and encourages female officers to keep their careers in perspective by maintaining friendships and relationships outside the job and cultivating police friends who are ethical in their duties. Her advice and observations apply equally well to her Australian colleagues.

In a research paper written for the Australian Institute of Criminology in 1996, Vicki Wilkinson and Irene Froyland (Wilkinson & Froyland, 1996) lament the gender imbalance in Australian police organisations, pointing out that only 13.5% of officers were female at that time. They blamed the three stages of recruitment for much of the imbalance, namely application (what would motivate women to join such masculine organisations?), selection (the physical qualities required were a challenge to many female applicants) and academy training where the emphasis on selection was on physical rather than intellectual and interpersonal attributes. The transition at that time for police organisations from "force" to "service" was considered by Wilkinson and Froyland to require aspects of the latter skillset, rather than only those of the former. The authors suggest that a 50% male to female ratio is not essential, but rather women police should reach a "critical mass" in such organisations to ensure the gradual demise of discriminatory practices then present.

The SAPOL Annual Report of 2014–2015 indicates that the percentage of female officers has risen in the intervening 21 years to 25.6%, and the present Commissioner has expressed the intention of increasing the percentage to 50% as soon as is practicable. The Deputy Commissioner of SAPOL is female, as are three of the six Assistant Commissioners. Three out of 30 Superintendents are women, 7 out of 24 Chief Inspectors and 7 out of 45 Inspectors. Some female officers expressed confidence in higher-ranked women to bring about change, "I would lie down on the ground for the female Assistant Commissioners. They have earned the right to be there" and from another, "Policing has changed as women in management become more involved in SAPOL politics, women are now less likely to be seen and not heard. The lower ranks are more likely to question things".

One such questioner from "lower ranks" (Paterson, 2014) argues, in the context of SAPOL "family friendly" work practices that encourage the retention of female officers, that only when women reach a critical mass in policing will female officers have a realistic choice around child-bearing and their careers. Paterson also points out that male officers, the fathers of the same children as their police officer wives, suffer no disadvantage in career terms, usually rising through the ranks unimpeded by parenthood. Many of the female officers interviewed in my research agreed that this is a significant issue in terms of staying in and enjoying "the job". Paterson highlights the disproportionate number of female members who resign from policing due to "the conflict between work and home commitments" (p. 1) arguing that SAPOL and police organisations elsewhere should allow greater access to flexible work practices, support parents of both genders and change leave and rostering arrangements for part-time members who are predominantly women. She points out that most senior female officers have "neither married nor raised children". The organisational focus, she argues, should be on the retention of female officers. Shift work, she also contends, has a greater impact on female officers who are more often primary caregivers when compared to their male colleagues. This argument is supported by the SAPOL Annual Report of 2011/12, which revealed that 93% of SAPOL officers are women. Paterson is clear that only "an almost complete rethink of what contemporary policing involves, is required" (p. 10). This will include changing the present SAPOL focus on recruitment to one that prioritises retention, which in turn ensures flexibility in permanent part-time work, career breaks and temporary transfer to non-operational roles for women and men in "the job".

A project named "Equitas", recently completed in SAPOL in conjunction with other Australian police organisations and the South Australian Human Rights Commission, considering the real needs of female officers may well be a vehicle for significant change for women in policing as they seek to balance their commitment to their career and family.

3.3 Women Police and Masculine Policing Culture

Female officers are more comfortable with expressing work-related emotions than their male colleagues and seem to have more freedom to do so (Nixon, 2012; Orrick, 2008; Vanstone, 2001; Wilkinson & Froyland, 1996). The recent Victoria police inquiry into bullying, harassment and predatory behaviour (Jenkins, 2015) and that more recently released in South Australia (Vincent, 2016) bode well for the future. Women in South Australian policing have come a very long way in the last 100 years, due to their commitment, determination and ability they have earned their future. The debate is no longer about whether women "fit" in contemporary policing; it is now more about what they bring to it from a female perspective. This inevitably has to do with rank, power and influence within police organisations (Nixon, 2012).

Retired Chief Commissioner of Victoria, Christine Nixon, was Australia's first female Chief Commissioner. She joined VicPol in 1972 and received her training at the Redfern Police Academy where 70 male and two female recruits were on the course. "I waded into a sea of men" says Nixon. "It was a proud, unapologetic, testosterone fuelled culture" (Nixon, 2012:29). She continued, reflecting the experience of her female colleague in 1972 and many women who followed "enduring that culture war with dignity, femininity and strength would prove the unending challenge of our careers, and without a sense of humour and an appreciation of the absurd I no doubt would have succumbed years ago" (p. 30).

Nixon and her fellow female cadet were excluded from weapons training and were allocated traffic duties and school visits after graduation entering a force with only 130 females in the job. At the age of 21, Nixon found herself "at the front-line of efforts to rethink conditions and roles for police women" (p. 34). Included was an insistence on expanded duties, opportunities for promotion, equal superannuation provisions, broader training and maternity leave, including return to work provisions. Such changes were resisted by older policewomen, who Nixon surmised were either jealous or threatened by the prospect of such change. Said one, "This is the most disgraceful thing! You will never be able to cope or do the job of a policeman" (p. 43). South Australian contemporaries seemed not to experience similar levels of conservatism from their fellow female officers (Higgs & Bettess, 1987; Paterson, 1984) at a similar time in Australian policing history, but faced significant problems at other levels including marriage and parenthood while in "the job", reflecting comments above and research from within (Paterson, 2014). Nixon comments re-parenthood from a female police perspective, climbing the promotional ladder at age 38, "the career I had committed myself to, didn't allow that kind of room" (p. 85). At her swearing-in as Victorian Chief Commissioner, Nixon summed up what many policewomen I interviewed felt, "First I am a woman….the female gender has brought its fair share of brains and imagination to policing, and femininity has, I hope, helped to nourish the caring and compassionate values and ideals that have always been at the core of good policing" (p. 126). This supports very clearly the views of my interview cohort, reflected in comments from officers of both genders that women in policing have come a long way far beyond mere acceptance from their male colleagues to a status of their own based on their achievements and what they bring to "good policing". Significant levels of resilience define Nixon's career and those of her female police colleagues around the globe. Women in policing have faced challenges above and beyond their law enforcement duties, as is well represented in both my interviews and the literature. Bullying, harassment and discrimination are routinely added to operational stressors in the lives of women who have chosen a career in policing. Recently in South Australia, the announcement that SAPOL has reached its goal of a 50% intake of women into the service indicates genuine progress towards a new era in policing.

Do these extra stressors make female officers more vulnerable to unwelcome trauma responses? The opinion is divided with Friedman (2015) arguing that women are more likely to be diagnosed with stress reactions noting that gender is a major risk factor. Do women identify more closely with victims at the expense of their mental well-being? Violanti and Paton (2006) argue in "Who gets PTSD?" that they do and this is borne out by many female officer comments in my interviews. Whether such identification is detrimental to their health is less clear. Orrick (2008) points out that female officers often demonstrate better communication skills than men, while Ménard and Arter (2014) argue from their research that women officers are more likely to engage in effective coping strategies. Women in my interview cohort bore this out, many arranging regular private debriefs with (usually female) colleagues and helping professionals as well as taking time off or changing roles when early signs of stress appeared. Maintaining exercise and a healthy lifestyle was another common coping mechanism among female officers.

There were however regular references among the policewomen interviewed to significant job-related challenges to their well-being. Bullying in the literature is defined as "sustained verbal abuse and hostility as well as more covert behaviours such as undermining a bullying target's position in the organisation" (Rafferty, 2001:4). Such bullying behaviours include verbal abuse, persistent and unjustified criticism, humiliating employees by using sarcasm, criticism or insults, particularly in front of colleagues, setting impossible deadlines or overloading the target with work, undermining work performance, failure to give credit where due and undue delays in the implementation of disciplinary action where it has been threatened. To constitute bullying behaviour, such actions must be persistent and ongoing (Zapf, 2001).

SAPOL, in an excerpt from the South Australia Police Equity and Diversity Employee Management Manual, defines bullying as follows:

> Bullying is a form of harassment. It is a behaviour that unreasonably interferes with the personal comfort, respect or dignity of others because of the actions of others, usually in positions of authority or power. Bullying occurs when a person inappropriately takes action to: coerce, intimidate, oppress or persecute others physically or morally by threat or physical force" (SAPOL, 2016:36).

The document goes on to explain that, "bullying does not include reasonable and justified demands for performance, justified, reasoned and constructive criticism and reasonable administrative action, taken in a reasonable manner" (p.37).

There is a surprising lack of literature addressing bullying behaviour in a policing context, considering the para-military nature and structure of such organisations as well as "command and control" approaches to management in police organisations such as SAPOL (Parsons et al., 2011) where bullying and harassment would seem to be more likely to be encountered. Many researchers refer to bullying in police organisations indirectly in the context of overall management and leadership practices as a source of stress more damaging than the day-to-day challenges of death and violence encountered routinely by operational officers (Donnelly et al., 2015; Ménard & Arter, 2014; Stinchcomb, 2004).

Cotton (2016) in his mental health review of Victoria police describes entrenched predatory behaviour, bullying and sexism as does a similar review conducted by the South Australian Equal Opportunities Commissioner (Vincent, 2016) who found a similar culture in South Australia police, making recommendations for urgent change. Both SAPOL and VicPol Executive Management have made a commitment to embrace these recommendations.

Sexual harassment within police organisations is also highlighted in the research literature (Cotton, 2016; Harrington, 2003; Kate, 2015; Prenzler, 1994; Prenzler & Hayes, 2000) and by many of the female officers interviewed in my study. Women serving in the 1970s and 1980s were particularly vulnerable. One woman said, "The 70s were the most challenging, with weekly sexual assaults by colleagues. The bosses were the worst offenders". This officer made a sexual assault complaint against a Superintendent, who "quietly resigned with his retirement benefits intact". A retired Senior Sergeant struck an optimistic note comparing her early and later career, "There was a lot of harassment and inappropriate comments back then. It is gradually changing".

The report described above on "Sex discrimination and sexual harassment, including predatory behaviour in Victoria police" (Jenkins, 2015) pulls no punches. Its author, Victorian Equal Opportunities and Human Rights Commissioner Kate Jenkins, paved the way for others to follow. A South Australian report (Vincent, 2016) one year later made similar revelations about harassment, assault and bullying against female officers in SAPOL.

In his initial response to Commissioner Jenkin's findings, a forthright and determined VicPol Chief Commissioner Graham Ashton declared:

> The results make confronting reading. When you read the report you will be left in no doubt there have been some terrible behaviours exhibited and some terrible experiences and ordeals have been endured by our staff (Jenkins, 2015:2).

Women in the job were clearly the main targets of such behaviours and male officers were the perpetrators. One female respondent said, "Men run this organisation, and they run it to suit other men. Women get intimidated, stood over, spoken over, excluded and overlooked-all day, every day-in this job. Because of their gender!" In the executive summary of the report, the authors concede that "Sex discrimination and harassment are widely regarded as 'non-events' within Victoria Police". Key findings included 40% of women and 7% of men answered "yes" to the question, "Have you ever personally experienced sexual harassment?" Two-thirds of women participants and half of the males reported they had witnessed at least one form of sexual harassment in the VicPol workplace in the last five years. The most common form of such behaviour was "sexually suggestive comments or jokes" and women were most likely to be harassed by "a colleague more senior in rank or grade". Gay men and lesbian women in the service were more likely than others to be sexually harassed.

Many of the female respondents to the VicPol survey reflected the comments of those in my interview cohort: "I felt betrayed and intimidated" and "I will never forget what has happened to me". Others reported feeling "humiliated and broken", a term commonly used by officers when referring to mental health challenges. The personal and professional costs of reporting harassment and assault were also high, including the loss of career prospects in terms of promotion or the termination of their police careers (Jenkins, 2015).

Commissioner Ashton concludes his response, "I give you my commitment we will bring about the necessary change in this organisation so that it becomes a more respectful workplace". The report recently released in South Australia (Vincent, 2016) will also have a significant impact and hopefully positive outcomes for present and future women in policing.

3.4 Women in Policing: The Data from the Interviews

The percentage of female officers involved in my interviews (23%) was almost exactly equivalent to the female/male ratio in SAPOL in 2016. Since their 1974 entry into uniformed service, involving the acquisition of equal duties and pay, female officers have progressed to the higher ranks with the present Deputy Commissioner, working with two female and four male officers at the rank of Assistant Commissioner under her command. Their journey has not been uneventful, "Basically Women police were Social Workers with no powers of arrest" (in late 1960s), recalled a now-retired Senior Sergeant.

There were also problems with male members of the general public as a retired Senior Sergeant recalled, "I remember the first guy I stopped for speeding. He made no eye contact. He wanted my (male) partner to take over". Female officers soon accustomed themselves to such responses and got on with the process of simultaneously doing their duty and working towards acceptance by their male colleagues.

When female officers sought to marry they were also confronted with even more challenges, "Getting married was the most confronting thing. Discrimination was rife. Just because I was married!" This officer went on to explain that SAPOL not unlike other organisations employing women in the 1970s and 1980s was concerned that once married, childbirth and child-bearing might pose serious impediments to the effective conduct of their policing duties. Having children while in the job did turn out to be very problematic for many, "after I returned to work after having my first child, I was yelled at by my Inspector in May 1983… 'There is no place in SAPOL for women with babies.' My uniform was drenched with tears during this confrontation".[2] Such incidents were not easily forgotten by the pioneering policewomen of that time. Another described issues around child-bearing during her early years in "the job" a decade later:

> There were issues with women in SAPOL, it was thought that women would just get pregnant and go…we were the main trainers for the new communication system and I applied for two positions, the second one when I was pregnant... I was the next most qualified person and didn't get the job. When I was on the road the male coppers looked after us…one day me

[2] I quote the same officer in more detail in the bullying and harassment data section below.

> and another probo {probationary constable} got into a spot of bother in Whitmore Square, everything went to shit so I called for back-up. There was still a stigma against women.

That stigma was also highly visible operationally, including problems around general patrol work and other duties, where "After 1974 we weren't particularly well accepted by male police. They didn't like taking us out (on patrol) with them". Another woman who retired in order to have children reported that "After my resignation, I tried to re-join SAPOL part-time. Full shift work with young children not possible". Current research undertaken by serving female officers continues to highlight such issues (Paterson, 2014). Contemporary female officers in 2018 still face a similar dilemma. From their perspective, there is still much room for change. As one young female officer explained, in response to the question, "are you comfortable in SAPOL?" "I will have to choose a career or a family…if you have kids and take leave its five steps backwards". A similar view was expressed by a female Sergeant, "Having kids is another major issue for women police. I was told, you have to decide whether you want to be a mum or a police Officer. Part time for me meant working four days and putting in six! Part-time contracts are negotiable and can be cancelled. You are not a dumb- arse because you have had children! Management don't understand that". As indicated above, a 2017 SAPOL project named "Equitas" has compiled a response to these and other equal opportunity-related issues and may impact positively on female officers who still face many challenges in common with their 1970s female colleagues (SAPOL, 2017).

Another female officer described her early career experiences thus commencing with a classic understatement:

> It was interesting times. Old school Sergeants didn't know how to deal with women. You needed to be strong and one of the boys to survive! I lived at back of Renmark police station and single women's quarters in Berri.[3] An older Sergeant had no idea how to make it work although as time passed, more blokes were willing to work with you. It was hard to have fun back then, there were plenty ready to be critical.

Dealing with "dinosaurs" such as this resulted in many women feeling pressure to change fundamentally, "we were encouraged to adopt a masculine persona. Many women got their noses broken on duty. You didn't have to be like the men. It was a female perception, none of the guys told them to be like that".

Changes to the masculine "tough it out culture" that underlines these comments are not yet at the stage where female colleagues can be comfortable about talking through trauma-related issues with their male counterparts. These are not conversations I have with male colleagues, more often with female colleagues, where I can say, "I'm feeling a bit wobbly". A female Sergeant recognised the progress that has since been made in this area, but added, "I think there is loads of room for women in SAPOL, but I don't see a lot of evidence that their part-time needs are being met. There are still some high ranking dinosaurs. It's sometimes hard to keep your head above all the crap". Recent SAPOL initiatives in this area through a yet to be published "women in

[3] In the Riverland of South Australia.

policing" report will address this issue more fully, building on the work already done by long-suffering female officers (Paterson, 2014). Recalling the early experience of working without direct male supervision, one Senior Constable commented, "In 1988 I was in an all-female crew. Our Sergeant got raked over the coals. He had faith in us. The boys still had a sense of responsibility for us (in terms of our physical safety) but it was a really good time". In this case, the Sergeant was ahead of his superiors in terms of female acceptance and paid the price as a result of his actions. Another recalled the early days (1986) in terms of challenging male partners on patrol:

> I've had some really good partners, supportive and happy to work with you. My first partner said I hate three things, WOPOS, {women police officers} people who don't know the streets and bad driving! He said if anyone goes for my gun, shoot the arsehole! I learnt the streets, never saw other females, I kept persevering. You felt like a leper. You're supposed to learn from these people! My second partner was old, he would drive all the time. My third partner was completely different, as we walked to the fleet {police car} he said do you want to drive? As we attended incidents we talked through what we would do when we got there. I learnt so much I married him!

This shows clear signs of change and acceptance at least from the younger generation of officers who were able to do more than just pay lip service to such an evolution 12 years after the initial female entry into full police service. The sense of isolation, the need to persevere and the barriers erected by older male officers are well described here as is an unexpected outcome for the young female constable and her more "with it" male colleague.

Other women officers were grateful to their female superior officers for paving the way: "Policing has changed as women in management become more involved in SAPOL politics, women are now less likely to be seen and not heard. The lower ranks are more inclined to question things". These "lower ranks" (Paterson, 2014) and all those women officers who enthusiastically embraced the opportunity to participate in this research, have certainly endured the worst of their journey towards credibility and acceptance in "the job". There is, it would seem, some way to go as a female Sergeant asserted, "I would let my son join SAPOL. My daughter? No fucking way!".

In terms of SAPOL management's prevailing perceptions of female resilience, a Detective Sergeant stated, "All female Detectives in family violence (section) are considered to be at psychological risk by management. 'We will move you for your own good'…we are usually moved when we are on annual leave". Such actions are rarely, if ever, taken out of similar concern for her male colleague's well-being.

A retired Deputy Commissioner reflected on his perception of the impact of the 1974 changes to policing in South Australia, "We had difficulties getting women to take the opportunities we offered them. I put a woman in charge of a patrol car with a male underling" and added, "Women were better educated and topped classes at the Academy". This comment reflects how progressive managers such as this one experienced setbacks in their attempts at change because the female officers in this case were nervous about the cultural impact of stepping up. It took courage for the female officer referred to here to accept such an opportunity.

3.5 Women in Policing: Bullying and Harassment (the Data)

Many officers interviewed remarked on a culture of bullying and harassment that they considered had been present in SAPOL for many years. A significant proportion of those highlighting these issues were female police officers. Other female officers were frank about the stressful implications of bullying behaviour, “I had been close to the edge but mainly because of sexual harassment. The psyches {police psychologists} had got me through those years. They understood because they were police officers before they became SAPOL psychologists”.

Others who referred to bullying in SAPOL as a significant issue made comments including “the enemy is within. Micro-managing and bullying is the central issue here”, commented a male Detective Senior Constable. Others were more philosophical about this issue, “I didn’t mind working in a bullying environment in SAPOL, it’s that kind of system. I kept a record of the bullying. Eight out of ten officers in my squad went out on stress”. This officer’s acceptance of the systemic bullying culture and his commitment to keeping a record of his experiences are indicative of the impact on his health and in the longer term, his policing career. He implies that his colleagues also succumbed, making stress-related claims.

Another female officer commented, “I had been off work three times in my career. Those periods adding up to almost a year”. She continued, “I was targeted by a bully who is now my manager again. When I took time off for the first time and saw a psychologist, what did SAPOL do for me? Answer, nothing!” Self-care under circumstances like this is a very difficult challenge. This officer organised her shifts to avoid the bully, worked in afternoon shift and weekends, took time off, sought support outside of SAPOL after her efforts to obtain it from within failed. She went on, “I love that I am a police officer, I know that SAPOL won’t look after me, so I have to look after myself”. In her present role, she commented that her female colleagues take similar measures to avoid the bully. In a previous role after she and another female colleague complained about bullying behaviour, “they transferred us and not the bully who stayed where he was”.

Such treatment by more senior officers of those beneath them was often taken for granted by those interviewed who saw it as an inevitable part of the combination of a male-dominated and para-military culture within SAPOL. One officer said, “I have accepted the fact that we have bullies in SAPOL, its part of the culture, you have to deal with it”.

Others, less accepting of such a culture, found such a response far more difficult. A young female officer was recently bullied whilst working at a suburban police station in Adelaide, “I didn’t want to go to work. I didn’t put anything on paper, when you are starting out you don’t want to rock the boat. Colleagues have said to me you should have gone to the Police Association {Union}. Sexual harassment and bullying is a big challenge in the job”. She continued, “Bullying is now in more of a mild form, it is now more subtle, the Police Association can’t do more about it than they are doing. There is a lack of positive feedback. I am really proud of much of what I’ve done. I've had some really bad managers, one resulted in a PASA complaint when a manager tried to drive me out because I was part-time". This is a clear reference to the importance of management-related stressors when considering the pressures of "the job". The women interviewed for this study had almost all experienced bullying and harassment in various forms. The observation that it now takes more subtle forms is of little comfort to them. More optimistically, a recently retired Senior Sergeant compared the present day to the 1980s, thus "there was a lot of harassment and inappropriate comments back then, but now it is gradually changing". This "gradual change" must accelerate, particularly in light of the various reviews and research recently conducted into Australian and foreign police organisations (Cotton, 2016; Hesse-Biber, 2011; Peters, 2009; Rafferty, 2001; Shane, 2010; Kate, 2015; Vincent, 2016).

A long-serving Sergeant made such issues very clear, "The hardest thing about the job is being bullied. I can handle guns, knives and bodies". She went on, "I was bullied for three years. I made a complaint. What followed was the worst twelve months of my life, when you're young and inexperienced, without a depth of knowledge about life you stand up and they knock you down". The same officer explained, "there is no system in place that works against bullying, I used to hyperventilate and vomit on the way to work. I would have preferred him to punch me!" The levels of resilience required to withstand this encultured behaviour are hard to imagine. Another female officer added describing her experience, "The bullying affected my whole family. I thought of all the things I have seen and done, I won't let this define my career. It made me stronger, more outspoken. That's the stuff in SAPOL you are not prepared for, the questioning of your credibility, overloading you with work, setting you up to fail. It's calculated and systematic". This is a graphic insight into what, for this officer was a career-defining experience that resulted in personal growth for her in the context of "calculated and systematic" bullying behaviour. This is somewhat bleakly summarised by a female Senior Constable, who during her interview stated; "SAPOL is a bullying culture, women have to adopt masculine traits to survive especially on the front line of policing". Adopting a masculine persona was an option for female officers in the 1970s and 1980s, many did so particularly in terms of not showing emotion. There is less pressure to do so in this century.

3.6 What Can Scholars Learn from the Experience of Women in a Police Force?

I was invited to address our daughter's police Academy course a few days before her graduation in late 2002. As I walked into the classroom, I was immediately aware of how much SAPOL recruits had changed since I first taught at the Academy in the mid-1970s. Then the room would have been full of young men, tall and robust, with a couple of young female cadets sitting at the back looking disengaged and isolated. Now it was a room with an equal number of female and male cadets, some in their late 20s and older, with male cadets of various shapes and sizes. They were a group in every sense, many had engaged in a tertiary study before police training, all were full of the excitement of the success of their course and they were soon to begin careers in policing. Our daughter had won the communication award and addressed the graduation ceremony two days later. There was no sense of the restless testosterone of the 1970s; it was clearly a more professional group ready for the challenges that awaited.

Women police interviewed in my cohort, who graduated in the 1970s and 1980s, had the extra responsibilities and challenges that accompany pioneers, especially those who are women. They faced sexual harassment and bullying that was a greater challenge than their duties, they realised that many male officers saw them as an encumbrance and an extra responsibility. They married at their peril in terms of career opportunities and decided on parenthood with the realisation that it would even further impede advancement and recognition. Younger women interviewed were still not immune from bullying and harassment but were no longer seen by all but the "dinosaurs" as anything less than colleagues in full standing. Many had achieved well-deserved promotion, most admired and respected by their female colleagues who had risen to the top of SAPOL, whilst recognising that parenthood was still an impediment to an upward trajectory. Much has changed in the organisation. There is now a real possibility of equality, with recent large-scale investigations of mental health, harassment and bullying in South Australia, New South Wales and Victoria police pointing clearly to the need for significant changes in culture, support and management for police of both genders. Commissioners (all male) in those states have made a strong commitment to such change which now seems almost inevitable.

Many female officers still serve in policing family violence, victim support and child protection, a legacy handed down by a determined group of female SAPOL Sergeants in the 1980s and 1990s, who trained male colleagues in attending such challenging events. "Real policing" is no longer just "catching crooks" but a far less violent, responsive, communicative process that depends on the many skills and attitudes that female officers bring to the job. Having emotional responses to confronting crime scenes and events is now more acceptable, at least when female officers are in each other's company. Empathic, supportive camaraderie as a central sustaining defence against trauma is modelled by women and less often by men in policing. Such responses, in the view of many women interviewed, are changing the masculine, stiff upper lip approach of the past to handling trauma. Women in policing seem to take better care of themselves emotionally than their male colleagues, often arranging private debriefs, friendships outside the job, regular exercise and self-care as part of their strategies.

The literature around women in policing still focusses on the extra problems they face as a legacy of their gender and ponders how far their acceptance as "real cops" has progressed. In line with the psychiatric PTSD literature, they are also seen as more likely to develop trauma-related symptoms. None of this was evident in the women I interviewed, whose resilience was beyond question and of heroic proportions.

3.7 Where Next?

There is now a clear road map for Australian police organisations with regard to bullying, harassment and discrimination against their female members in the early twenty-first century. Reviews conducted into Victoria and South Australia police into these issues have all reached the same conclusions and made similar recommendations (Kate, 2015; Vincent, 2016). In both reports, Commissioners Ashton (Victoria police) and Stevens (SAPOL) deplore the history of violence against their female officers and vow to institute change. Evidence of such change or strategies to bring it about are not yet revealed.

In this chapter, the voices of women police in South Australia are heard in the context of significant detailed interviews for the first time. Echoing recent reviews, these women have described careers in policing not primarily challenged by everyday crime and mayhem, but rather by systemic discrimination, bullying and harassment. Included in my interview cohort were women who had experienced sexual assault by senior officers, who had been bullied and harassed regularly, who had experienced discrimination as they married, had children and sought part-time or shared duties to fulfil family responsibilities. Their responses at the interview were more detailed than the questionnaires or focus groups used in the reviews described above. These are the voices of women who are intent on change that will allow future generations of their female colleagues to focus on their duties without the extra challenge of surviving bullying, harassment and discrimination so that they can continue in "the job". The level of resilience required to do so is almost unimaginable.

References

Blok, D., & Brown, J. (2005). *The gendered nature of policing among uniformed operational police officers in England and Wales*. School of Human Sciences, University of Surrey, November.

Brough, P. (2016). Women in policing: Exploring challenges associated with career progression and related health and well-being impacts. South Australia: Police Health.

Burke, R. J., & Mikkelsen, A. (2005). Gender issues in policing: Do they matter? *Women in Management Review, 20*(2), 133–143.

Charlesworth, S., & Robertson, D. (2012). Policing, gender, and working time: An Australian case study. *Police Practice and Research, 13*(3), 241–253.

Cotton, P. (2016). Victoria Police Mental Health Review. An independent review into the mental health and well-being of Victoria Police employees. Australia.

Donnelly, E., et al. (2015). Law enforcement officers and employee assistance programs. *Policing: An International Journal of Police Strategies & Management, 38*(2), 206–220.

Fleming, J., & Lafferty, G. (2003). Equity confounded? Women in Australian police organisations. *Labour & Industry: A Journal of the Social and Economic Relations of Work, 13*(3), 37–49.

Friedman, M. (2015). *Posttraumatic and acute stress disorders*. Springer.

Harrington, P. E. (2003). Advice to women beginning a career in policing. *Women & Criminal Justice, 14*(1), 1–13.

Higgs, P., & Bettess, C. (1987). *To walk a fair beat: A history of the South Australian Women Police, 1915–1987*. Past and present women police association.

Jenkins, K. (2015). *Independent review into sex discrimination and sexual harassment, including predatory behaviour in Victoria Police.* Victoria, Australia: Victorian equal opportunity and human rights commission.

Loftus, B. (2009). *Police Culture in a changing world.* Clarendon Studies in Criminology.

Orrick, D. W. (2008). *Recruitment, retention, and turnover of police personnel: Reliable, practical, and effective solutions.* Charles C Thomas Publisher.

Mckay, E. (2005). *Crime scene-true stories from the life of a crime scene investigator.* Viking (Penguin) Australia.

Moore, K. (2004). Bodgies, widgies and moral panic in Australia 1955–1959.

Ménard, K. S., & Arter, M. L. (2014). Stress, coping, alcohol use, and posttraumatic stress disorder among an international sample of police officers: Does gender matter? *Police Quarterly, 17*(4), 307–327.

Neil, B. (2014). *Under siege.* Australia: Harlequin Mira.

Nixon, C. (2012). *Fair cop,* Victory Books.

Paterson, A. (1984). Women Police in South Australia in 1974: The beginnings of a chequered career. Unpublished mini thesis.

Paterson, K. (2014). Modern, motivated, progressive and professional? Flexible work practices and the retention of female members in SAPOL. *Australasian Policing, 6*(1), 21.

Parsons, A., et al. (2011). Effective policing: Management influence and the commitment of senior police personnel. *Policing & Society, 21*(1), 1–26.

Peters, R. F. (2009). *Police under pressure (A donkey on the edge).* HEAS Publications.

Prenzler, T. (1994). Women in Australian policing: An historical overview. *Journal of Australian Studies, 18*(42), 78–88.

Prenzler, T., & Hayes, H. (2000). Measuring progress in gender equity in Australian policing. *Current Issues Crim. Just, 12,* 20.

Rafferty, C. (2001). Health and safety guidelines to address bullying at work. In *Bullying-from backyard to boardroom.*

Shane, J. M. (2010). Organizational stressors and police performance. *Journal of Criminal Justice, 38*(4), 807–818.

Stinchcomb, J. B. (2004). Searching for stress in all the wrong places: Combating chronic organizational stressors in policing. *Police Practice and Research, 5*(3), 259–277.

Vanstone, A. (2001). No longer lady policemen: the changing role of women in law enforcement in Australia. *EDITORS: JAN VAN DIJK, 1*(2), 119.

Vincent, N. (2016). *Sex discrimination, sexual harassment and predatory behaviour in South Australia Police. Independent review.* Equal Opportunity Commission.

Wilkinson, V., & Froyland, I. D. (1996). *Women in policing.* Australian Institute of Criminology.

Winlow, S. (2001). *Badfellas: Crime, tradition and new masculinities,* Bloomsbury Academic.

Zapf, D. (2001). European research on bullying at work. In *Bullying: From Backyard to Boardroom* (pp. 158–167).

Chapter 4
Death and Bodies

Abstract Death is the constant companion of an operational police officer, whether it be attending uncomplicated sudden deaths in the community, suicides, fatal road crashes or violent homicides. This chapter explores the unusually violent and tragic deaths that test the coping strategies of officers, the impact of suicide within their ranks and how they cope with this challenge. There are significant international literature works around "confronting jobs" and the impact they have on the well-being of officers who attend them. The qualitative interviews at the centre of this research are an ideal opportunity for the officers to graphically describe the death-related situations that challenged them and on occasion required significant time and reflection to be effectively and permanently dealt with. Their accounts describe the nature of resilience with clarity, how they learn to distance themselves from tragedy and the resources common to their capacity to continue to cope. Suicide in a police organisation has a significant impact on colleagues left behind. Often the act leaves many questions in its wake and is a point of reflection for many in the job. This chapter examines the international literature and focusses on a study conducted by the Queensland Police Service referencing suicide over a 30-year period as well as the rich data from interviews with SAPOL officers and six psychiatrists and psychologists who treat and assess them. A common theme from the interviews is that of smell and its long-term impact on traumatic memory.

Managing death and dead bodies in various states of decay, injury and mutilation is given in terms of police experience throughout an officer's operational career. Much of the policing and trauma literature focusses on this constant theme as a major stressor of operational and retired police officers (Amaranto et al., 2003; American Psychiatric Association, 2013; Burke, 2016; Burns et al., 2008; Cotton, 2016; Dollard et al., 2003; Donnelly et al., 2015; Green, 2004; Henry, 2004; Huddleston et al., 2006; Kroes, 1976; McFarlane, 2011; Mckay, 2005; Moss, 1999; Nievas, 2015; Paton, 2009; Toch, 2002; Verity, 2014; Violanti & Paton, 2006). At the centre of my research was an assumption that the negative impact of these experiences would form a critically important part of the interviews. The police officers I interviewed spoke of their exposure to death in surprisingly positive ways, largely due to the development of the capacity early in their careers to accommodate and appropriately

A. Paterson, *Trauma and Resilience in Contemporary Australian Policing*,
https://doi.org/10.1007/978-981-16-4416-0_4

distance themselves from the negative aspects of that experience. It became clear as the interviews progressed that the occasions when such distancing became difficult usually had some personal ingredient as far as the officers were concerned. For example, the dead person may remind them of a relative or a family member or in a rural setting they may have known the deceased person and his or her relatives socially. Contact with dead children was almost always reported as more stressful and difficult to deal with. As a young police Senior Constable said, "Death is part of this job. During training you get told of the good things, not the bad things. The academy seems to assume that we know about the dangers".

4.1 Death and Bodies. The Informing Literature

Every sudden death that occurs outside of a hospital in South Australia is attended by a police patrol. Added to such taskings are those related to crime scenes, suicides, road crashes and natural disasters that result in death and sometimes grotesque disfigurement. Henry (2004:3) describes his research aim as examining "the psychological struggles and transformations urban police officers experience as a result of their routine work related exposure to the deaths of others". Henry refers to this process as "psychic numbing" which creates distance between the confronting event and the officer's personal (as opposed to professional) response to it.

All of the officers interviewed in my research made reference to the ways in which they came to terms with this aspect of police work. This is a transition that must be made at the beginning of a police career if it is to achieve longevity. Often, particularly in the second half of the twentieth century in South Australia, this transition was forced upon young officers as they were routinely assigned patrol duties that included regularly transporting bodies to the city morgue, identifying them, cleaning and washing them, and preparing them for viewing by grieving relatives. The clear suggestion from my conversations with officers who had this early career experience was that it constituted a form of "flooding", a very high level of exposure to a potentially damaging stressor at an early stage in a police career which set the bar to a height in terms of stress responses that puts subsequent exposure to less challenging situations into a more comfortable context. There is a sense here that those who can cope with such exposure continue in their careers and those who find such experiences overwhelming leave policing at an early stage.

Henry (2004) considers death exposures a constant reminder of the individual officer's own mortality and outlines in his research the strategies that officers use to deal with such issues. "Psychic or professional numbing" is one such strategy that involves the creation of a level of detachment that balances operational efficiency and appropriate responses to crime victims and the general public against over-identification with the situation that may be damaging to the individual's well-being. Yuan et al. (2011) and Bourke et al. (2006) argue that research has focussed excessively on the possible pathology of such death encounters, suggesting that "protective factors" including temperament and personality, attitudes that develop in officers over time that reinforce a personal sense of competence and coping, social support through the "family" culture of policing, and, against all odds, the development and maintenance of a positive view of the world contribute to more positive outcomes for the officers involved. These researchers highlight the development of resilience and coping strategies in the context of such experiences that contribute to post-traumatic growth (Schiraldi, 2011; Seligman, 2012; Tedeschi & Calhoun, 1995).

Much of the quantitative police-oriented literature examined in my research is unable to drill down to such detail. Henry's qualitative work (2004) includes interviews with "rookies" (officers who recently graduated from the police academy) patrol Sergeants, who are required to visit most crime scenes in a supervisory capacity, and homicide detectives who attend few death scenes than patrol officers. The death scenes they do attend are, however, at the more confronting end of the scale comprising homicides, suicides and those resulting from accidental or more often intentional violence. Henry also interviewed crime scene examiners or technicians who attend such scenes to gather and preserve forensic evidence as well as creating a record of the scene. He found that these groups experience such situations differently, each developing with experience and exposure, their own strategies of self-protection from the traumatic impact. For example, with reference to crime scene examiners, he found that they typically perceive each situation with "scientific detachment" (p. 181) and that they often find their duties "intellectually stimulating". In answer to a question posed by Henry to one such officer regarding his ability to cope with horrific crime scenes, he responded, "what you see is a person {in this case a murdered rape victim} I see a very interesting piece of evidence" (p. 185). The officer continued, "If I looked at this as a person, I'll never see the evidence, and I'll never do my job". This task focus was evident in many of the interviews I conducted as evidenced in the interview data below.

A constant theme in much of the biographical and grey literature explores how the experience of such scenes builds resilience. A typical comment regarding this issue is "It's not the dead ones you worry about, they can't hurt you". The confronting aspects of operational policing, including a constant and intimate contact with sudden death are aspects of the job that most officers learn to deal with in a variety of ways, including conscious distancing strategies, the ability to focus on duty and process and a capacity to compartmentalise experiences into those that are personal and professional. Cultural realities of policing are prominent in this area, where officers gain comfort and capacity from the aspects of these confronting experiences that are not shared with the general public. This is what police do and what they are expected to do. In performing such duties officers focus on process and outcomes and when well managed, derive satisfaction and growth from their role. To assume inevitable negative outcomes from such duties, as is common in much of the literature (Carlier et al., 1998; Faust & Ven, 2014; Green, 2004; Kates, 2008; Kroes, 1976; McFarlane, 2011; Paton, 2009; Peters, 2009) is not borne out by this research and fails to account for the individual officer's capacity to thrive regardless of the presence or absence of perceivable organisational support and in the presence of high levels of personal and peer professionalism, experience and cultural wisdom. As I argued earlier, major stressors are more likely to arise from other factors central to policing, including the way officers are managed and led.

4.2 Confronting Jobs: The Literature on Policing and Trauma

Research into policing and trauma responses often focusses on operational stressors such as exposure to grotesque death and physical danger at the expense of the less obvious organisational and management influences on individual well-being. Debriefs after confronting taskings, positive feedback from superior officers for a "job well done" and informal debriefs with colleagues after difficult shifts are seen by many officers as all that are necessary to deal with the emotional side of policing.

Pole et al. (2006) use the term "passive coping" to describe the same phenomenon, warning against the hazards of not squarely confronting the possible negatives of such operational experiences. Others (Elntib & Armstrong, 2014; Flannery, 2015; Ménard & Arter, 2013; Rees & Smith, 2008) sound similar cautionary warnings around such strategies which were frequently described by those officers I interviewed as a positive and effective stress management tool with no discernible negative outcomes. This may well be an example of the effectiveness of a qualitative, interview-based approach where, instead of responding to a questionnaire, interviewees are able to describe effective trauma techniques that work for them in significant detail, referring to the need to develop a focus on "protective factors" and coping skills rather than pathology.

Yuan et al. (2011) reach similar conclusions around coping, drawing attention to the need to develop "basic attitudes to self and the world" that were observed in those officers I interviewed. Put simply, officers develop the capacity to accommodate this level of challenge by repeated exposure and a sense of purpose and achievement as well as the cultural support offered by colleagues. Hadass et al. (2014) in a study of coping mechanisms of paramedics in the context of "difficult jobs" refers to the learnt skill of "striking a balance between emotional connection and detachment". This raises the question as to whether such strategies involve the repression of emotional responses, which according to some, raise the spectre of repressed events and responses "bursting through" in a major trauma response later due to what Kirschman calls "maladaptive coping" (Kirschman et al., 2015: 30). Others (Elntib & Armstrong, 2014; Flannery, 2015; Ménard & Arter, 2013; Rees & Smith, 2008) sound similar cautionary warnings around such strategies which were referred to frequently by those officers I interviewed as a positive and effective stress management tool with no discernible negative outcomes. Repeated exposure, particularly to death and bodies in the context of police duties, builds the capacity for those who stay in "the job" to deal with such experiences without trauma. Delivering countless bodies to the city morgue early in his career said one Chief Superintendent, "taught me resilience in one respect".

4.3 The Data from the Interviews: Death and Bodies, Confronting Jobs

All of the officers interviewed described duty-related exposures to sudden death that accompany a career in operational policing. The experiences they chose to recount were therefore the most challenging. In line with the policing and trauma literature, the accounts covered incidents that challenged the individual officer's resilience, often re-assuring them the ability they possessed to cope.

The death of children is always significant for even the most experienced and resilient officers. A Senior Constable of 12 years, said, "Sudden Infant Death Syndrome death scenes were another cause of trauma for me. I had two in two weeks at one stage. In one a twin was crushed by her mother when she rolled on to her while asleep. I felt sorry for the remaining child". This is a very clear example of how an out of ordinary tasking can be traumatic. The close proximity of two such deaths in this officer's experience challenged her capacity to "bounce back". Without departmental support or assistance she did so, utilising the social support of her close colleagues, family and an "on call" non-departmental helping professional. Echoing a similar insight, a Detective Senior Sergeant of 30 years experience commented, "you look at dead bodies as humans but you repress your feelings", adding, "Dealing with families where young children had died was always difficult". Repressing feelings in such situations is a learned and essential skill. Recognising the humanity of the deceased is in this context professionally respectful but never overwhelming.

Another officer, a recovery diver, referring to a career-long exposure to dead bodies said:

> I've seen a lot of bodies, I don't remember many. I remember retrieving the body of a five year old boy from the Murray {river}. He had drowned when he jumped off a boat without his life jacket. I had been playing with my five year old son that morning before I went to work. Stroking and cuddling him as you do. I was on the bottom waiting to be raised holding the child and touching him. He felt just like my son a few hours earlier. That was fairly trying.

Again there is clear evidence here of a personal connection that makes such an experience challenging, but not threatening. In this case, the officer went on to recount how typically, the personal connection, once "trying" became a non-intrusive memory after a few days.

Grotesque deaths, dismembered, disfigured bodies were even more confronting. A Chief Inspector described a tasking earlier in his career where he and his partner attended a suicide, "She had burnt herself to death with petrol and we found her body in the back of a burnt out car", and the officer described the scene, "It was just a skeleton with the organs intact inside it. My junior partner said it's the worst thing I have ever seen". There is here, evidence of the cultural aspect of such experiences, where the more junior officer, clearly challenged, was able to safely express his discomfort. Another officer referred to his perception of the ways in which such "horrendous things" threaten to build up over the length of a career. His solution was to "Build an iron wall, so that it didn't affect me. My experience as twenty one year old recruit, dealing with dead bodies at the start of my career stood me in good stead". This interviewee also referred to his successful long-term marriage, indicating his capacity to lower the "iron wall" when not on duty. Early experiences in police careers with the metropolitan patrols that were tasked with delivering bodies to the then morgue which was located in the West Terrace Cemetery[1] seem important in terms of officers developing the capacity to accept death and disfigurement. One such officer after a very long career said, "We collected the keys as a twenty year old constable to the West Terrace morgue. We stripped and washed bodies. They were ghastly conditions totally chaotic, with bodies on the floor. There was no coronial section then, that was my introduction to death". A retired Chief Superintendent, referring to his early experience of death and working on the same patrols said, "You could spend a whole shift at the morgue on West Terrace or delivering bodies to the morgue. Cleaning, checking ID and laying them out". Another experienced retired officer described the same situation and its challenges:

> We took bodies to the morgue, murder victims, burnt bodies, car crash victims, and decomposed bodies. That was just part of it. We washed and cleaned bodies, cleaned clothing and valuables, arranged ID's. Covered bodies with sheets to hide injuries and comforted the families. Some cops tried to avoid these duties. We just went and did it. For those who could incorporate it, it wasn't an issue. We often had three or four bodies a shift.

The retired Detective Chief Inspector went on, "I think the experience in the mortuary set me up for the future". This was a form of "flooding" where intense, early career, unavoidable exposure to death on a large scale, either halted that career or encouraged individual officers to recognise that they possessed the resilience to cope with such challenges often to the benefit of their capacity to cope with later challenges. This is clearly a learning process, more to do with culture than training. Another retired Chief Superintendent commented, recognising the challenges to his "wall", "Dead bodies didn't bother me, although young kids the same age as ours was a challenge. I was probably involved with two hundred post mortems during my career. They sometimes trigger things but it doesn't stay with me. You develop an attitude that helps you deal with visually traumatic things". The "attitude" ensures that memories of such experiences when dealt with are controlled and not intrusive.

However, on some occasions, the challenges are beyond immediate comprehension and present obstacles that are very difficult to manage. The "Snowtown" murders commonly known as "The Bodies in the Barrel murders" (Marshall, 2006) were a significant challenge for the police team that was tasked with dealing with them. A senior officer involved in that investigation said, "Snowtown set a new scale for human depravity. Vasilakas murdering his stepbrothers, Bunting torturing victims who were forced to make recordings before they died. The putrification of the bodies, the property room, the stink on your clothes, the longevity of the investigation". All these factors were beyond even the most extreme duty-related experiences of death and bodies that most would meet during their careers. SAPOL management recognising

[1] Near the centre of Adelaide in South Australia.

this made extraordinary efforts to assist those involved to cope, with regular debriefs and easy access to professional support over the 6-year period of the investigation.

An officer "bagging" a decomposed body, which had been in the open and exposed to high temperatures for some time, took a great deal of time to recover from the experience. He said of the scene:

> I took responsibility, twisting him around trying to fit him into the bag .We took him back to the Country Fire Service in the back of the ute. We went through his pockets for ID. I found his wallet. Dollar bills were covered in slime from the decomposition. We bagged him again. I was pushing his head trying to get him into the bag. It reminded me of my five year old's head. We make jokes, tried to laugh it off. I pulled the police car over to the side of the road later, and just broke. I called in sick the next day.

A PTSD diagnosis followed. The officer, just weeks before had been involved in a succession of fatal motor vehicle crashes, receiving just one phone call from SAPOL Employee Assistance to enquire about his well-being. He is recovering and hopes to return to full operational duties.

A Senior Sergeant recounted a double motor vehicle fatality that he and his partner witnessed at Ramco in South Australia's Riverland, some 30 years ago. The accident involved two 18-year-olds who were in a car identical to that of the police officer's partner. He said:

> It was a cool morning. One of the bodies was half out of the car window. Half his head was missing and there was steam coming out of his brain cavity. My partner lost it and was vomiting. The family of the dead men rocked up at the scene, one brother sprinting toward the car. I rugby tackled him to the ground. We got the bodies out. I picked up the brain matter and put it in a plastic bag. We cleaned the bodies up for ID. I knocked off at 18:00 the next day. I was twenty years old then. The next day I saw the tow truck driver in the main street. He said 'I haven't slept for three days, all I can see is you picking up the brains off the road.

The challenge for a 20-year-old was to find a way through the experience in the absence of departmental intervention which was at that time extremely rare in such circumstances.

Other officers had made clear distinctions between the difficulties of confronting death and their capacity to deal with that as well as the confronting aspects of, for example, picking up body parts of the deceased. One commented, "Picking up body parts isn't the difficult bit, telling the relatives is the most difficult. I remember my first one. I asked, can I do this one? I felt myself taking on their grief. I said to myself it's not my grief. I can't take this on and that has always worked for me since". The capacity to be desensitised was apparently mentioned during training at the police academy but can only be learned according to this officer and his colleagues through the experience. There is again clear evidence here of the need to learn from experience that over-involvement with grief and grieving can be costly. Not "taking it on" is at the centre of this aspect of coping, learning to be numb (Henry, 2004) but still being able to be professional when dealing with the death scene, is central. This is at the heart of professional policing. One said, "My first crime scene shocked me. You can't collapse in a heap, it's not the body that gets to you, it's the emotions of the family. I was able to compartmentalize the horror and be professional and clinical while still showing enough empathy to the family members". This level of professional expertise is essential to a resilient officer, having the capacity to establish distance, to "compartmentalise" to find a non-threatening location for the experience in memory and to recognise the developing expertise and resilience that results.

A Senior Constable described his coping mechanism as, "Although you are apprehensive every time you attend a death scene it's always nowhere near as bad as you thought it would be. I remember retrieving the body of a person who had been dead for five weeks in an apartment and I can remember the smell vividly, but I am fascinated by the human body and a black sense of humour helps". What he learned from this experience was not explained, but his capacity to cope was clear.

A young water operations member of Star Group offered this response to his first body recovery off Granite Island in South Australia. "We were in Mt Gambier training when we were called in and arrived at Victor Harbor at 3:00 am. We spotted the body quite quickly. I wasn't affected until I looked at him. Crabs and lice had eaten his lips, eyes and neck". Recognising the visual effect of such disfigurement was a learning experience here, and the capacity to deal with it was encouraged by the policing culture that surrounded this individual early in his career. Such experiences were to become part of his profession, part of his "assumptive world" (Janoff-Bulman, 1989).

Some officers with many years in "the job" recognised that this distancing process, for them had gone too far, an ex-United Kingdom officer commented: "I am quite desensitized. I am kind of indifferent. When in London I was attending a drug overdose in a stairwell and I thought to myself I am watching a human being die and I am feeling nothing".

It was not always that easy to avoid taking constant death-related experiences home. A retired Major Crime Detective Chief Inspector told of how "I used to go into the kids bedrooms when I returned home off duty while they were asleep to touch them, to make sure they were warm". A Senior Sergeant described clearly the impact of such exposure at another level where it intruded into his personal life in a different way, "When my parents died, I just got on with it" describing how the impact of their death was blunted on him by constant exposure to duty-related deaths he had encountered during his career.

A Senior Sergeant was not so desensitised, "Dead bodies are always a challenge, car accidents for example. Only one situation came back to me eight weeks after it had happened. A twenty year old girl committed suicide with a shot gun to her head. Her father came home and in the darkness trod on her brain matter on the floor. I thought about that for quite a while. Other members at the same crime scene vomited". Processing such experiences "for quite a while" is part of the learned capacity to cope and bounce back. The absence of an emotional response to the scene described here would indicate levels of distancing behaviour that could preclude meaningful interaction with victims. Clearly, a departmental response to such incidents including debriefing and continued individual support where required would be a significant aid to processing an out of the ordinary experience. In this case, none was offered.

Experiences in childhood dealing with death may have assisted in such circumstances according to one interviewee, "Maybe growing up on a farm helped me deal with death. I struggle more dealing with injured people, an old man who was badly burnt affected me. Suicides when the family is there. I think of a Dad who hung himself. His daughter was in matric.[2] I felt like I was intruding". Such feelings are not uncommon, particularly among officers in their early career. Opportunities to express such feelings without career repercussions are rare. When provided, the impact of well-being, coping and resilience were positive and considerable.

In response to the question "how did you handle death experiences", an officer of 15 years experience thus responded:

> The academy training course didn't prepare us well. It was more focused on law and procedures. When we graduated the older police told us don't believe the bullshit they told you at the academy. In terms of the death experiences we had it was a matter of luck where you were at the time. The mortuary and fatal motor vehicle accidents could not be prepared for in the Academy. You simply learned that you had to cope and move on.

Such "simple learning" is clearly not that simple. The absence of even the most rudimentary preparation at the Academy for such experiences, which apparently continues, can only be explained by the expectation that such skills will be learned "on the job", that culture and the passing down of wisdom learned from experience is expected to suffice.

Commenting on his first death encounter, a young officer said of seven years on "the job", "It was a bit surreal, the simple death scenes are no problem for example an older person dying out of hospital. You try to detach yourself. It doesn't affect me much. The youngest death so far I have had was a teenager. I expect a young child would be difficult".

4.4 Suicide and Policing: The Literature

The issue of suicide as an aspect of police service permeates much of the policing literature at cultural, political, organisational, industrial and, of course, personal levels (Blum & Blum, 2000; Chae & Boyle, 2013; Chopko et al., 2014; Gilmartin, 2002; Kirschman et al., 2015; Marzuk et al., 2002; Peters, 2009; Schaffer, 2014; Silverii, 2014; Sparkes, 2013; Stone, 1999; Sutton, 2005; Violanti 2014; Violanti & Paton, 2006). The reasons for such an emphasis rest on the wider interest in police mental health in the light of contemporary trauma, resilience and workplace safety, often expressed in the context of the rigours and challenges of policing outlined in detail above (Chopko et al., 2014). At the heart of the discussion is the incidence of suicide in police organisations. Officers themselves are heavily impacted when a colleague suicides (Schaffer, 2014), this being partly due to the "family" culture in most police organisations as well as the deep bonds formed working in "the job".

[2] Final year of secondary school in South Australia.

Police hierarchies are often unsure of how to respond to suicide in the ranks, which complicates the issue further. The studies considered here reflect that confusion and uncertainty. Assumptions that suicide rates among police officers are much higher than the societal norm are often based on perceptions of the challenging nature of police work and the failure of management to adequately care for the mental health of those who serve (Cotton, 2016; Marin, 2012, Peters, 2009) and there are of course difficulties in obtaining such very sensitive information. Reviews of police organisations from the "outside" have come to differing conclusions. One strategy is to explore "suicidal ideation" among officers by survey (Chae & Boyle, 2013) the obvious other is to obtain statistical data by examining police and other records which often are unclear about the cause of death, and if indicating that a suicide has taken place fail to include information regarding known contributing factors (Cantor et al., 1995; Chae & Boyle, 2013; Marzuk et al., 2002).

Marin (2012) Ombudsman of Ontario Canada, on the advice of an Ontario Provincial police psychologist, was drawn to the conclusion that the Ontario Provincial police organisation has lower rates of suicide than in the population at large, due in part to rigorous psychological selection processes at entry and also argues that candidates for entry into police services are broadly aware of the challenges and confronting aspects of the job as they join the profession. The suicide rate in the Ontario police service was reported to be 12 per 100,000 which was lower than the 17–21 per 100,000 rates for males between the ages of 20 and 55 years in the general Canadian population. In sounding a cautionary note regarding the above conclusion, Marin argues that police officers should be compared only with similar demographics as the general population includes the most vulnerable, for example, those with mental health issues, who may be more prone to suicidal ideation and completed suicide. Marin also makes a clear link between a diagnosis of PTSD and an increase in the risk of suicide among those diagnosed, this may apply particularly to police officers. I will consider this again in the New South Wales autobiographical accounts below, but there seems to be a direct link between a PTSD diagnosis received by a police officer and a sense of failure and betrayal of the fundamentals of policing culture, the ability to be tough and to cope as "good coppers" do.

O'Hara and Violanti (2008) while evidencing in their research higher rates of suicide among US police officers suggest that rates among police officers should be lower than the general population (agreeing with Marin above) in that police are a fully employed, healthy and thoroughly psychologically tested group, at least at the time of recruitment. They also argue that the general population includes the unemployed, the mentally ill and institutionalised who cannot be compared in this context to the police cohort. In their web surveillance study, O'Hara and Violanti (2008) concluded that within US police organisations, 92% of completed suicides are male officers with 6% female officers. The 40–44-year-old age group has the most prevalent cluster of suicides. Death by firearm (usually the officer's own service weapon) was the method used in 91.5% of suicides. Personal problems were the most common reason for the act in 83% of cases, with work associated legal problems (such as being under departmental investigation for breaches of ethical standards or facing criminal charges) accounting for 13% of incidents. Among other conclusions, the researchers observed that 64% of officers who completed suicide showed no warning signs of distress to colleagues before the act, this being attributed to the ever-present fear of being perceived as "soft or weak" by close colleagues as well as their management hierarchy.

US psychologist Stephen Curran (2003), in a study reviewing death certificates of New York police officers, concluded that police are 26% less likely to suicide when compared to a similar demographic and have lower rates of alcoholism and divorce than the general population. The title of his study "Separating Fact from Fiction about Police Stress" is a clear indicator of his position in this debate. Understandably, other researchers (Violanti, 2004 and Toch, 2002) disagree, arguing that their research shows that policing is the most dangerous job in the world resulting in an increased risk of physical and mental health issues.

Another study of the New York Police Department (Marzuk et al., 2002) concluded that an examination of the death certificates of the 668 operational officers revealed a suicide rate of 14.9 per 100,000 compared to a similar demographic of New Yorkers at 18.3 per 100,000. Male officers suicided at rates close to their comparable population, while female officers rates were lower than their comparable demographic. Marzuk also reported no increase in suicide rates in recent years among NYPD officers. Violanti in 2004 wrote to the editor of the American Journal of Psychiatry to express his dissatisfaction with studies such as Curren's and Marzuk's which he argued, failed to accurately compare police populations with those of the general community. In a later study, Violanti et al. (2013) concluded that detectives, criminal investigators and police generally had an 82% increased risk of suicide over the general US working population.

An Australian study of suicides in the Queensland Police Department produced similar findings to Curren (2003) and Marzuk et al. (2002). Cantor et al (1995) had the unique opportunity to study a register of all death records of police members in that department between 1843 and 1992, arguing that many such studies into suicide in policing rely on small samples and "fail to recognise the cultural context of specific police populations" (p. 499). The authors concluded that suicide rates of this police population actually declined over the 49-year period, from rates of 60 per 100,000 to 20 per 100,000 in the latter years of the study. These later rates are similar to employed general populations in Queensland at the time. The contributing factors including physical and psychological ill-health, alcohol abuse and "domestic problems" were common as were those connected to "disciplinary events" within the police organisation. These factors are commonly described in many studies into police suicide rates and causation (Violanti, 2009, Marin, 2001, Marzuk, 1995). 79% of the Queensland police suicides over the study period were completed with the Officer's own firearm. The mean age of death was 36 years, 58 of the 59 recorded suicides over the period were committed by male officers, and the average length of service prior to the suicide was 11.73 years. Interestingly, although there were no reliable indicators of diagnosed psychiatric conditions, there were mentions in the records indicating "depressed" states, "alcoholic, nervous disorder, personality change" which the researchers classified as "psychiatric disorders inferred" (p. 503).

34.5% of the circumstances of the death described "separation" from the wife of girlfriend as a factor and "service problems" accounted for 50% of cases already referred to above, involving suspensions from duty, demotions, reprimands and involuntary transfers.

Chae and Boyle (2013) employed a "best evidence synthesis approach" to researching suicide risk and protective factors for police officers by studying the best available empirically sound research on the topic. They describe much of the available research as "limited because few studies have employed methodologically sound research designs to test risk and protective factors related to police suicide" (p. 91) but identify risk factors including organisational stress, critical incident trauma, shift work, relationship problems and alcohol abuse. In gently criticising much of contemporary research which investigates whether police are at a higher or lower risk of suicide than the general population, the authors argue for a greater focus on risk and preventative factors rather than the incidence of such events. Protective factors proposed by the authors include psycho-education and suicide prevention programmes, social support (a central factor in police culture), family connectedness and friendship networks (with other than fellow police officers) resilience training and easy access to psychological support and services external to police organisations. Chae and Boyle are also optimistic about the impact of resilience training and post-traumatic growth approaches in terms of the well-being of officers, arguing that "helping to provide meaning, structure and perspective" (p.103) to operational and management issues may help personal growth. Peer support programmes and counselling are also seen as a critically important protective factor, being an effective alternative to the culture of not acknowledging stress-related problems in most police organisations for fear of organisational and personal repercussions. The authors quote Stinchcomb's (2004) recommendation that organisational and management factors are of critical importance and that three important approaches can contribute to change in this area; these being, commitment (to the individual well-being of their staff), participation (staying involved at the operational level of policing) and action (for change in management approaches) by executive police management.

Chae and Boyle recommend from their research that police organisations encourage officers to employ "active coping styles" that facilitate engagement with the process of confronting job trauma and life stressors that can and should lead to post-traumatic growth. The emphasis on prevention and early intervention in contemporary police management through training of managers and cultural change among them in terms of moving away from "command and control" to Cotton's (2016) "person centred management approach" is also central to such a strategy.

Peters (2009) writing from the perspective of a long-serving police psychologist in New South Wales, Australia has a more "hands on" perspective of suicide and policing, suggesting that rather than focus on suicide as a predictable and threatening reality in policing, attention should instead be given to the management of police, the development of resilience and the avoidance of "burnout". His challenge is to change the basic culture of policing and to go "upstream" from the predictability of PTSD and depression among officers to a new era of openness, prevention and a culture of support. This has profound implications for present and future management strategies for police organisations.

Violanti and Paton (2006:167) strike an optimistic note where he argues that researchers should consider that the "persons who survive traumatic experiences without pathological outcomes can provide important clues to interventions and treatment of those who suffer from PTSD".

There is clearly much more research to be done around the incidence of police suicide as well as the contributing factors from within and outside "the job". Lester et al. (eds.) (2014), in a collection of essays relating generally to male suicide, argue that men kill themselves in relation to problems of work and financial issues and that bullying in the workplace is also a significant issue. Men, they argue, are more often than women self-defined in terms of their occupation and by their intimate relationships, particularly at the point of breakdown. "Not perceiving or admitting anxiety" (p. 16) is a significant factor as is loneliness and isolation, particularly for older men. Risk factors identified include alcohol use and abuse, childhood abuse, loss of a parent by suicide, mental health issues, isolation, combat exposure, substance abuse, family conflict and helplessness and hopelessness. Protective factors include social support, positive coping skills, life satisfaction, resiliency, hopefulness and self-efficacy.

Silverii (2014:28) argues that police culture itself adds to the risk of suicidal ideation among officers, "seeking help when stressed is breaking the code of silence" and refers to the common fear of being revealed as weak, leading to rejection by police peers and the loss of the "law enforcement identity" (p. 136). This was clearly supported by the officers interviewed for my research. They agreed that the decision to reveal that they were struggling with duty-related stress involved a careful choice of the confidant.

Schaffer (2014:25) in an autobiography covering a long policing career in the United States argues that officers who complete suicidal acts are called cowards and weaklings by some colleagues who focus at such times on the wrong aspect of the tragedy, "we should ask what's wrong with us, not what was wrong with him" blaming this in part on broken organisational and leadership cultures in contemporary law enforcement.

4.5 Suicide and Policing: The Data from the Interviews

Most of the officers I interviewed knew of colleagues who had killed themselves and most expressed the view that SAPOL and other police organisations did not openly address what they saw as the "elephant in the room". Because of the culture of policing, when a "family" member dies by his or her own hand the ramifications are significant. Fellow police officers deal with the scene of the death, usually those close to the deceased are spared that ordeal unless the situation occurs in a country or regional setting. According to those interviewed the departmental response is usually the same, "Suicides in the job are usually kept quiet", meaning that SAPOL makes no reference to the nature of the event apart from acknowledging the passing of the dead officer. Whether this, in fact, is a process of keeping suicide quiet or it reflects an ambivalence or uncertainty among police organisations about how they should respond to these incidents is open to question. This was well reflected by a Detective Sergeant who responded to a question about suicide in policing by describing an incident that occurred behind his police station in a Southern suburb of Adelaide, "He shot himself in the car park at the rear of the station. He was a lovely chap. I asked when told what's that about? There was no official departmental response, I have no recollection of being approached by colleagues. Those sorts of situations hit hard". Referring to the same event, another Senior Constable commented, "After the suicide at Sturt, we heard nothing from SAPOL". Clearly when a colleague suicides within an occupation such as policing those who know him or her personally, those that have worked with the individual professionally and the rest of his or her police colleagues wonder what contributed to that final act.

"When I attended the funeral of a colleague who had suicided" a Senior Constable reported, "no-one talked about the fact that it was suicide. There is a strong message from SAPOL that police don't suicide more that the general public." He added, "There's no way I'd ever do it. I wouldn't want my offsider to find me!" Referring to a widely held perception among police members that SAPOL is ignoring the issue one officer commented, "In the seven years I've been in SAPOL there have been three suicides. That has pushed the organisation and PASA {the police union} into thinking about welfare and resilience. They don't know what to do, they don't have a policy". A retired Senior Constable addressed the same issue that "I don't know how many people I know who have committed suicide". The actual incidence of suicide among SAPOL members was of little interest to the police officers I interviewed but the departmental response to such events has their attention. Many felt that suicide as an issue was swept under the organisational carpet and that the response to suicide within the organisation was inadequate without having a clear idea of what a more appropriate response might entail.

I was told of an officer who suicided in a southern Adelaide police area. Many of his colleagues, who were his personal friends, commented that in the days following his death, senior officers made no attempt to communicate with police colleagues who may have been impacted by his death. Few were surprised that no senior officers offered support to their junior colleagues. This reinforced a perception among these officers that the department had no immediate response to such situations that they thought adequate, "They don't know what to do, they don't have a policy". This lack of a management strategy in such circumstances serves to reinforce the view among SAPOL officers that senior management is uncaring and unsure when one of their colleagues suicided. The lack of any intervention only adds to their grief and uncertainty.

There was, however, one exception to that rule. An officer, deeply concerned about the suicide death of a colleague and in contravention of departmental regulations, sent an email directly to the Commissioner. The Commissioner then called him at home and discussed the situation. The officer concluded, "Suicide is a serious problem in SAPOL". Such a problem will not be solved by SAPOL management ignoring such incidents. Any outcome of this discussion with the Commissioner was not obvious to this SAPOL member.

One long-serving Detective Senior Sergeant dismissed the issue in terms of his own beliefs, "I don't do suicide, you ride the waves". This is a clear reference to the need to be resilient in the face of the ups and downs of a long police career as well as an expression of the more traditional cultural insistence that "toughing it out" was the only alternative. In this Sergeant's experience, such a strategy had served him well through a long and eventful career, his younger contemporaries may need to benefit from more contemporary departmental interventions and strategies.[3]

Attending deaths by suicide was seen by many officers interviewed as challenging. One who served in the APY Lands[4] of South Australia described his duties:

> There was domestic violence, assaults with weapons were common, extreme suicide attempts and threats, petrol sniffing in those days caused a lot of that, suicide threats got the communities attention, there were many suicides, always by hanging. Fatal road crashes were common. Alcohol plus all the normal stuff, just more and worse! SAPOL were aware of these issues, we needed a psych assessment to go up there. I never saw a psych while I was there. One really rough suicide involved a young woman who hung herself after seeking help, I performed CPR for forty five minutes. SAPOL sent the Chaplain up. I was there for another twelve months.

The isolation of such postings is well illustrated here. Challenges such as dealing with death by suicide are magnified by the distance from potential support services.

Other officers interviewed were aware of implications of suicide not addressed by the literature and not considered in other aspects of my research. For example, one who was a Detective Sergeant involved in the investigation of child sexual abuse commented on a couple of cases where a paedophile who had been under investigation had committed suicide after being questioned by this officer and her colleagues. Her comment was, "having some input into another person's decision to die is difficult".

Clearly, the officers I interviewed were concerned about suicide not only out of a feeling of camaraderie with the colleagues who chose that form of death but also because it added to the level of anxiety they feel in the present context around the damage that may or may not be done to them by their policing careers. In the context of a societal expectation that emergency service workers including police are more vulnerable to stress-related conditions such as PTSD and depression, operational officers need the reassurance of an organisational support system when suicide becomes a part of their professional experience. This is clearly an argument for preventative mental health strategies such as those that may result from a nationwide "Beyond Blue" research project that commenced at the beginning of 2017. Police, Fire, Ambulance and Correctional Services officers were surveyed about their levels of stress and the direct or indirect contribution that they might make to suicidal ideation in their experience (Lawrence et al., 2018).

---

[3] See recommendations in my final section.

[4] These are Aboriginal lands in the far North West corner of South Australia.

4.6 Suicide from the Psychology/Psychiatry Interviews

Suicide in the ranks was an issue raised by several of the clinicians interviewed. A psychiatrist said, "The rate in SAPOL is lower than the general population but no effort is made to deal with this issue when it happens. Management generally try to ignore the issue". This confirms vividly the observations of the officers I interviewed.

Another was more personal in referring to a former Commissioner, and said, "**** was detached from the troops. Management should be better prioritising well-being among the troops these days. We should be moving away from that level of remote executive management".

A psychologist responding to this issue was clear that part of the departmental response should be to "Get rid of bullying and harassment! The suicide rate in South Australia is high by Australian standards. SAPOL's suicide rate is lower than the general population".

Another veteran SAPOL psychologist confessed that "Suicides used to rattle me. Often they were related to issues outside of policing. I remember a woman who killed herself was lesbian, had just been refused a Commission. It saddens me that no effort is made to deal with this". This clinician makes another reference to the unwillingness of SAPOL executive managers to engage with police members when a suicide occurs within the ranks or to facilitate any preventative measures through consultation with outside agencies such as Beyond Blue.[5] Another was clear about the appropriate departmental response to such events, "After a suicide they should get the psychologists in. We should provide the hug. We psychologists need to engage with the senior Commissioned Officers about this". Across all the interviews with officers for this research, there was no evidence that such a strategy had been employed, much to the dismay of many affected by such incidents.

Exactly how a police organisation could and should respond to such incidents is an important question not addressed in detail in the literature. The debate around suicide in policing generally addresses the incidence of suicide, with a passing reference to other factors that may contribute to such decision-making usually cloaked in operational terms. Much of the discussion (Horner, 2011; Kirschman et al., 2015; Paton, 2009; Violanti & Paton, 2006, Violanti, 2014) focusses on operational aspects such as the trauma encountered in everyday policing but rarely shed light on other factors that may contribute. As discussed above, these might include relationship difficulties, issues pertaining to disciplinary action taken by the organisation, depression diagnosed or otherwise, and a raft of other factors that may or may not have a direct relationship to the officer's professional activities. It is clear from the interviews I conducted that among officers there is more than a general awareness of the issue and a clear assumption that it is a significant factor presently ignored by SAPOL.

[5] Beyond Blue is a national suicide prevention organisation that also focusses on "first responders" and trauma reactions.

4.7 Death Messages: The Data from the Interviews

Several of the officers interviewed referred to the challenges around the delivery of death messages. Police officers are called upon to undertake this task as they are authority figures, particularly when in uniform and also directly involved in incidents such as fatal accidents and other forms of sudden death. Unsurprisingly, this is a task not relished by operational police who prefer to be confronted by the death itself rather than having to convey the news to close relatives. A Sergeant, referring to the uncertainty of such situations, made this clear, "Death notices were always difficult. You never knew how people would react". A vivid example of such a response was described by an experienced Senior Constable, then working in a Regional setting: "I dealt with exposure to death very easily apart from delivering death notices, for example woman whose husband died on mining site. I'll be OK she said, then collapsed and wailed".

Another officer, referring to a profound learning experience during an early career challenge of delivering his first death message, made this comparison, "picking up body parts isn't the difficult bit, telling the relatives is the most difficult. I remember the first one. I asked can I do this one, I felt myself taking on their grief. I said to myself, it's not my grief, I can't take this on. That has always worked for me since". This is the evidence of an early career lesson coping very well with the ability to create distance and to some extent become "numb" (Henry, 2004).

Such a learning approach was common, as officers created their own capacity to deal with the raw pain of those who have been recently bereaved; "its second hand trauma, you can be detached if you don't know them. We were desensitised at the Academy, talked about it, were shown videos and attended autopsies". Such detachment is a skill learned from career beginnings and is only violated when officers encounter situations that break through their usual defences, for example, when the deceased is known to them. A retired Sergeant recalled an example of such a situation, "My first fatal Motor Vehicle Accident involved a car hitting a stobie pole at high speed. Three people were dead. Identifying the deceased was very difficult. I will never forget it. There were dismembered bodies and their car boot was full of Christmas presents. I had to tell the children of those who died".

The timing of such duties is also beyond the control of those officers involved. A Sergeant remembered, "A lad was killed on the Eyre Highway. I had to deliver a death message to the family in the middle of their Grandchild's birthday party". Delivering death messages was a point of high stress for one retired officer, only comparable to his perception of other unavoidable sources, "What stresses us most is the organization. Dead bodies and death messages is the other stress point".

Another retired Senior Sergeant echoed the comments of her colleagues. The most stressful activities were death messages and high-speed chases. For example, I was comforting a young guy who had crashed his car and killed his sister. He asked, "what about my sister? I knew she was dead. When delivering the death message to the rest of the family, I was punched by the Mother. You take on board their pain for a while. I used to debrief with my partner".

4.8 The Smell of Death: Data from the Interviews

Smell and trauma were seen by many of those interviewed to be closely linked, particularly when the officer was confronted by a decomposed corpse. This is in line with much trauma-related research (Henry, 2004; Kates, 2008; Kirschman et al., 2015; Kitaeff, 2011; Pietrzak et al., 2014; Rees & Smith, 2008) and the autobiographical accounts discussed above and in later chapters (Mckay, 2005; Neil, 2014; Sparkes, 2013). Many officers interviewed for this research referred to the challenges posed by effectively dealing with the smell of death. There were also, however, other sources of such memories that were similarly persistent, "You never got over the smell of attending neglect cases, smells are traumatic!".

Another officer had adopted well-known defences against such challenges, "use of Vicks vapour rub inside face mask helps when dealing with decomposed bodies". And "I often have to have long showers to get rid of the stink of decomposed bodies". Another made a similar comment, "I used to put Vicks up my nose for the smell. We survived the horror" adding, "there was no disrespect for the dead".

The notorious multiple murders of 12 people in South Australia between 1992 and 1999 (Marshall, 2006) referred to above was a major challenge to the team of police investigators from this perspective. "The putrification of the bodies, the property room, the stink on your clothes" was a major challenge to the investigators.

A Detective Senior Sergeant had an early career experience involving smells of another kind. He described the first "standout" trauma that occurred while still a cadet that involved an isolated, mentally ill woman. He and his partner broke into her house through a back door that had been barricaded with ten-gallon drums full of human excreta. They searched the house which was full of empty food tins, finding it hard to describe the stench! The woman jumped up in his face, wearing a Nazi helmet and soiling herself as she did so. This he said, "Was confronting experience for a seventeen year old boy. I can still smell it!" This may well be an example of how resilience in such situations is built. This cadet probably measured many of his more confronting taskings against this one; as his career progressed, he was confident that they offered a lesser challenge to his well-being.

A Detective Senior Constable, after a career-long exposure to homicide crime scenes, made a distinction between traumatic images and the smells, thus, "the death and injury images don't bother me, the smell is worse, I try not to link the smell to a crime scene". Trying not to make such a link in terms of controlling memories is at the centre of this comment. The smells involved clearly make such control more difficult. A Senior Constable agreed when asked about the trauma of death and bodies remained with her and commented, "Not for me, you develop a strange sense of humour…when a person is dead on the ground I can separate myself from them. It's easier if it doesn't look like a person…the smell is always difficult". This is a clear expression of this officer's ability to create distance between herself and such experiences and move on. This is resilience, learned and practised. A Senior Sergeant added, "It's the smell rather than the things you see that sticks with you". A retired Superintendent made a distinction between physical and emotional stressors, "bodies, death smells are the physical side. Emotional is the organizational side".

4.9 Death and Bodies: Conclusions

All of the officers interviewed for my research referred to their experience of death, bodies, smell and the delivery of death messages to the relatives of those killed in out of the ordinary circumstances. Death is a part of policing, and it populates the duty-related experience of every officer in a variety of forms from the routine attendance to a home where an elderly person has died, to grotesque mutilation caused by accident or human intent. All long-serving officers learn to accept the centrality of death and dying to their duties and develop strategies that distance them from emotional responses to the death scenes they encounter. This is always learned on "the job", as more experienced officers and supervisors pass on strategies that are effective in creating and maintaining a distance that ensures operational competence and avoids long-term impacts. Some officers, early in their careers, were subject to patrol duties that involved multiple experiences with dead bodies on most shifts and attributed such "flooding" to their capacity to cope well as a result. This was a "make or break" management strategy that clearly contributed to individual officers continuing in or leaving policing.

Some death scenes stood out and were clearly recalled by those interviewed. The deaths of children, of those known by the officers involved often in rural areas, grotesque injury, extreme violence, or long-term decay were all described in detail by many who were interviewed. They took pride in doing their duty with regard to the dead, realising that as police officers they made a unique societal contribution in such circumstances. Many of their most challenging recollections related to early career experiences, indicating clearly the importance of learning to cope. Some recalled short-term traumatic responses to particularly demanding events, where all was well after a few days of contemplation. Humour was often identified as an effective coping strategy, usually shared with colleagues.

Female officers felt more able to express emotional reactions to out of the ordinary death scenes than their male colleagues and more ready to seek support from each other and from outside of "the job" when needed. It is clear that most viewed their contact with death as an inevitable consequence of their duties and had come to terms with their capacity to deal with it. When such experiences were "out of the ordinary" by policing standards (Janoff-Bulman, 1989) they had no reservations about seeking support and the opportunity to debrief usually from colleagues within and resources such as social workers and family members from without the organisation.

The issue of suicide within SAPOL was often mentioned usually in the context of a lack of organisational response when officers killed themselves. Most officers interviewed thought suicide rates in SAPOL were high and expressed concerns that were based on their confusion and uncertainty when a colleague completed the act. SAPOL policy of "non-intervention", despite advice to the contrary from clinicians within the organisation undoubtedly contributes to such concerns from those at the front line.

4.9.1 Where to from Here?

A recent front-page article in the *Adelaide Advertiser* (Kemp, 2017) entitled "Fight for our force: The black cloud that hangs over police" outlined the stressful nature of policing, describing the emotional challenges faced by South Australian police officers, including "Violent confrontations with the public, delivering news of death and dealing with domestic and child abuse" (p. 1). These were described in an accompanying editorial as "a potent cocktail of emotion laden incidents that require significant resilience to manage" (p. 56) in the context of the release of a self-help booklet by the police union, with the support of SAPOL management and the South Australian Government (Carroll, 2017). This is a step in the right direction, clearly recognising the emotional challenges posed by constant duty-related contact with among other things, death. Although almost all of those officers interviewed for this research had developed effective coping strategies in this area, public attention to such challenges and their long-term well-being is important in terms of organisational responses from their management cohort. This is especially so in terms of the provision of support services for out of the ordinary duty-related experiences of officers who need timely support and encouragement. I will refer to this again as I make recommendations for change in my final chapter.

This chapter has featured the voices of the police officers interviewed describing how they have coped with many forms of death encounters as they have carried out their duties. For most, this was the first time they had told their story, although all had reflected on the development of the skills and insights that had built their resilience. This research has demonstrated clearly the value of detailed interviews and how they contribute to the literature of policing. The importance of police culture, learning from experience on "the job" with input from more experienced officers rather than during academy training, was highlighted as was pride and satisfaction that came from becoming proficient and professional in the context of such challenges. Many of those interviewed saw challenges to their mental health in issues other than those related to their duties. For most of them, it is "SAPOL" that causes them stress far beyond that of death encounters. Management approaches based solely on risk and "command and control" and a culture of bullying and harassment from above were the ingredients offering most challenges to their well-being. This was particularly true for the female officers interviewed.

References

Amaranto, E., et al. (2003). Police stress interventions. *Brief Treatment and Crisis Intervention, 3*(1), 47.

American Psychiatric Association. (2013). *Diagnostic and statistical manual of mental disorders (DSM-5®)*. American Psychiatric Pub.

Lawrence, D., Kyron, M., Rikkers, W., Bartlett, J., Hafekost, K., Goodsell, B., Cunneen, R. (2018). *Answering the call: National survey of the mental health and well being of police and emergency services*. Detailed report. Perth: Graduate School of Education, The University of Western Australia.

Blum, L. E., & Blum, L. N. (2000). *Force under pressure: How cops live and why they die*. Lantern Books.

Burke, R. J., & Mikkelsen, A. (2005). Gender issues in policing: Do they matter? *Women in Management Review, 20*(2), 133–143.

Burke, R. J. (2016). *Stress in policing: Sources*. Routledge.

Burns, C. M., et al. (2008). The emotional impact on and coping strategies employed by police teams investigating internet child exploitation. *Traumatology, 14*(2), 20.

Chae, M. H., & Boyle, D. J. (2013). Police suicide: Prevalence, risk, and protective factors. *Policing: An International Journal of Police Strategies & Management, 36*(1), 91–118.

Chopko, B. A., et al. (2014). Prevalence and predictors of suicidal ideation among US law enforcement officers. *Journal of Police and Criminal Psychology, 29*(1), 1–9.

Cantor, C. H., et al. (1995). A historical survey of police suicide in Queensland, Australia, 1843–1992. *Suicide and Life-Threatening Behaviour, 25*(4), 499–507.

Carlier, I. V., et al. (1998). Disaster-related post-traumatic stress in police officers: A field study of the impact of debriefing. *Stress and Health, 14*(3), 143–148.

Cotton, P. (2016). Victoria Police Mental Health Review. An independent review into the mental health and well-being of Victoria Police employees. Australia.

Curran, S. (2003). Separating fact from fiction about police stress. *Behavioural Health Management, 23*(1), 38–38.

Dollard, M., et al. (2003). *Occupational stress in the service professions*. CRC Press.

Donnelly, E., et al. (2015). Law enforcement officers and employee assistance programs. *Policing: An International Journal of Police Strategies & Management, 38*(2), 206–220.

Elntib, S., & Armstrong, T. (2014). Critical incidents' impact on front-line South African police personnel in light of the current briefing and debriefing strategies. *South African Journal of Psychology, 44*(4), 416–425.

Faust, K. L., & Ven, T. V. (2014). Policing disaster: An analytical review of the literature on policing, disaster, and post-traumatic stress disorder. *Sociology Compass, 8*(6), 614–626.

Flannery, R. B. (2015). Treating psychological trauma in first responders: A multi-modal paradigm. *Psychiatric Quarterly, 86*(2), 261–267.

Gilmartin, K. M. (2002). Emotional survival for law enforcement. *ES Press, PMB, 233*, 2968.

Green, B. (2004). Post-traumatic stress disorder in UK police officers. *Current Medical Research and Opinion, 20*(1), 101–105.

Henry, V. E. (2004). *Death work: Police, trauma, and the psychology of survival*. Oxford University Press.

Horner, P. (2011). *Jack knife: The crashing of a policeman*. New South Wales, Australia, Zeus Publications.

Huddleston, L. M., et al. (2006). Conceptualizing traumatic stress in police officers: Pre-employment, critical incident, and organizational influences. *Traumatology, 12*(3), 170–177.

Kates, A. (2008). *Copshock: Surviving Post Traumatic Stress Disorder (PTSD)*. Holbrook Street Press.

Kirschman, E., et al. (2015). *Counselling cops: What clinicians need to know*. Guilford Publications.

Kitaeff, J. (2011). *Handbook of police psychology*. Routledge.

Kroes, W. H. (1976). *Society's victim, the policeman: An analysis of job stress in policing*. Thomas Springfield.
Marin, A. (2012). In the line of Duty. Ombudsman's report. Ontario, Canada.
Marshall, D. (2006). *Killing for pleasure: The definitive story of the snowtown serial murders*. Random House.
Marzuk, P. M., et al. (2002). Suicide among New York city police officers, 1977–1996. *American Journal of Psychiatry, 159*(12), 2069–2071.
McFarlane, A. C. (2011). *Many paths, one purpose. Expert forum*. Australian Centre for posttraumatic mental health.
Mckay, E. (2005). *Crime scene-true stories from the life of a crime scene investigator.* Viking (Penguin) Australia.
Ménard, K. S., & Arter, M. L. (2013). Police officer alcohol use and trauma symptoms: Associations with critical incidents, coping, and social stressors. *International Journal of Stress Management, 20*(1), 37.
Moss, I. (1999). Officers under stress: A special report for Parliament under section 31 of the Ombudsman's Act. New South Wales, Australia.
Neil, B. (2014). *Under siege*. Harlequin Mira.
Nievas, V. (2015). Posttraumatic stress Disorder and Police Officers. *Australian Police Journal*, 69(4).
O'Hara, A. F., & Violanti, J. M. (2008). Police suicide, a Web surveillance of national data. *International Journal of Emergency Mental Health, 11*(1), 17–23.
Paton, D. (2009). *Traumatic stress in police officers: A career-length assessment from recruitment to retirement*. Charles C Thomas Publisher.
Pietrzak, R., et al. (2014). Dimensional structure and course of post-traumatic stress symptomatology in World Trade Center responders. *Psychological Medicine, 44*(10), 2085–2098.
Peters, R. F. (2009). *Police under pressure (A donkey on the edge)*. HEAS Publications.
Pole, N., et al. (2006). Resilience in retired police officers. *Traumatology, 12*(3), 207–216.
Rees, B., & Smith, J. (2008). Breaking the silence: The traumatic circle of policing. *International Journal of Police Science & Management, 10*(3), 267–279.
Schaffer, B. (2014). *Way of the warrior*. Self- published.
Silverii, L. S. (2014). *Cop culture: Why good cops go bad*. CRC Press.
Schiraldi, G. R. (2011). *The complete guide to resilience: Why it matters how to build it and maintain it*. Resilience Training International.
Seligman, M. E. P. (2012). *Flourish: A visionary new understanding of happiness and well-being*. Simon and Schuster.
Sparkes, A. (2013). *The cost of bravery*. New South Wales, Australia: Penguin Group, Australia.
Stone, V. (1999). *Cops don't cry: A book of help and hope for police families*. Creative Bound.
Sutton, S. R. (2005). *True blue: Police stories by those who have lived them*. Macmillan.
Tedeschi, R. G., & Calhoun, L. G. (1995). *Trauma and transformation: Growing in the aftermath of suffering*. Sage Publications.
Toch, H. (2002). Stress in policing. *American Psychological Association Journal*.
Verity, W. (2014). Our shameful silence on police Suicide. The Drum, Australian Broadcasting Corporation: 20 minutes.
Violanti, J. M. (2014). *Dying for the job: Police work exposure and health*. Charles C Thomas Publisher.
Violanti, J. M., & Paton, D. (2006). *Who gets PTSD?: Issues of Posttraumatic Stress vulnerability*. Charles C Thomas.
Yuan, C., et al. (2011). Protective factors for posttraumatic stress disorder symptoms in a prospective study of police officers. *Pshychiatry ResearCh, 188*(1), 45–50.

Chapter 5
Keeping Well. Coping

Abstract Police organisations across the globe have not been well known for offering any form of resilience training to officers at the beginning or during their careers. Most officers have therefore relied on natural coping skills and a culture of toughness in the face of the challenges of the job. Police operational culture has reinforced such an approach but change is in the wind. Some officers become emotionally "numb" when on duty; this often transferring into their private lives with devastating consequences. This chapter examines how the traditional use of alcohol as a coping mechanism by police officers is changing, how humour promotes resilience, how some officers rely on life partners to debrief and how others never take their work home. Critical incident debriefing, the so-called Mitchell model, has been the focus of much debate in recent years among the helping professions. The arguments are described in this chapter as well as the impact the absence of debriefs has on police officers challenged by events that are out of the ordinary for them. The interviews add much detail around how officers stay well in a "command and control" management environment described by one psychiatrist as "toxic".

A central theme emerging from the 50 interviews with SAPOL officers highlighted strategies they used to cope and keep well in the context of operational policing. Resilience and wellness are closely associated in practical terms. Resilience is the capacity to recover between challenging duty-related events and wellness is the continuing benefit of being able to do so as officers reap the ongoing benefits of self-care. Coping is the long-term outcome of resilience and wellness (Donnelly, 2015; Pole et al., 2006; Stinchcomb, 2008). Those who responded to the invitation to be involved in my interviews expressed a variety of motivations for doing so, which ranged from their experiences in the job that pointed to the need for changes in management and operational practices, as well as an awareness of the personal costs and benefits of their career choice in the long term. The information sheet provided to participants prior to the interview and the advertisement placed in the *SA Police Journal*[1] seeking their participation stated:

[1] See Appendix A.

A. Paterson, *Trauma and Resilience in Contemporary Australian Policing*,
https://doi.org/10.1007/978-981-16-4416-0_5

Andrew is researching how exposure to the trauma encountered in the day to day events of policing is handled by members and the organisation and how members might stay healthy on the job.

Without exception, the officers arrived at the interview having given much thought to these research aims. Across a very broad range of experience and challenging duty-related incidents, they described their coping strategies, often in the context of an awareness that their organisation (SAPOL)[2] had little to offer them in this regard, apart from annual reviews which in theory are undertaken by officers working in key areas, and SAPOL's Employee Assistance Programme which many viewed with deep suspicion.

The literature around operational policing and stress is often more negative in its focus (Amaranto et al., 2003; Barron, 2010; Blum & Blum, 2000; Henry, 2004; Kates, 2008; Kroes, 1976; Violanti, 2014). Little attention is given to the more personal aspects of coping mechanisms developed by police officers to stay well. Flannery (2015) describes a "limited awareness" of self-care strategies among "first responders" that was not evident in those interviewed in this study. Some officers I interviewed, who were aware that their resilience was wearing thin, applied for transfers out of more stressful roles into less challenging ones, while some embraced comprehensive change to their eating habits and exercise regimes. Many officers revealed during an interview that they maintained a clear demarcation between duty and family by arriving at work in civilian clothes, then changing into uniform before commencing their duties. At shift's end, they reversed the process, often showering before their homeward journey. Another aspect of the same approach to keeping well was the effort many undertook to maintain friendships outside of the "job" as well as having community engagement with schools, sporting clubs and many other non-policing activities. Such strategies are not mentioned in the literature addressing "protective factors" apart from more general references to "isolation" (Ménard & Arter, 2013) although Chae and Boyle (2013:105) refer to the importance of "friendship networks in the community".

The ability to deal with exposure to trauma by compartmentalising it was referred to by many of those interviewed who reported that they are able to "maintain a clinical distance and not buy into it". Other references to "forcing oneself to be detached" do reflect the literature (Chapin et al., 2008; Henry, 2004). A focus on the importance and significance of the outcomes of police work is also important to individual wellness (Burns et al., 2008; Shane, 2010; Stephens & Pugmire, 2008). A good result where no one is hurt and justice is done creates and maintains satisfaction and well-being, particularly when it is accompanied by positive feedback from a senior officer.

The lack of attention in SAPOL to training in areas related to maintaining "wellness" and building resilience was often referred to by those interviewed. This is also a frequent theme from the literature with reference to the possibility of building resilience in first responders through training and development programmes (Bannink, 2014; Burke, 2016; Cornum, 1993; Honig & Sultan, 2006; Neocleous,

[2] See Chapter 2: "Power, organisational and police culture:'the job'".

2012; Pole et al., 2006; Schiraldi, 2011; Seligman, 2012; Shochet et al., 2011; Violanti & Paton, 2006; Yuan et al., 2011).

5.1 Not Dwelling on Things: A Way of Coping. The Informing Literature

Many of the officers interviewed commented on how they avoided "dwelling on things" when talking about the coping strategies they employed to stay well. Most were well aware that the continual revisiting and thinking about stressful and challenging events, whether they be operational or management related, was not beneficial. It was always better, according to one of those interviewed, "to move on and put things behind me". There appears to be a common-sense and learned understanding of effective responses to stressful experiences among officers, which may have its source in Academy training programmes, or more likely a part of the generational knowledge passed down from more experienced officers, or the result of personal research done by officers into coping strategies as their careers progress.

Gilmartin (2002) warns against officers worrying about or dwelling on aspects of their duties over which they have no control. Using an example of a fictional newly appointed Commissioner, who has an obsession with officers wearing uniform hats when on duty, Gilmartin asks the question, "What will you do in response to such a hat-related general order?" The immediate response from the police audience was: "I will wear my hat!" This is, according to Gilmartin, a healthy coping response that should be applied to more operational aspects of policing as well.

Post-traumatic growth theorists and researchers (Berger & Weiss, 2009; Harms, 2015; Jackson, 2007; Tedeschi & Calhoun 2006; Shakespeare-Finch et al., 2013) warn against avoidance mechanisms such as excess alcohol and drug use among police officers who have been regularly confronted by traumatic experiences. They instead see "rumination" or "cognitive emotional processing" (Tedeschi & Calhoun, 2006) as the process of "the construction of a narrative that bridges the "before and after" and that culminates in Posttraumatic Growth" (Berger & Weiss, 2009). By not dwelling on things, the officers I interviewed meant that once the process of "meaning making" (Jackson, 2013) was over they felt free to move on in their personal and professional lives. This aligns with Tedeschi and Calhoun's (2006:230) concept of "the meaning of work" as a factor in increasing the possibility of duty-related post-traumatic growth rather than PTSD. Many of the officers interviewed for this research found great meaning in what they did despite constant exposure to dysfunction, violence, death and their experience of the 90/10 rule in policing.[3]

Some researchers identify traits such as perfectionism as risk factors, (Gilmartin, 2002; Kirschman et al., 2015) advising officers and those offering them support to counsel against levels of perfectionism that mitigate against "moving on". This is

[3] See ..., Plantinga, (2014: 183).

well represented in the data from the interviews below, where officers aware of that tendency take action to counteract its negative impact.

The actual mechanisms used by officers to avoid dwelling on things and to encourage "moving on" are difficult to define. Very few of those interviewed attempted to do so. If PTSD is "a disease of time which permits past memory to relive itself in the present" (Young, 1997:7), and if remaining healthy involves a capacity to retain such memories in their appropriate place in time (the past) then officers who can repeatedly achieve such control may well thrive and consistently avoid the emotional hazards of their chosen career. Pole et al. (2006), researching retired police officers, concluded that "passive coping" which includes responses such as those quoted above, "I didn't let it get to me" and "I refused to let myself think about it" is an ineffective coping mechanism and links it to other negative coping strategies such as the abuse of alcohol, drugs, food, smoking and medication. Stone (1999:50) in addressing the same issue, quotes an officer, "I make it a rule not to let the ghosts haunt me. Sometimes they try. When they turn up, I pat them on the shoulder and show them the door. My concern is for the living". The literature and the officers interviewed agree that the capacity to deal with repeated trauma-related experiences is a combination of learning and experience. Police officers are drawn into their profession by a desire to help and protect citizens as well as the anticipated enjoyment of the unpredictability and immediate relevance and importance of "the job". This ability is complex and involves the capacity to locate challenging events in their time and place and move on.

5.2 Not Dwelling on Things: The Data from the Interviews

The mechanisms that officers use to cope are clear when explained in terms of their experience, and were taken for granted by them once they have achieved the capacity to consistently apply them and then incorporated into their professional and personal routines. Those officers who participated in this study did so for various reasons. Some because they had an intense, personal interest in resilience and coping and some because they felt that SAPOL (the organisation) should and could do more to support and foster the development of coping skills among its members. Others saw external research as an opportunity for a conversation that could lead to changes in the conditions and challenges of policing away from the traditional "we weren't supposed to show weakness or emotion" to a different approach to the job where it could be acceptable to express emotion and deal with it openly without being judged as weak.

A significant number of police officers interviewed revealed they had developed strategies that enabled them to avoid dwelling on challenging experiences such as grotesque death scenes, violence and issues that might threaten longer-term coping. Often they recounted the importance of having "outside" interests and activities that allowed them to refocus after duty-related experiences that required processing. Some researchers might classify such responses as "avoidance" (Carlier et al., 1998;

Evans & Coccoma, 2014). The interviewees who touched on this theme had a more positive view.

A Senior Constable of over 30 years' experience in "the job" saw her capacity for resilience to stem from several sources, "I have always been able to handle stress, I didn't dwell on the past". "Not dwelling on things" was often mentioned by those interviewed, and clearly involved developing the ability to move on after challenging incidents, to intentionally stop thinking about what might have been, in the case of taskings that didn't turn out well and to dismiss images of crime and accident scenes that threaten to linger. This officer continued, "When I came across challenges like dead children, I didn't let it affect me. Helping others helps me. I enjoy my life, friends and family. I have served on school committees throughout my children's education. I have friends outside of SAPOL and played lots of sport". This comment reveals a skill developed around resisting the impact of in this case "dead children" particularly threatening to an officer who is also a parent. Friends, family and outside interests add to and develop such a coping skill.

A Detective Sergeant, a veteran of years of homicide investigations, spoke of the effort involved in dealing with challenging emotions: "You can't let your emotions get in the way, for example, repressed rage. You need to have outlets so that things don't dwell on your mind". Outlets are here seen as defence mechanisms, not against intrusive trauma-related thoughts, but against intense anger generated in the face of bad things happening to those who don't deserve such a fate.

Those "outlets" can also be within the police profession, as was well expressed by a Sergeant who pioneered domestic violence awareness training for police Sergeants in the 1980s, "Prosecutions and DV work were my obsession…trying to get coppers to understand that DV can't be ignored". Her efforts succeeded as along with female colleagues of similar rank she was able to change domestic violence policy and practice within SAPOL. She saw such success as a major contributor to her capacity to cope. A strong sense of achievement, particularly in terms of cultural change within SAPOL, contributing to her coping with other job-related challenges.

A retired Detective Senior Sergeant described how an interest in and a commitment to outcomes from complex investigations of homicides provided such satisfaction: "It was always interesting work which was challenging, frustrating, rewarding, emotional, and traumatic. You pretty well were working with someone's grief every day. We weren't supposed to show weakness or emotion, we grew up in a different era". The major focus here is not on the confronting aspects of the crime scene itself but on the need for investigators to deal with other factors such as the emotional outpourings and experiences of secondary victims. This is a profound commentary on an era in policing where there was a clear albeit unspoken, expectation that officers would cope and where emotional responses were seen as weakness particularly among those on the extreme sharp end of policing.

A retired Detective Chief Inspector said, in response to my question, "Have there been any costs to you as a result of your career?" "There have been difficult periods in my career. I'm a bit of a perfectionist. You need to dust yourself off and move on. I have sometimes dwelt on things for too long…did I make the right decision?" This reveals both an often used coping mechanism ("moving on") as well as a high level of self-awareness around a character trait often associated with the development of problematic trauma-related responses and referred to above (Gilmartin, 2002; Kirschman et al., 2015). A retired Detective Senior Sergeant revealed a similar level of self-awareness, "I have a personality type that makes me vulnerable. I am an obsessive worrier with massive attention to detail. A perfectionist!" This level of self-awareness contributed to both these officers ability to cope with their duties. Their recognition of such a trait and its potential negative impact on their well-being was recognised and taken into account and dealt with as a part of their coping.

Healthy processing of out of the ordinary traumatic experiences was also evident in many responses to my questions around coping mechanisms employed by officers, "I have had periods when it's been difficult due to the impact of situations that stick in your head for a while. I had a serious motor vehicle accident in police car. You think about them a lot for a week or so, then less the following week and so on…". Here the Detective Senior Sergeant is referring to a "normal" reaction to extreme trauma exposure, defined in DSM 5 as "Acute Stress Disorder" (Association, 2013:275) which, as he describes, experience diminishing in severity over a period from three days to one month after such a traumatic event. Even the most confronting death-related experiences in the line of duty were dealt with in a similar way. A retired Senior Sergeant described her coping mechanism in this way, "Challenges included delivering death messages, taking bodies to the mortuary, I remember the most awful one where a motorcyclist who had been incinerated. We had to weigh him and try to remove his leathers that were stuck to his body and take his helmet off. It doesn't sit with me though. Life's too short to let that happen". The research focus on the perils of PTSD among police rarely focusses on this phenomenon, the learned capacity to move on after out of the ordinary experiences.

Growing in resilience through such experiences was the key to meeting such challenges, and that was well expressed by a Senior Sergeant after 30 years of service, "I saw horrible things that happened to victims. It helped me grow and develop defence mechanisms and resilience". He added, "Suck it up, and move on!" This is a clear rebuttal to those who warn of the inevitable consequences of prolonged trauma exposure. This is growth, not disorder. Further evidence of such insights came from two other officers of similar mind. Referring to traumatic memory fading with time, another officer added, "You think about them a lot for a week or so, then less the following week and so on…" and "You process all this over time".

A STAR group recovery diver, regularly exposed to traumatic events through his duties, saw his genes and upbringing as the key to his resilience and optimism, "I don't dwell on things. My parents are low stress people. My brother (a police officer) always sounds cool and calm headed on the police radio when things are going to shit and I'm the same I think". Such predispositions are referred to in the literature around resilience. Yuan et al (2011) include personality and temperament in their list of protective factors as do Bourke et al. (2006). A Major Crime Detective confirmed the learning process referred to here by his colleague, as well as one of the sources of such skills, "As far as trauma goes I have compartmentalised it, maintained a clinical distance… you don't buy into it…I probably taught myself to do that, I have always had other interests outside the job". He added, "There were some real legends in

Major Crime who were usually good at giving advice on how they coped". Intergenerational skills of coping are the focus here. Despite a culture of keeping a "stiff upper lip" and "toughing it out", there was room for experienced officers to have such conversations with younger members around the realities of policing and effective coping strategies.

Coping sometimes involved the realisation that it was time to move on and to seek a different field of activity within policing. One retired Major Crime Detective said, "After five years in Major Crime, I had had enough. I learnt people were being killed for ridiculous reasons! I went into crime prevention to try to stop that, I enjoyed the preventative side, I had a different attitude from then on". Whether this officer received advice to this effect or he arrived at his decision alone was not revealed, but this is very clearly a decision to take advantage of the breadth of roles available in SAPOL to aid longevity in "the job" and long-term coping.

Sometimes on duty experiences become unexpectedly personal. At such times, officers must perform their duties without the "shield" of emotional distance to protect them. I asked a long-retired Senior Sergeant, "Were you ever close to the edge?" He responded: "Sometimes I had this hard feeling. I attended a motor vehicle accident where two young kids were killed. Someone said there's supposed to be a baby here. We found the baby dead, wedged up under the dash…I had a five year old at that stage". The "hard feeling" here described did not linger and allowed this officer to continue his long and fulfilling career.

Coping strategies included creating a clear demarcation between work and private life, developing the ability to move on after confronting incidents, not dwelling on things, having friends and interests outside of SAPOL, playing sport and keeping fit through limiting alcohol intake and eating healthily. After confronting, out of the ordinary events, some officers observed that it took a short while for them to move on and locate the trauma in their past experience. The process of not dwelling on things is therefore part natural, as other taskings and outside of policing activities distract the officer, and part practised as the officers use effective patterns of thought that shift her/his attention from the event to other, more pleasant ruminations. "Not dwelling on things" is, therefore, a skill, a learned response to events that creep under the "shield" of even those officers who are vastly experienced. This, according to those interviewed, is not avoidance as in the use and abuse of alcohol or other risky activities, but a pro-active practised routine and more like Tedeschi and Calhoun's (2006) "cognitive processing".

5.3 Alcohol and Coping. The Informing Literature

Much of the research literature into policing has a focus on the perils of self-medication and, in particular, the part played by alcohol consumption as a means of debriefing and dealing with the stresses of the job. Pole et al. (2006) refer to excessive alcohol use by officers as "escape /avoidance coping", which in the long term, they unsurprisingly conclude, is an ineffective strategy. Burke (2017) agrees, describing alcohol abuse as "maladaptive coping" in the context of anger outbursts, emotional over-eating and driving dangerously as similarly ineffective strategies. Chae and Boyle (2013:116), addressing issues around police suicide in terms of prevention and risk management, argue that police culture "encourages drinking as a means of stress relief" and also identified an outcome which is reflected in my interviews, that older, more experienced officers in their research cohort, were less stressed and consumed less alcohol than their younger colleagues. A number of officers I interviewed revealed how alcohol had been a significant problem for them when they used it to self-medicate in destructive and career-threatening ways. This was often in response to self-diagnosed depression in the context of what one described as "a self-medicating culture covered up by a social culture". Others recounted how in the 1980s officers, after finishing a seven straight night shift roster, would gather at the Police Club in the centre of Adelaide to drink to excess, often being taken home the next morning by colleagues who had replaced them on the same roster. These gatherings were referred to as "barbecues" or in the police jargon of that time, "choir practice".

Associating, as one retired Detective Senior Sergeant puts it, with "very social police" became a major problem for many officers with the introduction of the highly controversial drink-driving legislation and more specifically, Random Breath Testing in South Australia in October 1981 (Homel, 1989). As the enforcers of such legislation and as the initially negative community reaction to RBT changed, some police officers had no choice but to abandon their drinking practices, or to transfer them on a much smaller social scale to other settings such as their private homes.

The five police autobiographies (Henry, 2004; Horner, 2011; Mckay, 2005, 2010; Rogers, 1999; Sparkes, 2013) reveal a consistent theme of alcohol dependence and abuse in that group prior to their PTSD diagnosis. All described a gradual increase in their alcohol consumption, usually in private, which became less and less effective in terms of repressing their unrecognised symptoms which included significant bouts of depression, outbursts of anger, nightmares and various forms of avoidance. All five accounts focus on the highly encultured emphasis on alcohol use and abuse within police organisations at the time these officers served.

Schiraldi (2016) argues in the context of creating and maintaining resilience in policing that alcohol abuse is a significant threat to a healthy approach to a policing career as does Henry (2004) in the Epilogue to his "Death Work". Garner (2008) reinforces this in his advice to police Sergeants to be vigilant about "signs of being under the influence" among team members as they report for duty.

5.4 Alcohol (A Coping Mechanism) Data from the Interviews

The officers interviewed for this research were very aware of the changes that have occurred in the drinking culture within SAPOL over the last 25 or so years. These, to a significant extent, have been brought about by changes in the South Australian Road Traffic Act (Homel, 1989) with regards to blood alcohol content and driving and also what appears to be a growing realisation, particularly amongst younger police, that alcohol use and abuse is an ineffective way to cope with the stresses of policing.

One officer of 30 years experience said of the history of alcohol use in SAPOL, “I had three sudden infant death syndromes to attend on one shift at one point. We use to go to the Police Club after night shift and drink too much. We used to work seven night shifts straight and then have a barbie. This was in those days a good way of debriefing. It’s not possible now”. Another commented, “male cops in particular dealt with stress by drinking and partying. If you didn’t drink you were an outsider”. Another related that “some colleagues stayed at the police club for twenty four hours after night shift ended. The night shift that had just started would take them home for the next morning”. Debriefing with the aid of alcohol, telling “war stories” in an atmosphere of non-judgemental acceptance over whatever period of time it took may well have been an effective, albeit short-term coping mechanism for the police of those days. In the longer term, the health benefits were less obvious, impact on family life pronounced and career threats through the possibility of drink driving charges brought an end to the public aspect of this cultural activity.

In confirming this set of behaviours, a recently retired Detective Sergeant continued this theme,

> I was a really heavy drinker at that time, I associated with very social police. There was a lot of drink driving. Piss is very destructive, bad behaviour, violence and adultery is the result. Nobody told me to stop being angry. Half of every working group went to the pub. Alcohol was effective self medication. When random breath testing came in and the blood alcohol legislation that was the end of the drinking culture. The whole culture was gone. We used to stand around telling war stories for hours.

Such activities were not confined to male “social” police. A female officer of many years of experience commented, “I saw many shitty things, we used to drink, kill brain cells, write yourself off, go to work the next day and start again”. Another continued the negative focus on the earlier days of policing, “The major coping mechanism was to go to the Police Club with people who understood. Some colleagues were alcoholics, who used alcohol to shut it all out”. There is, however, clear evidence from the interviews that there have been significant changes to this level of alcohol use. A Detective Sergeant commented, “We have a team of eight detectives, we try to look after ourselves, alcohol doesn’t work”. Here it is clear that this team has a clear view of the impact of alcohol abuse on well-being, as well as a collegial approach to staying well and coping without reliance on alcohol as a coping strategy. A young Senior Constable encountered problems around alcohol consumption and had to take action to change his situation, “My main issue has been that around alcohol. I was depressed and self medicating with alcohol. I am now off the drink”.

Another officer, acknowledging his history of alcohol abuse, approached SAPOL for assistance, “I went to a GP re my alcohol issues and then I contacted the Employee Assistance Program of SAPOL eighteen months ago. My partner convinced me to go to management. I am a highly functioning alcoholic". He went on in a less positive but insightful mode, "Policing is still a self medicating culture covered up by a social culture. We now have quiet beers now in people's houses". This answers the question asked around what replaced the 1980s "choir practice and barbies behind the police club". In support of this comment, alcohol was mentioned as an issue by only two of the clinicians interviewed. In reference to the impact of drink driving legislation enacted in South Australia in the 1980s, one said, "SAPOL's historic drinking culture now happens in their homes". Another added, "People drink to deal with their symptoms. In some ways that helps, although often not in the long-term".

A Detective Sergeant, commenting on the complexities of modifying the historic drinking culture, said, "We were supposed to be tougher and stronger, we coped by having a drink. It was the culture of the time and we were all in the same boat and knew what each other was experiencing". She went on, "I am aware that policing exposes me to things that I normally would not be exposed to. Drinking is not helpful, exercise is helpful but not always practical". One of the issues addressed throughout this research connects strongly with what is being said here. If exercise is "helpful, but not always practical", what more could SAPOL do for its officers to encourage exercise in the context of shift work and the rigours of police work? As well, this officer shows a profound understanding of the impact of her chosen career and the difficulties encountered in the process of coping as well as a clear awareness of historic strategies that were and are ineffective.

On a more positive note, an officer who began his career with the London Metropolitan Police commented, "My response to traumatic incidents in London was to get pissed and smoke. SAPOL is much less of a drinking culture, in London, pubs were close to public transport". This could well constitute evidence that the comments of the officers above concerning the change in SAPOL's drinking culture may well be accurate and that change may have more to it than simply access to public transport to avoid drink driving offences.

A younger officer commented with regard to alcohol, "I don't drink much alcohol, it's not the best way to go about it. There is not a positive relationship between alcohol and coping with the job. Although I'm all for a beer at the end of the day", where such an insight originated in this officer's career was not made clear. It is, however, a direct indicator of a process of change in attitude to the historic and traditional self-medicating police culture where such attitudes can be expressed without negative responses from divergently minded, more traditional colleagues. As if in support of such an insight, a long-retired Detective Sergeant was more positive commenting, "Throughout my career I had no alcohol issues, I hardly ever drank, I never smoked".

5.5 Humour. A Cultural Way of Coping. The Informing Literature

Many officers interviewed made reference to the common use of dark or gallows humour to relieve tension and to express their discomfort in acceptable ways in situations that were extremely challenging. Pogrebin (1988:183/184) argues that through humour officers share common experiences, which in the context of "not putting your hand up" after confronting taskings can allow the expression of emotion with little risk of criticism. Humour promotes cultural solidarity, says Pogrebin, generating "feelings of implicit understanding and camaraderie", as well as a coping strategy in the face of negative operational outcomes. This was well evidenced in the interviews as officers talked directly of humour that aided their coping strategies.

Garrick and Williams (2006:169) identify humour as a factor in coping responses to challenging events, describing it in the police context as a "powerful healing tool", going on to point out that such humour is common in policing. Widera-Wysoczanska (2016), arguing that in terms of developing and maintaining resilience in the face of challenge, agrees a sense of humour is a positive asset. Rowe and Regehr (2010) describe dark humour as giving vent to feelings, drawing social support from colleagues and creating emotional distance from confronting situations such as those encountered in operational policing. Such humour, they argue, ensures effective function during and after such events. They also point out humour has a role in reinforcing group cohesion and a sense always present in policing of difference and distance from the general public. Kuhlman (1988) describes laughter as having a cathartic function and Kuiper (2012) argues that humour also indicates and cultivates positive, resilient responses to traumatic experiences.

From this research and the data below, we can conclude that officer's use of humour in unusually confronting situations is part of the cultural glue that holds police officers together and that they utilise such humour as a traditional means of coping passed down through policing generations.

5.6 Humour: The Data from the Interviews

One veteran officer was very clear about a direct link between humour and resilience, "We relied on humour good or black. You learn not to take things too seriously and each time you do that you build resilience. There is a hell of a lot of trauma there in my career. Black humour is a part of it". Again there is evidence here of learning to cope, in this case by creating distance from other's trauma by seeking out factors that offer alternatives to being emotionally drawn in. This officer continued with some reservation, "I have been guilty of it myself". Other officers were more forthright, "Humour is helpful, taking the piss, and black humour is a marvellous medicine", said a retired Senior Constable. This refers to an aspect of camaraderie, "taking the piss" where officers communicate with each other in the context of serious situations without actually being serious.

A Senior Sergeant retired from the force for some years gave a specific example of black humour at a scene of suicide, "Black humour helped. We found a guy who had set up a rifle in a shed, shot himself over a pool table. All the blood went into one pocket". Many officers when interviewed revealed that attending such death scenes was usually challenging. Here the team (in private) perceived the scene on their terms as they deal with it.

When asked, "Has exposure to death been a problem for you?" one Senior Constable replied, "Not for me. You develop a strange sense of humour. When a person is dead on the ground I can separate myself from them, it's easier if it doesn't look like a person". This "strange sense of humour" is well illustrated by an officer who commented, "You sometimes lose the ability to laugh" and used as an example a situation in which he and a colleague had attended a suicide by hanging. The body was swinging in the breeze from a tree that lent out over a reservoir South of Adelaide. The officer and his colleague sat eating fish and chips while waiting for colleagues to arrive to help retrieve the body. His comment describing that time was, "it was peaceful". The humour here is not present in the scene itself, as with the pool table above, but rather in the casual eating of fish and chips in a situation where civilians might be aware of something other than the "peacefulness" of the scene. Such a description sets this officer and his colleague apart and underlines their "difference".

Humour as bonding was clearly indicated by one officer who said, "We used humour a lot, we enjoy ourselves as a team. We often have lunches as a group as well as team days and barbecues".

Sometimes, however, officers on duty realised that their use of black humour points to a level of desensitisation that may not be acceptable. One ex-London officer referred to the death of a teenage female cyclist, "She had a tattoo on her breast. We made jokes about that as she lay on the morgue slab. I knew we had gone too far, we had become ruthless with less empathy and less compassion". This was a very clear admission that there are limits to the efficacy of such humour as a coping tool. Such "ruthlessness" for this officer was ethically unacceptable and an indicator of his need to recalibrate the balance between "coping" and empathy. The same attention must be paid to the extent of "numbing" used in similar circumstances where being too unresponsive can lead to a lack of appropriate engagement when dealing with crime victims and members of the public.[4]

Another officer referred to what he saw as his career journey towards the essential contradictions between tragedy, experience and humour, "I have had some highs and lows, often things are tragic but humorous at the same time". This balance between tragedy and humour has a private, cultural component for the police officers involved. In this sense, it mirrors the need for them to create distance between themselves and tragedy. Humour obviously has no place in their dealings with victims and other civilians. A high-ranking Commissioned Officer summed this up, "I'm not sure it's

---

[4] See also "numbing" below.

the gruesome experiences that get to you. You get through that with black humour and support from colleagues and a few beers after work".

There is clear evidence that officers interviewed were well aware of their use of humour as a coping mechanism. This awareness is strongly embedded in SAPOL culture as "a marvellous medicine", as bonding and demarcation from mainstream society, "we use humour a lot, we enjoy ourselves as a team" and as a means of "not taking things too seriously", and "each time you do that, you build resilience". Black or gallows humour is a mechanism, however, that has its limits and is recognised as a part of coping but not by those interviewed, as a central component of their coping and wellness strategies.

5.7 Relationships, Marriage and Coping

Policing research literature abounds with references to "protective factors" that mitigate against officers falling prey to unwanted stress reactions. Prominent among them are social support, caring attachment to others, work/life balance, sufficient time with family, positive relationships and the experience of love and acceptance (Bannink, 2014; Chae & Boyle, 2013; Chopko, 2011; Stephens & Pugmire, 2008; Yuan et al., 2011).

Gilmartin (2002) highlights the importance of reducing duty-related hypervigilance so that off-duty officers can usefully relate to their families and friends, while Tedeschi and Calhoun (1999) emphasise how the transition from work to home for emergency service workers should facilitate coping strategies when engaging in social support outside of that provided by the police organisation. Kirschman (2007) stresses the importance of "family support' in encouraging the "police face" to make a healthy transition from duty-related activities to those that provide time and opportunity to debrief. Plantinga (2014:182) argues for a similar creation of distance between policing and home, "the distance you create between these worlds, keeps you from floundering, keeps you balanced, keeps you sane". Schaffer (2014:105) advises officers to, "Continue to educate yourself about the world around you and cherish your loved ones".

5.8 Relationship Issues from the New South Wales Police Autobiographies

Allan Sparkes (Sparkes, 2013:136) describes his relationship with his wife Deborah as being strong and supportive, although he says, "I kept my mental state from her". Her support, Allan believes was central to his later recovery after a PTSD diganosis. Horner (2011) experienced a marriage breakdown in mid-career, as did Esther Mckay. She described her subsequent partner as "extremely sensitive and comforting" in terms of her battle with the trauma that was then a challenging part of her everyday experience. Belinda Neil had a similar experience, as did Geoff Bernasconi (Mckay, 2010:74) where he describes his marriage as "weakening under the strain". After being absent from home for four days involved with the forensic investigation of a plane crash scene (during which time he made no contact with his pregnant wife) on arriving back to his hometown he went straight to the hotel, got drunk and called his wife, suggesting she joins him for dinner. The relationship did not survive.[5]

5.9 Relationships and Coping: The Data from the Interviews

Police officers have a reputation in the literature for over-indulging in alcohol, eating junk food, being unfit and in particular, handling personal relationships badly (Davis, 2013; Gilmartin, 2002; Kirschman, 2006; Littles, 2011; Ménard & Arter, 2013; Plantinga, 2014). Many of the officers interviewed, particularly those nearing the end of their careers, were thoughtful about the impact of "the job" on personal relationships. Being "married to the job" in early career was not unusual for many of the male officers, and this was often a challenge to their life partners. Some were aware that their wives had been responsible for more than their fair share of parenting, many confided in partners about duty-related stressors as a way of debriefing, some were careful never to do so. They reflected a clear view that being able to rely on support from loved ones who understand the challenges of policing was of critical importance. Said one, "My wife and I talk a lot about work. She is an ex-member. We debrief". Several of those interviewed were married to police officers or to partners who had been in "the job". All saw great advantage in debriefing with a person "who has that understanding". Another in a similar vein added, "My wife could smell if I had been to the mortuary. I could discuss things with her". A Detective Sergeant, describing such conversations that had continued throughout his long career, said of his wife, "She is my rock, my greatest sounding board".

A STAR group officer, who was single for the first 13 years of his career, was clear about the difference between departmental debriefs and the process that occurred within his relationship with his wife, "I cannot overestimate the importance of my wife, and the stable family life I have had largely due to her and her readiness to talk with me about my police experience at crucial times". Such appropriate and timely interventions kept this officer well and were crucial to his coping ability. He was careful to make it clear that the stability she brought to the relationship, as opposed to the exposure to chaos and tragedy through his duties, was of equal importance to his well-being and that of their relationship.

Keeping the work–life balance can be challenging as expressed by a young Detective Senior Constable, "As far as my wife is concerned, I want to be human for her.

---

[5] See more detail regarding these officers in Chapter 9 "PTSD and policing".

She will say sometimes, you've lost your balance". Sometimes, however, such a balance is not possible. A retired officer of 45 years experience described an incident where a young woman died in a road crash, "I remember how she moaned and groaned. All we had then was our wives to talk to". A clear majority saw the importance of personal relationships as a strategy for keeping grounded and maintaining a life outside of policing which contributed directly to their capacity to cope (Plantinga, 2014). Those who were in relationships with police officers saw great value in debriefs based on a clear mutual understanding of the challenges faced, while some expressed relief that their marriage to a civilian provided them with incentives not to take work home. Keeping duty-related activities and home-life separate was important to others. Leaving the "emotional side of things at work" and "I sometimes took work home in the early stages, then I decided not to talk about it", said a Detective Sergeant.

Older officers whose careers reached back to the 1970s found that their duties had a significant impact on their relationships. "I was a full-time cop" said one. "In the 70s, when we were young, we were married to the job". Another was clear about the personal cost of his career, "My first marriage of fourteen years failed because of the job. I wasn't a copper when we got married. She hated the job".

Some had regrets about the demands of policing that had impact on their family life, "I spent a lot of time away from home at this time" and "my wife raised the boys. You've got a job to do. Life work balance is very important". The latter, retrospective comment was with the benefit of hindsight and some tangible regret.

A Sergeant, married to a civilian and working in child abuse investigation saw her relationship as pivotal to her well-being and resilience, "I have a great relationship with my husband and plenty of connections outside of work". The experience-based assumption here is similar to that of the officer above. Being "human" and "grounded" for a partner was crucial to the survival of the relationship and to the "emotional survival" (Gilmartin, 2002) of the officer in that relationship.

Gilmartin (2002) in his "Emotional survival for law enforcement" book and lectures delivered to hundreds of South Australian officers and their families speaks directly about being "fully present" when off duty and at home. In terms of the issues that police officers can control, Gilmartin places officer's personal lives at the top of that list, arguing that the "non-police support systems" (family and community) determine the success or otherwise of her/his police career. Many of those I interviewed agreed, one was frank as she ruefully commented, "I lost a marriage along the way. If only someone had given me this book when I was a cadet!".

Shift work and being on the call were seen by many as significant challenges to family and social interaction. A young officer said, "I find being on call at home difficult. It makes me agitated waiting for something to happen". Another had a positive view of shift work, "Shift work is good and bad, good for family and extended family". Shift work was not seen as an issue that disadvantaged family or social life. Some saw it as a positive opportunity for quality interaction.

5.9.1 Critical Incident Debriefs and Coping

All of the officers interviewed had an opinion about the importance or otherwise of debriefs after critical incidents that cause "unusually strong emotional reactions" (Mitchell, 1983). Such critical incidents may involve the death of a child, grotesque death or injury, a lack of a positive outcome or some aspect of the situation that was able to bypass the "emotional shield" or "numbing" that officers learn to construct (Henry, 2004).

The ongoing, academic debate concerning the effectiveness or otherwise of the Mitchell model of Critical Incident Stress Debriefing (Alexander, 2000; Bledsoe, 2003; Greenberg et al., 2008; Hunt et al., 2013; Kennardy, 2000; Malcolm et al., 2005; Raphael & Meldrum, 1995; Whybrow et al., 2015) was of little interest to those police officers interviewed in the present study, particularly those at the rank of Sergeant, whose focus is more on the health and well-being of their "troops" and practical ways to limit the number who are "broken" by the impact of their duties and other life challenges outside of "the job". They saw debriefing as an effective and logical approach to duty-related events they considered to be challenging and out of the ordinary.

5.9.2 Debriefs and Coping. The Informing Literature

Critical Incident Management and Critical Incident Stress Debriefing have been much discussed in trauma-related literature (Al-Shahi & Warlow, 2000; Alexander, 2000; Amaranto et al., 2003; Dyregrov, 1998; Greenberg et al., 2008; Raphael & Meldrum, 1995) and have particular relevance to maintaining the well-being of police officers and other emergency service personnel.

Mitchell (1983: 36) defines a critical incident as "any unplanned, unexpected or unpleasant situation faced by emergency services personnel that causes them to experience unusually strong emotional reactions and which have the potential to interfere with their ability to function either at the scene or later". Mitchell developed clear protocols for Critical Incident Stress Debriefings (CISD) and an overall organisational approach Critical Incident Stress Management (CISM) which outlined the structures and practices that organisations might put in place to facilitate effective management of emergency personnel after critical incidents. Mitchell has a PhD in Human Development from the University of Maryland, USA, and is presently the President Emeritus of The International Critical Incident Stress Foundation. He is not part of the international psychological or psychiatric establishment and his CISD approach has been much criticised by many in those professional communities (Malcolm et al., 2005; Bledsoe, 2003. Kenardy, 2000). In his own defence, Mitchell (2004) argues that CISD is a crisis intervention strategy, a psycho education tool as well as a form of early intervention, with a particular focus on critical incidents and emergency worker's responses to extreme manifestations of them. Quoting Dyregrov

(1998:12), Mitchell argues that "the debate on debriefing is not only a scientific but also a political debate. It entails power and positions in the therapeutic world. As a technique, (debriefing) represents a threat to the psychiatric elite". Mitchell also published a list of 50 of his professional detractors (2004) showing that only one had undergone CISD or CISM training offered by his organisation, the International Critical Incident Stress Foundation. His argument here is that if CISD is critically evaluated, it should be the product offered through training by his organisation and not simply an approach his detractors evaluate which may or may not comply with the protocols of the Mitchell model.

Roger Peters, an Australian clinical psychologist, expresses outrage at Mitchell's treatment by some of his international colleagues that "It is hard to believe that such infighting in any profession could have been as hostile and embarrassing as it has been in mine". As a supporter of the CISD process, he goes on to outline his, and Mitchell's understanding of the purpose and nature of debriefing. Peters argues that CISD is intended for tertiary victims of such incidents, that is those tasked with dealing directly with the incident as professional emergency service workers and not for primary or secondary victims, such as bank staff held up by an armed robber or members of the general public who may have observed such an event from a distance. He concludes that such debriefs are intended to "normalise and legitimise the feelings of the participants and to accelerate their return to usual functioning as well providing psycho-education around normal reactions to trauma" (p. 52). CISD says Peters should include monitoring and follow-up of those involved.

Bledsoe (2003:272) does not hold back, criticising the fundamentals of CISD as the province of "pseudo mental health workers" and suggesting that "CISD may inhibit natural recovery and prevent workers from talking to their families and may be a breach of confidentiality". Another issue addressed by Bledsoe is the capacity of CISD to prevent PTSD, which is clearly a claim not made by Mitchell and his supporters. In his review Bledsoe also takes pains to explain Mitchell's financial interest in CISD training in the context of his Presidency of the International Critical Incident Stress Foundation. His motivation is clear and not always scientifically based.

Kenardy (2000:231) in the British Medical Journal briefly reviews the state of the CISD debate, surmising that the lack of published randomised trials of a consistent version of the approach, coupled with the possibility that those who are debriefed "might develop an expectation that they might become unwell" and also outlines his concerns that CISD might "medicalise trauma" concluding that, "there is little evidence to support current debriefing practices". Mitchell's response to this and similar criticisms are contained in "Critical Intervention and Critical Incident Stress Management: A defense of the field" (2004) and comprise a detailed critique of randomised control trials, controlled studies, meta-analyses, literature reviews and case studies.

The impact of this sometimes hostile debate has been two-fold. First, there is evidence of a retreat from offering any form of debriefs by police and other emergency services (Horner, 2011; McKay, 2005, 2010; Sanford, 2003), and secondly, alternative, more conservative approaches such as "Psychological first aid" (Australian Red

Cross, 2009) have been adopted that focus more on practical support and a "wait and see" whether trauma symptoms develop. Trauma Incident Risk Management (TRiM) programmes (Greenberg et al., 2008) criticise the Mitchell approach as "of no use and at worst harmful" and adopt a peer-based "watchful waiting" regime to monitor the possible development of post-trauma symptoms in those affected, rather than implementing an early intervention strategy such as CISD.

Raphael suggests that on the basis of a lack of controlled experimental evaluation of well-sampled individuals exposed to trauma and then debriefed using the Mitchell model, caution should be displayed in drawing conclusions around the efficacy of CISD or otherwise. In an example of such a study Addis and Stephens (2008), in a study of New Zealand police officers response to a police shooting five years after the event, surveyed 74 police employees, most of whom had no direct contact with the event, some of whom were unsworn and some who had not received debriefing although it was at the time mandated by New Zealand police. The debriefs in this instance took three forms, some officers and employees were debriefed in groups, some received individual attention from a psychologist and some received both services. No description is given by the researchers of the debriefing approach employed. Nor was there any evidence of follow-up of those who were debriefed, although measurement of subsequent traumatic experience was attempted. Unsurprisingly, no positive outcomes were measured although all those debriefed reported the experience of receiving the intervention as helpful.

Chae and Boyle (2013) argue in support of CISD that re-experiencing the trauma in the context of expert debriefs may lead to post-traumatic growth and the reinterpretation of the incident in positive rather than negative terms. Such an argument is in part based on the view that such debriefs may reproduce the widely acknowledged benefits of Cognitive Behaviour Therapy, an approach used by many clinicians in their treatment of PTSD (Calhoun et al., 1999; Flannery, 2015; Garrick & Williams, 2006; Kitaeff, 2011; Raphael & Meldrum, 1995; Seligman, 2012). Tehrani (2009) after a quantitative study of 276 first responders concluded that debriefs when conducted by peers or "caring professionals" increase "sense making" of critical incidents by those involved. Marin (2012) mounts a similar argument, supporting the use of trained police peers as "mental health professionals don't always understand police culture". Flannery (2015) argues that formal debriefs following critical incidents offer police organisations an opportunity to focus on self-care and psycho education among officers as well as feedback, positive or otherwise about operational outcomes in that context. Such an approach may well allow police managers to combine operational and stress-related debriefs to overcome the cultural reluctance of many officers to participate, believing that such measures are "only for wimps who can't cope with the job, and not for real men".[6] Rees and Smith (2008) see peer-presented debriefs based on the Mitchell approach, as offering an important opportunity to break down this culture, as well as the typical police "code of silence" around emotional reactions to trauma. Silverii (2014:28) agrees asserting that "seeking help when under stress

[6] This is an insight that will be considered in the recommendations in the final chapter of this research.

is breaking the code of silence". Raphael and Wilson support this assumption as well, arguing that effective critical incident stress debriefing "may lead to learning" about useful coping mechanisms among police officers. Asken makes a similar point asserting that the previous "get over it" or "deal with it" culture should be replaced in contemporary policing with "learn to get over it and how to deal with it". Tedeschi and Calhoun (2006) describe other potential benefits of debriefs when well conducted, including those of offering opportunities for management to underline the "positive meaning" of much of the work that emergency service personnel undertake and thus contribute to their post-traumatic growth and well-being.

Malcolm et al (2005) provide a comprehensive approach to the debate around who should conduct debriefs in the form of a literature review focussing on the importance of police culture on the impact of debriefing. They outline the difficulty when a debriefer, as an outsider enters the "closed" police culture with the expectation that those officers will be relaxed about divulging personal information, particularly in the context of what Mitchell would call "unusually strong emotional reactions". The presence of senior officers during debriefs and the proximity of the activity to shift changes are among other issues that need to be considered and if possible controlled for in such evaluations. In this study, a literature review of 12 academic evaluations of debriefing concluded that "this lack of useful and valid assessment tools permeates CISD research in general" (p. 9) and goes on to question differences in the application of the CISD protocols as laid out by Mitchell affirming that the CISD model was designed to be used in the context of an overall management approach including the thorough training of the CISD facilitators and subsequent follow-up through the support services of the organisations involved. The majority of the studies around CISD considered by Malcolm et al. indicate that the debriefs were well received by the police officers involved who all reported satisfaction at very high levels. This, although a common response from those being debriefed, did not convince these researchers with regard to the efficacy of the CISD approach.

A more positive example of a CISD approach is provided by Honig and Sultan (2006) in a study of the Los Angeles Police Department's response to an officer involved in a mid-1980s plane crash. Four hundred personnel participated in mandatory debriefs using the Mitchell model, and Sergeants were trained to detect early symptoms of trauma responses in their teams, and referrals were made for "troubled" officers to other counselling and support agencies. Subsequently, no workers compensation claims were made in connection to the incident. The LAPD continued to use the Mitchell model for many years including on-scene psychological first aid, resiliency training, supervisory intervention where indicated, at risk assessments and follow-up for individuals, pre-incident briefings where possible and ongoing psycho education programmes that are built into departmental practice. Police psychologists, peers and Chaplains are utilised in the delivery of the programmes and all officers closely involved in the disaster were required to "show up" for an individual debrief with a clinical psychologist.

The real possibilities of more positive trauma-related outcomes as a result of effective debriefing and support are revealed in a significant study by David Alexander, "Debriefing and body recovery: police in a civilian disaster" revealing how effective preparation, management and recognition of the possibilities of traumatic responses can lead to positive long-term outcomes for police personnel involved in tasks that could otherwise lead to career-limiting responses such as PTSD. In this case, officers in two groups were tasked with body retrieval and identification after the North Sea Piper Alpha oil rig disaster of 1988. A total of 167 men died on-site, and 105 were entombed in an accommodation module which was located under 120 m of water in the North Sea. It was raised to the surface some three months later and transported to the nearby island of Flotta. The first team of officers searched the module, retrieved and bagged the bodies of the deceased which were then transported to a mortuary close to the Aberdeen Airport where the second team were responsible for the stripping washing and identification of the bodies. All officers who volunteered for the mission had previous experience with sudden death. Preference was given to experienced officers and those who exhibited a sense of humour! The police teams worked in pairs, usually a more junior officer with a more experienced colleague.

A small group of civilian mental health professionals was available to the police teams throughout the operation. These were known to the officers as they had conducted a well-being study with the groups some months earlier. The use of "black humour" was encouraged, regular defusing and debriefings were conducted, talking with colleagues about the process was commonplace and regular "chats" with the health specialists were seen as normal. As well, high-ranking police commanders visited regularly and expressed their appreciation of the team's efforts. The officers involved reported positive outcomes from the experience when surveyed 3 months and 3 years later. All felt that their contribution had been significant. "Keeping things to oneself" (Alexander 2000:118) was seen by the teams as "neither helpful nor popular". Sick leave taken in subsequent months by the officers involved was also below average when compared to a similar control cohort of other officers not tasked to the post-disaster operation. It is of note that this study reinforces the practical "Post Traumatic Growth" possibilities of such a difficult undertaking given the opportunity to introduce some of the strategies referred to above. The PTG strategies employed here were basic but obviously effective. This situation offered a rare opportunity to conduct a "before and after" study due to the previous involvement of the researchers in the well-being review of the officers involved which was conducted a few months prior to the disaster. Clearly, the positive organisational response to those working in the retrieval and identification process was of crucial importance to the positive outcomes achieved.

5.9.3 Debriefs and Coping: The Data from the Interviews

Some officers at interview complained about the absence of debriefs in the context of their perception of the Department's lack of concern for their welfare, while others because their experience of the process had been positive and seen as valuable to their "wellness" and ability to cope. More traditional, "old school" officers had reservations about debriefs from the perspective of the "just get on with it" approach to the challenges of policing, also expressing doubt about the capacity of those without a SAPOL operational background ("the psyches") to make a useful contribution in such circumstances. Younger officers were very positive, welcoming the provision of such support as well as expressing its benefits to their well-being. One long-serving officer, recently diagnosed with PTSD commented, "Debriefs are usually operational, not about you. When there is no relief {as achieved in an effective debrief} things build up. I didn't know until I was broken".

Another officer interviewed was involved in domestic violence-related murder where two of his colleagues gave CPR to the victim. He commented, "No one said anything to them until I did. We had firearm training every year but no mental health training and no debriefs". This is an articulate and effective indicator of where SAPOL's priorities lie. In this officer's view, both firearms training and (the absent) mental health training are of equal importance to his and his colleague's well-being and survival when situations get tough.

A member who is attached with the Special Task Force and Rescue Group as a recovery diver in reference to a recent double child murder/suicide in Port Lincoln, South Australia, described the formal debrief that followed the incident as, "We were all invited. A psych sat with us in silence for a while, and then said 'right who wants to start?' I didn't want to know the details. I wasn't there. It turned out to be an incident debrief they gave us brochures". This is a very obvious example of an approach to debriefing that fails to meet the requirements of even the most basic trauma management. Mitchell makes it very clear that those uninvolved in critical incidents, such as this officer, should not have any involvement in the debriefings that follow. Even those most critical of Mitchell and in favour of alternatives to CISD would agree.

When interviewing a Senior Detective Sergeant who had recently retired I asked the question, "Have you been offered debriefs during your career?" He responded by laughing and said:

> I have been offered debriefs twice in the last ten years, four times since I joined SAPOL. The yearly psych assessments are okay, they are better than nothing. They are routine, you know where they are going. The best psych that I saw was outside of the organization. She could tell what I was thinking. I felt I didn't hide things from her. SAPOL psyches' are young, inexperienced. I don't need anything more than informal debriefs.

Such a need is rarely met despite SAPOL management's assurances to the contrary. Informal debriefs, where officers support and comfort each other, were commonly referred to where "you're with your mates, they know what you're going through" summed up the intention and the outcome. Such debriefs were a feature of policing in the 1980s and 1990s before the impact of Random Breath Testing legislation (see above) and are less likely to take place especially in public in contemporary policing. An officer talked about his way of dealing with confronting death scenes suggesting, "we had our own debriefs over pizza and beer, camaraderie was and is very important. I have always had close police friends".

Female officers were more supportive of a debriefing approach and were more comfortable expressing emotion openly than were their male colleagues. One recounted a situation where a child, known to her and her rural colleagues had committed suicide, "I ended up sobbing behind the police car. The SAPOL blokes showed no emotion. There was no formal debrief only a cup of tea". Often, officers reported that little or no attention was paid to formal or informal debriefs after such critical incidents. A Detective, referring to informal debriefs as a result of her duties in family violence investigations, responded saying, "There have been very few formal debriefs, we do it every day as a team. There are many manifestations in that situation, anger, laughter, singing. My colleagues make it all possible". This comment testifies to the importance of the family culture of SAPOL, particularly evident more in the recent fields of Family Violence and Child Protection. These usually under-resourced areas of police duty breed an intense level of mutual care and support as described by this officer.

The provision of annual mental health reviews to officers deemed by management to work in unusually challenging areas, such as major crime, major crash, family violence, child exploitation and special task and rescue, were either viewed as "window dressing" by recipients or noted for their non-provision despite well-publicised SAPOL policy in this area of employee assistance and well-being maintenance. The delivery of such services, including formal debriefs and offers of support, is at best inconsistent within SAPOL. A young female Senior Constable commented, "In my six years of policing I've never had a debrief. After we dealt with a dead baby our Sergeant rang my partner who was a mother to see if she was okay but didn't ring me".

Sergeants outlined their involvement in early intervention approaches to unusual stress reactions in their teams, as well as their regular provision of "hot debriefs" in the context of a common-sense approach rather than one involving any formal in-service training. Leadership in this context is the province of Sergeants who provide such debriefs regularly and also keep a close eye on their team's well-being and is aware "that every time I send them out on Patrol they could be killed". This is the management level within SAPOL that is most relevant to the development and maintenance of coping skills as well as the observance of operational safety. Those at this rank during the interview showed how seriously such responsibilities were taken.

One interviewee confirmed this interpretation, stating, "I watch team members that go quiet (after an incident) very carefully. I always debrief staff after a critical incident, for example a suicide…I talk about what might happen to them with regard to sleeping patterns and emotions". In the view of many of those interviewed, operational Sergeants are best placed to offer debriefs, usually out of concern for their troops and with no organisational support or training. These are "insiders" with credibility stemming directly from their operational engagement and their closeness to their teams. With basic training in early detection of trauma symptoms and Critical Incident Debriefing, Sergeants could be the key to significant culture change within SAPOL. Such change is long overdue as evidenced by a less than engaged Sergeant who when he encountered a weary Detective Sergeant in a corridor offered her $5 and the advice, "You look tired! Take this and buy yourself a cup of coffee!".

Officers interviewed made it clear that Sergeants are a critically important factor in terms of the well-being of operational police. Throughout the interviews those officers who had been debriefed often referred to the importance of their Sergeant to that process. It is more likely, for example, that individual officers will receive positive feedback about operational outcomes in that context from their Sergeant rather than from higher-ranking officers, who most operational police perceive as being risk-averse and less positively responsive. Sergeants, usually without training in the procedural and psychological aspects of debriefing take care of their troops, "We are required to do debriefs, once upon a time the psyches would come out". The "psyches" that this Sergeant is referring to are the three psychologists (all sworn police officers), who were employed by SAPOL up until ten years ago. They were accepted and respected by fellow officers because of their history in operational policing. Those referred to as "psyches today" are psychology graduates who offer police officers debriefing services without the perceived benefits of operational police experience.

An officer who had vast experience commented, "Face to face debriefs have to be with the right person. It shouldn't be a psych". This is an expression of the clear view that people in "the job" were preferred to offer debriefs on the rare occasions they occurred. "Psyches" were too young and inexperienced and even though employed by SAPOL were seen as outsiders.

A Senior Constable described a debrief that took place with a Sergeant after a critical incident thus, "It was really good, we talked through what had happened and we were given time to deal with the experience. This has been a common experience with my Sergeants. Some Sergeants don't look after their troops that well. Where do Sergeants learn to be effective in these areas?" The latter question assumes no SAPOL involvement in the acquisition of such skills.

The academic debate around the benefits or otherwise of CISD, Trauma Risk Management or Psychological First Aid is entirely lost on the cohort of police officers interviewed for this research. Like many officers studied by researchers, they see the value of debriefs from their own experience in "giving us time to deal with incidents" as well as "talking through the experience and taking time to digest its implications". This is particularly important when outcomes are not positive; for example, when despite officers best efforts, members of the public or colleagues are physically injured or worse. The intense criticism of CISD from academic researchers belies the intention, typically in line with treatment strategies such as cognitive behaviour therapy of providing a context among police in which they are able to come to terms with experiences outside of their normal experience and to consider them without fear of criticism. This is a function within SAPOL that such debriefs still fulfil.

Structured peer support programmes are unpopular with SAPOL executive management. A locally organised, pilot peer support programme was recently undertaken in an Adelaide Police Local Service Area. It was, according to a Sergeant, "canned by higher command" this being confirmed during a later interview conducted with a Chief Superintendent who confided that in his view that kind of thing is not helpful and just leads to "group whinging". The Senior Sergeant went on, "Many people come to talk to me informally", the informality of such approaches bearing witness to the cultural stigma attached to such formal conversations.

Many officers interviewed saw the lack of debriefs as symptomatic of SAPOL's lack of concern for their mental health, particularly those who are aware of their personal vulnerability to traumatic situations. This was often expressed in the context of a general lack of positive feedback around operational outcomes from senior officers above the rank of Sergeant. A clear example of this was expressed by an officer who had served in the far North of South Australia:

> Domestic violence, assaults with weapons are common as are extreme suicide attempts and threats. Petrol sniffing in those days caused a lot of that. There were many suicides always by hanging. Fatal road crashes were common. Alcohol and all the normal stuff. I just saw more and worse. SAPOL were aware of these issues. We needed a psych assessment to go there. I never saw a psych while I was there.

The "psych assessment" was seen by this and other officers as window dressing or even worse "arse covering" by the Department. Well-conducted debriefs, by the right person, would have meant a great deal more in practical terms.

Another officer referring to three Sudden Infant Death syndrome taskings during one shift pointed out, "We used to go to the Police Club after night shift and drink too much. This was an effective way of debriefing then, it is not possible now". A further reference to a culture of informal debriefs was made by a retired Senior Sergeant who said "In the 1970s the end of night shift barbies were the go. At "Nelsons Beach" behind the Police Club we would talk about work. They were therapy sessions". A colleague explaining the reluctance on the part of some police officers to seek debriefs and support within the police organisation said, "psychs were also available, but it wasn't really an issue, you dealt with it in your own way". Another observed, "SAPOL needs to acknowledge the need for this kind of support. There is still a high level of discomfort about saying 'I need to see someone".

A retired Sergeant referred to informal debriefs in the context of family members describing his environment during his service in the Riverland of South Australia, thus "I saw some horrific accidents there including five really bad ones. I came across a smoking engine block in the middle of the road. A young woman had been thrown out. I remember how she moaned and groaned. All we had then was our wives". Progress has been made since that time in the provision of support to officers after such experiences, there is room for much more.

A retired Detective Chief Inspector referring to an experience early in his career commented, "I was first on scene at a motor vehicle accident where a police officer had been killed. His partner administered CPR. That added another dimension to the trauma. There were no debriefs in those days. A Sergeant asked me and my colleagues 'are you blokes alright?" This officer was clearly ahead of his time to even contemplate asking such a question. This incident was outside the normal range of most officer's experience and should have resulted in a far more effective response.

A Special Task and Rescue Group officer commenting about the increasing incidence of debriefs in his experience said, "We've had more debriefs recently. The chaplain drops in for a bit of a chat. Debriefs don't do much for me. We talk about it openly with our peers. You're into overtime, have a bit of a chill we are all bonding, offloading without being judged". An experienced officer in the same group commented, "I am happy and comfortable with what I have seen. We talk about things at work in a casual way after a big job. Formal debriefs are a waste of time. Just people from outside wanting to get into our heads. We have a laugh when no one is looking and relieve the stress in a casual humorous way in our truck". Such informal debriefs were highly valued by many, relieving stress "in a casual humorous way" on the understanding that responses to out of the ordinary trauma were not being judged by colleagues in the process.

Debriefs after critical events that are outside of the usual experience of operational police are valued by younger members as long as they are conducted by debriefers who are "in the job". Older, more experienced officers doubt the value of formal debriefs, preferring to "get on with it". Sergeants have adopted a debriefing role as well as a watching brief regarding the well-being of their operational teams albeit without training in this area of management. One Sergeant expressed this role clearly: "If I saw changes, I would call them in for a chat". They adopt a "common-sense" approach to this aspect of their duties, largely motivated by their concern for their teams after confronting events such as suicides and grotesque death encounters. Said one, "We don't get any training, but use common sense". Clearly, more needs to be done by SAPOL to augment this common sense with relevant training input.[7]

5.9.4 Numbing: A Way of Coping

Much of the research literature in the field of policing and trauma focusses on the challenges officers face with the constant exposure to death and injury in various forms. Henry (2004) considers such exposure a constant reminder of the individual officer's own mortality and outlines in his research the strategies officers use to deal with such issues. "Psychic or professional numbing" is one such strategy that involves the creation of a level of detachment that balances operational efficiency and appropriate responses to crime victims and the general public against over-identification with the situation that may be damaging to the individual's well-being. Yuan et al. (2011) and Bourke et al. (2006) argue that research has focussed excessively on the possible pathology of such death encounters, suggesting that "protective factors" including temperament and personality, attitudes that develop in officers over time that reinforce a personal sense of competence and coping, social support through the "family" culture of policing, and, despite all odds assist in the development and maintenance of a positive view of the world. The latter is well summed up by one officer I interviewed, "I wouldn't be the person I am with all these challenges" and another commented, "I have enjoyed my career so much, the good outweighs the bad".

[7] See recommendations in the *Conclusions* section.

5.9.5 *Numbing, a Way of Coping: The Data*

South Australian police officers learn very early in their careers that numbing is an essential strategy when dealing with the more confronting aspects of policing (Henry, 2004). When in the presence of out of the ordinary death scenes, such as plane and vehicle crashes, horrific injury and disfigurement, smell of decayed human flesh or the death or injury of children, they "numb" their emotional responses to both facilitate their duties at the scene and to protect themselves from later uncontrolled responses that may impact on their well-being. They are all aware that they cannot afford to "dwell" on such experiences. Commenting on the need to balance such distancing, a retired Chief Superintendent added, "Numbing starts early in your career, but you can get too cold. You need not to get too close personally to victims, but not too far removed so that you can't show empathy". Developing such a balance is a skill learned by most outside of the Academy as illustrated when a young Constable, early in her career was found by her Sergeant looking at family photos on the wall during a routine death attendance of an elderly person in her home. The Sergeant cautioned the younger officer, "You can't afford to be that involved". This was an early lesson in creating appropriate distance from such taskings to ensure long-term survival in "the job".

A Senior Sergeant in the STAR group after 25 years of exposure to death and gross disfigurement, "I'm affected, I'm saddened, I feel for those involved, I have had tears, but it doesn't affect me, I don't let it affect my life. It's like watching a movie!" This insight and its expression is a very clear indicator of how self-aware this officer is of his coping skills. His levels of empathy have been high, to the point of shedding tears, but he is aware also that he is part of the audience to such events, a spectator.

And a colleague of his stated, "The Whyalla plane crash was horrific,[8] the bodies had been attacked by lice which had eaten their eyelids and lips. They were grinning and their eyes bulging out of their skulls. I thought I don't know who they are! So I didn't have any connection with them. They were just dead bodies in my eyes". Creating emotional distance is here achieved by enhancing a focus on duty and by underlining where possible a lack of emotional connection with victims of crime or misfortune. The challenge, particularly for investigators such as Detectives who need to maintain a relationship with families and those close to victims, is to balance empathy with their own personal needs. This STAR group recovery diver, although confronted with the images he describes was able to create and maintain an effective distance from them that enabled him to be resilient, to move on.

A Detective Senior Sergeant of some 30 years experience commented, "You look at dead bodies as humans but you repress your feelings", adding, "Dealing with families where young children had died was always difficult". An ex-United Kingdom officer commented, "I am quite desensitized. I am kind of indifferent. When in London I was attending a drug overdose in a stairwell and I thought to myself I am

[8] A light passenger aircraft en route to Adelaide crashed into the sea. It took some time to recover the bodies, one of which was never found.

watching a human being die and I am feeling nothing". A Senior Sergeant described clearly the impact of such exposure at another level where it intruded into his personal life, "When my parents died, I just got on with it" describing how the impact of their death was blunted on him by constant exposure to duty-related deaths he had encountered during his career. Numbing, the ability to be appropriately present at times of great challenge, is critically important to a long and successful police career as long as it is a skill that can be suspended at times when off-duty relationships require being as Gilmartin (2004) puts it, "fully present".

Those interviewed were clear about the challenges in this area. Some in their personal relationships were reminded from time to time to regain their "balance" by vigilant partners, responding by making necessary changes to the on and off-duty behaviours.

What have we learnt?

At the heart of my research is the question, "how do South Australian police officers remain resilient, how do they "cope" with their sometimes traumatic duties?" In this chapter, I have examined some of their strategies. Much of the literature around policing and trauma focusses on the hazards of the profession (Barron, 2010; Blum & Blum, 2000; Burke, 2016; Gilmartin, 2002) and this is consistent with the intention of recognising the danger of traumatic responses to the confronting aspects of the occupation, often with little respectful attention paid to the officers own awareness of the hazards and the actions they take to maintain their health and enthusiasm for "the job". Much research into the traumas of policing focusses on the possibility or sometimes the inevitability of post-traumatic stress or of "sub-threshold" reactions that don't justify a full diagnosis (McFarlane, 2011, 2017). Police officers it seems, can't win and much of the quantitative research pays little attention to effective strategies they use to cope with operational and managerial challenges. In this context officers are identified as almost hapless victims of the traumas of their profession, while (Kemp, 2017) those interviewed here were not. The officers interviewed for this study were clear about how they were able to distance themselves from horror and grotesque death and injury. Many described this as "building a wall", "creating a distance", thus reminding themselves that they have no personal emotional connection with victims of traumatic injury or death. Much of this is learned from senior colleagues and refined as their careers unfold.

Humour and camaraderie were also mentioned with an accompanying recognition that cultural influences on trauma were not always positive, particularly in terms of the traditional macho cultural imperative around not displaying or acknowledging feelings or emotion. A sense of humour, particularly in the most confronting situations was highly valued, a coping mechanism that simultaneously provided a sense of distance from horror and the reassurance of the support and presence of colleagues.

Alcohol abuse as self-medication in the face of trauma was regularly mentioned, particularly by older officers who were operational and "social" before the drink driving legislation of the 1980s put an end to "choir practice" and 24-hour "barbecues behind the Police Club". Younger officers were very clear that there was no positive relationship between alcohol abuse and coping.

Access to SAPOL-provided Critical Incident Debriefs was valued but rarely experienced by those interviewed. The debate around the Mitchell model (Addis & Stephens, 2008; Burke, 2016; Flannery, 2015; Malcolm et al., 2005; Raphael & Meldrum, 1995) had little or no impact on the Officers interviewed who interpreted a lack of debriefs as a sign of indifference on SAPOL's part, many laughingly aware of their lack over the best part of their careers. Officers valued such debriefs as a means of putting critical incidents into perspective, coping and "moving on". Sergeants in particular, who were acutely aware of the stress levels of their teams provided such debriefs. "We don't get training" said one, "we operate out of common sense".

Where next?

How these officers coped and their awareness of the need for such skills contradict many of the negative predictions of researchers in the trauma industry. McFarlane's assertion that "Even the healthiest of individuals, when exposed to enough trauma will become unwell" (McFarlane, 2011, 2017) with specific reference to "first responders" is not supported by my interview data. If SAPOL took more seriously its officers capacity to perform their duty whilst acknowledging the personal arrangements they have made to stay well and cope and made it easier for such coping to occur, executive management would benefit from the increased optimism and decreased cynicism that would inevitably follow. A clear SAPOL mental health strategy would be a very good place to start. Improved access to stigma-free support services, both internal and external to the organisation, meaningful debriefs or psychological first aid after critical incidents, relaxation of "command and control" management practices, the provision of externally sourced management training for Sergeants and Commissioned officers, peer support programmes, the inclusion of coping and resilience training at the academy and an in-service training would all contribute to a cultural health revolution within SAPOL. These needs will not be met by the regular importation of "experts" such as Dr. Kevin Gilmartin (2002) or by self-help booklets such as "Head Notes" and "A cop in the family" (Carroll, 2017/2018) but by a change in policy and practice that is imbedded into SAPOL. Such a change is long overdue.

Police officers interviewed for this research were not hapless individuals whose duty-related experiences sentenced them to a PTSD diagnosis. They clearly coped with the challenges of their chosen profession in a variety of ways that indicated their awareness of the need to take responsibility for their own mental health. Most were clear that SAPOL, although offering internal resources such as the Employee Assistance Programme, had little or nothing to offer in that regard. Many felt that the lack of consistency in the provision of debriefs after challenging critical incidents, as well as the absence of annual reviews of their mental health, indicated a lack of practical concern for their welfare.

Therefore, most benefitting from the wise counsel of more experienced colleagues learned to create distance between themselves and the carnage they witnessed, to build "walls", to emphasise the difference between their off and on-duty lives. Sergeants out of concern for the welfare of their teams built "common sense" strategies to take care of them, again with no input, training or support from "SAPOL".

There was an acknowledgement of the need for change and the nature of such change is revealed in the interview data. The need for a clearly articulated mental health strategy, access to support services both internal and external to SAPOL, the provision of debriefs after particularly challenging incidents, the provision of training for team leaders in early intervention mental health strategies and a change in management protocols encouraged coping and recognised achievements in the field of duty. Such strategies, generated from within SAPOL and not imposed from above, will enhance coping and build resilience in this and future generations of SAPOL members.

References

Alexander, D. (2000). Debriefing and body recovery: Police in a civilian disaster. *Psychological debriefing: Theory, practice and evidence* (pp. 118–130).

Amaranto, E., et al. (2003). Police stress interventions. *Brief Treatment and Crisis Intervention, 3*(1), 47.

Al-Shahi, R., & Warlow, C. (2000). The current status of psychological debriefing. *BMJ, 321*, 1032–1033.

Australian Red Cross. (2009). Psychological first aid: An Australian guide. *Australian Psychological Society.*

Bannink, F. (2014). *Post traumatic success: Positive psychology & solution-focused strategies to help clients survive & thrive.* WW Norton & Company.

Barron, S. (2010). Police officer suicide within the New South Wales police force from 1999 to 2008. *Police Practice and Research: an International Journal, 11*(4), 371–382.

Berger, R., & Weiss, T. (2009). The Posttraumatic Growth model: An expansion to the family system. *Traumatology, 15*(1), 63.

Bledsoe, B. E. (2003). Critical Incident Stress Management, (CISM) benefit of risk to emergency services? *Prehospital Emergency Care, 7*(2), 272–279.

Blum, L. E., & Blum, L. N. (2000). *Force under pressure: How cops live and why they die.* Lantern Books.

Burke, R. J. (2016). *Stress in policing: Sources.* Consequences and Interventions: Routledge.

Burns, C. M., et al. (2008). The emotional impact on and coping strategies employed by police teams investigating internet child exploitation. *Traumatology, 14*(2), 20.

Calhoun, L. G., et al. (1999). *Facilitating Posttraumatic growth: A clinician's guide.* Routledge.

Carlier, I. V., et al. (1998). Disaster-related post-traumatic stress in police officers: A field study of the impact of debriefing. *Stress and Health, 14*(3), 143–148.

Carroll, M. (2017). "Head notes" A social and emotional well- being/mental health initiative for South Australian police officers. Police Association of South Australia. Adelaide: SA Government and SAPOL.

Carroll, M. (2018). "A cop in the family" Police Association of South Australia. Adelaide: SA Government and SAPOL.

Chae, M. H., & Boyle, D. J. (2013). Police suicide: Prevalence, risk, and protective factors. *Policing: An International Journal of Police Strategies & Management, 36*(1), 91–118

Chapin, M., et al. (2008). Training police leadership to recognize and address operational stress. *Police Quarterly, 11*(3), 338–352.

Chopko, B. A. (2011). Walk in balance: Training crisis intervention team police officers as compassionate warriors. *Journal of Creativity in Mental Health, 6*(4), 315–328.

Cornum, R. (1993). *She went to war: The Rhonda Cornum story.* U.S.A: Presidio Press.

Davis, K. M. (2013). *Sinister intent.* Australia: Simon and Schuster.

Dyregrov, A. (1998). Psychological debriefing—An effective method? *Traumatology, 4*(2), 3.
Evans, A., & Coccoma, P. (2014). *Trauma-informed care: How neuroscience influences practice.* Routledge.
Flannery, R. B. (2015). Treating psychological trauma in first responders: A multi-modal paradigm. *Psychiatric Quarterly, 86*(2), 261–267.
Garrick, J., & Williams, M. B. (Eds.). (2006). *Trauma treatment techniques: Innovative trends.* The Haworth Maltreatment and Trauma Press: Birmingham.
Gilmartin, K. M. (2002). Emotional survival for law enforcement. *ES Press, PMB, 233*, 2968.
Greenberg, N., et al. (2008). Trauma risk management (TRiM) in the UK Armed Forces. *Journal of the Royal Army Medical Corps, 154*(2), 124–127.
Harms, L. (2015). *Understanding trauma and resilience.* Palgrave Macmillan.
Henry, V. E. (2004). *Death work: Police, trauma, and the psychology of survival.* Oxford University Press.
Homel, R. (1989). Crime on the roads: drinking and driving. In *Alcohol and crime: Proceedings of a Conference,* held 4–6 April 1989.
Horner, P. (2011). *Jack Knife: The crashing of a policeman- NSW police and PTSD.* New South Wales: Australia, Zeus Publications.
Honig, A. L., & Sultan, S. (2006). Reducing trauma through maximizing resiliency: A departmental case study. *Traumatology, 12*(3), 217–219.
Hunt, E., et al. (2013). TRiM: An organizational response to traumatic events in Cumbria Constabulary. *Occupational Medicine, 63*(8), 549–555.
Jackson, C. A. (2007). *Posttraumatic Growth: Is there evidence for changing our practice? Australasian Society for Traumatic Stress Studies (ASTSS), 2006.* Adelaide: SA, Australia, Massey Univ.
Kates, A. (2008). *Copshock: Surviving Post Traumatic Stress Disorder (PTSD).* USA: Holbrook Street Press.
Kemp, M. (2017). Fight for our force: The black cloud that hangs over our police. The Advertiser. Adelaide, South Australia.
Kennardy, J. (2000). The current status of psychological debriefing. *British Medical Journal, 321.*
Kirschman, E., et al. (2015). *Counselling cops: What clinicians need to know.* Guilford Publications.
Kitaeff, J. (2011). *Handbook of police psychology.* Routledge.
Kroes, W. H. (1976). *Society's victim, the policeman: An analysis of job stress in policing.* IL: Thomas Springfield.
Kuhlman, T. L. (1988). Gallows humour for a scaffold setting: managing aggressive patients on a maximum-security forensic unit. *Psychiatric Services, 39*(10), 1085–1090.
Kuiper, N. A. (2012). Humour and resiliency: Towards a process model of coping and growth. *Europe's Journal of Psychology, 8*(3), 475–491.
Littles, M. (2011). *The police wife: Bullets in the washing machine.* USA: Self.
Malcolm, A. S., et al. (2005). Critical incident stress debriefing and law enforcement: An evaluative review. *Brief Treatment and Crisis Intervention, 5*(3), 261.
McFarlane, A. C. (2011). *Many paths, one purpose. Expert forum.* Australian Centre for Posttraumatic mental health.
McFarlane, A. C. (2017). Improving internal practices to support emergency services. Mental Health strategy for first responders: Tackle stigma & enhance prevention strategies. Melbourne Australia: Criterion Conferences.
Mckay, E. (2005). *Crime scene-true stories from the life of a crime scene investigator.* Viking (Penguin) Australia.
Mckay, E. (2010). *Forensic investigator.* Viking (Penguin) Australia.
Ménard, K. S., & Arter, M. L. (2013). Police officer alcohol use and trauma symptoms: Associations with critical incidents, coping, and social stressors. *International Journal of Stress Management, 20*(1), 37.
Mitchell, J. T. (1988). CISML: A new era in crisis intervention. International Critical Incident Stress Foundation.

Neocleous, M. (2012). "Don't Be Scared, Be Prepared" Trauma-anxiety-resilience. *Alternatives, 37*(3), 188–198.

Plantinga, A. (2014). *400 things cops know-Street smart lessons from a veteran patrolman*. USA: Quill Driver Books.

Pole, N., et al. (2006). Resilience in retired police officers. *Traumatology, 12*(3), 207–216.

Raphael, B., & Meldrum, L. (1995). Does debriefing after psychological trauma work? *BMJ: British Medical Journal, 310*(6993), 1479.

Rogers, L. K. (1999). *Post Traumatic Stress Disorder: A police officer's report*. USA: Proctor Publications.

Rowe, A., & Regehr, C. (2010). Whatever gets you through today: An examination of cynical humor among emergency service professionals. *Journal of Loss and Trauma, 15*(5), 448–464.

Sanford, L. L. B. (2003). Critical incident stress and the police officer a pro-active approach.

Shakespeare-Finch, J., et al. (2013). A qualitative approach to assessing the validity of the posttraumatic growth inventory. *Journal of Loss and Trauma, 18*(6), 572–591.

Shane, J. M. (2010). Organizational stressors and police performance. *Journal of Criminal Justice, 38*(4), 807–818.

Schiraldi, G. R. (2011). *The complete guide to resilience: Why it matters how to build it and maintain it*. Resilience Training International.

Schiraldi, G. (2016). *The post-traumatic stress disorder sourcebook, revised and expanded second edition: A guide to healing, recovery, and growth: A guide to healing, recovery, and growth*. McGraw Hill Professional.

Seligman, M. E. P. (2012). *Flourish: A visionary new understanding of happiness and well-being*. Simon and Schuster.

Shochet, I. M., et al. (2011). The development and implementation of the Promoting Resilient Officers (PRO) program. *Traumatology, 17*(4), 43–51.

Stephens, C., & Pugmire, L. A. (2008). Daily organisational hassles and uplifts as determinants of psychological and physical health in a sample of New Zealand police. *International Journal of Police Science & Management, 10*(2), 179–191.

Sparkes, A. (2013). *The cost of bravery*. Penguin Group, Australia.

Tedeschi, R. G., & Calhoun, L. G. (2006). Expert companions: Posttraumatic growth in clinical practice. In *Handbook of posttraumatic growth: Research and practice* (pp. 291–310).

Violanti, J. M., & Paton, D. (2006). *Who gets PTSD?: Issues of posttraumatic stress vulnerability*. Charles C Thomas.

Violanti, J. M. (2014). *Dying for the job: Police work exposure and health*. Charles C Thomas Publisher.

Widera-Wysoczanska, A. (2016). *Trauma treatment: Factors contributing to efficiency*. United Kingdom: Cambridge Scholars Publishing.

Whybrow, D., et al. (2015). Promoting organizational well-being: a comprehensive review of Trauma Risk Management. *Occupational Medicine, 65*(4), 331–336.

Yuan, C., et al. (2011). Protective factors for posttraumatic stress disorder symptoms in a prospective study of police officers. *Psychiatry Research, 188*(1), 45–50.

Chapter 6
Asking for Help

Abstract **Police culture and putting your hand up.** Most officers who recognise the early symptoms of stress-related problems don't ask their organisation for help although universally encouraged to do so. The reason both from the interviews and the reviewed literature is simple. To do so, despite organisational reassurance to the contrary is seen as career ending or at best limiting. Most, therefore, seek assistance confidentially outside of their police organisation or ignore the mounting symptoms. The psychologists and psychiatrists interviewed for this chapter agree that early intervention is, thus, compromised and the inevitable outcome of a PTSD diagnosis follows. Reference is made here to biographical accounts of police officers in New South Wales whose careers followed such a trajectory. This chapter concludes with an examination of contemporary treatment approaches and how they might apply to police service and traumatic outcomes and how this culture of secrecy might change through academy training and timely interventions in the operational field of policing.

Police officers enjoy their chosen careers for a variety of reasons. Many join "the job" to make a difference and to ensure the good order of their society. Some make very clear a desire to contribute to a safer world, some simply to help others. The excitement, the adrenaline, the periods of boredom, the challenges of shift work and the satisfaction of contributing to positive outcomes all contribute to a fulfilling police career. But when stress-related difficulties arise, either personal or to do with "the job", it is difficult for many officers to seek support from within their police organisation. This chapter explores that tension and seeks to define a new reality for officers where asking for help within the organisation might become free of stigma.

6.1 The Informing Literature

Police organisations are characterised in the literature as male dominated, macho cultures where seeking help for developing stress-related problems are seen as a betrayal of the code of silence and where "complaining is not seen as acceptable

A. Paterson, *Trauma and Resilience in Contemporary Australian Policing*,
https://doi.org/10.1007/978-981-16-4416-0_6

behaviour and where seeking mental health counselling is not likely to be thought about" Flannery (2015:262). This chapter will discuss how police cultures including that of SAPOL have been characterised by a clear stigma around officers seeking help for duty-related stress responses. Officers like those whose experience is well described in the five autobiographies and reinforced in the interview data for this study suffer such reactions in silence, often with little or no understanding of what is happening to them as they lose their previous capacity to cope with trauma. Macho attitudes of toughing out these challenges and the culture of secrecy and shame around trauma responses and challenges are well researched in trauma and policing literature. Chae and Boyle (2013) argue that in terms of preventing suicide and posttraumatic stress in police organisations, a more proactive approach involving psycho-education and critical incident debriefing should be integral within policing in the future. Rees and Smith, (2008:277) reinforcing this insight, describing police culture as embodying defensiveness, lack of emotions and resistance to change, pointing out how police usually refrain from engaging in counselling, debriefing services or access to Chaplains. Those services "are there for wimps, those who can't cope with the job and not something for real men". Hesketh et al., (2014:158) agree, describing their UK study findings that "hiding feelings was a badge of courage" and that policing embraces a "culture of toughness". Malcolm et al. (2005) take this concern further arguing in agreeing with Volkman (2007) that the introduction of Critical Incident Stress Debriefing (Mitchell, 1988) may be a pathway through the traditional resistance shown by (male) officers to any form of psychological intervention and may be an instrument to shatter the code of silence that discourages them to reveal trauma-related problems. This, they argue would be more likely if such debriefs and follow-up services are provided by trained police peers or professionals who have a solid understanding of police culture and are respected as a result.

In terms of the need for psycho-education in police organisations as a means of encouraging timely help-seeking, Blum and Blum (2000:14) mount a clear argument that such education should include resilience training for officers, making it clear that in their view "the traditional avoidance of (police) training around resilience must be changed". There was no evidence of reticence in seeking support and informal debriefs in the Alexander (2000) study of officers involved in the retrieval of bodies after the North Sea Piper Alfa oil rig disaster outlined in Chap. 5.

6.2 Asking for Help: Data from the Interviews

There is little doubt that officers in SAPOL have been well aware of the dangers of "putting your hand up" when stressed in terms of career longevity and promotion. Said one, "Shit happens and you just get on with it. It was seen as weak to ask for help in SAPOL. If you did you were then sidelined".

A lack of trust in internal helping services such as the SAPOL Employee Assistance Programme (EAP) was also clearly expressed, "No-one went to welfare when things like that happened {critical incidents}, they leaked!" This is in line with the findings of Donnelly et al. (2015) who found that only 16.2% of the officers studied were aware of their organisation's EAP and had accessed it for support services. Another ex UK officer now in SAPOL expressed a view that involved his distrust of his EAP, "I don't trust the organisation. I wouldn't go to them if I had problems. SAPOL needs to use confidential external services, then coppers would use them". A Sergeant confirmed this after dealing with some mental health issues. In answer to the question, "Did you use the EAP?" he replied, "No! They work for SAPOL, not for our welfare. I went to an outside psych". Another retired Senior Sergeant added, "I have never spoken to anyone in the welfare section of SAPOL. There's no safe place to say, 'I'm not doing very well". This highlights the divide between those on the frontline and "SAPOL" which many officers see as a different organisation to theirs. Within the Special Task and Rescue section, the response was similar, "When {after a critical incident} the psychs ask 'do you need help?' The usual response from my team is "Nup!".

A retired Superintendent, in line with the literature, saw a clear need for change, "SAPOL needs to acknowledge the need for this kind of support. There is still a high level of discomfort around saying I need to see someone". A colleague was clear about the same issue, "You've got your mates, you need to deal with it yourself" and, "You're with your mates, they know what you're going through".

A retired Detective Senior Sergeant was extremely blunt in his response, "You survive or get out of the job". Describing the early days of his career in the 1970s, a Detective Sergeant said, "We didn't have psych units to go to (not that you would anyway), no special leave days or urgent necessity days or part-time work. You had to go to work and cope or you would get moved out". An officer diagnosed with PTSD, said from his own experience, "Police are reluctant to get help…".

A Senior Sergeant in the Major Crash unit was very clear about the results of seeking help from within SAPOL, "There is still a stigma about going to health or welfare sections. If you say I have PTSD forget your career!" Pressure also came from within the organisation in a different way as officers considered the response of their peers to such a disclosure, "My main friends were other police, I didn't want to bother them, we have a tendency not to show any weakness. When you go off on stress, you know what the others are thinking". But some officers interviewed drew attention to signs that such attitudes may be changing. Women officers have fewer concerns about showing signs of stress and taking action than their male colleagues. A veteran Senior Constable outlined how she had an "on-call" social worker with whom she made contact "when I need to". She had also had several sessions with departmental psychologists who she found "down to earth and very helpful". Another female Senior Constable was very clear about the benefits of such services, "I used to be dead set against psychologists and social workers. I was referred to a psych by my GP, which probably saved my life". A recently retired Senior Sergeant described a change in the traditional "stiff upper lip", masculine culture of SAPOL, "Some members may still think that if you put your hand up you will be discriminated against, overlooked or kicked out. There is a lot of support and empathy now".

Another told of a fortnight early in her career when she attended three sudden infant deaths. After the third tasking, deeply distressed and in tears, she was comforted by her (female) Sergeant with no suggestion that her reaction was anything but a normal response to very challenging series of events. No concerns were raised about her reaction or her subsequent duty-related performance. This may have implications for the macho "tough it out" approach, which has been a central aspect of SAPOL culture. With the progress made in the assimilation of female officers into operational policing since the 1970s[1] when male officers saw them as a burden and hoped they would be up to the challenges of the job, there is now evidence that policewomen have a softer and more realistic approach, which includes the capacity to show emotional reactions to some situations and a greater awareness of the need for self-care to foster resilience. This was clearly evidenced in the interviews with officers of both genders and revealed that it is no longer seen as necessary by most female officers to become "one of the boys" to succeed in the job. A female Senior Constable, serving in a rural area reacted to a suicide involving a young person she knew well, "I ended up sobbing behind the police car. The SAPOL blokes (her colleagues) showed no emotion". This is a sign of progress from the early days of women in uniform, when such an emotional response would have resulted in much criticism and scorn from male officers. In this case, none was given.

Doubts about the way SAPOL values its staff as individuals surfaced in many ways. One officer commented: "SAPOL sees you as an FTE[2] not a person. They are completely allergic to risk. This causes a great deal of stress. I have never spoken to anyone in the welfare section of SAPOL". And again, doubts about the usefulness of helping professionals who lack experience as police officers were expressed thus by a Senior Constable, "I don't like the present Psych unit. The psychs[3] revolve through it and are too young and don't understand Policing". In response to the question, "have you ever asked the department for help in terms of you coping with the job, or looked for help outside" some of those interviewed gave different answers.

The assumption in much of the literature and common among officers interviewed that officers don't trust their own organisation if they "put their hand up" to ask for stress-related support is not always valid, as revealed below. A retired Commissioned Officer, heavily involved in the notorious Snowtown "bodies in the barrels murders" (Marshall, 2006) pointed out progress in departmental support during particularly challenging investigations, "I had no extra psych support. I went to the interviews {debriefs} with everyone else. We had 360 degree support, a good team and great support from the Commissioner down." A Sergeant, who recently successfully returned to work after being diagnosed with a significant anxiety disorder, commented:

> I became anxious and obsessional, had to take time off. I couldn't get away from work. It was hard to talk about it being an issue for me. If I talked about it I knew I could be in trouble so I let it fester. I read a journal article that described a different form of anxiety. I did nothing for two to three years then took leave and went to doctor. It was a blur although

[1] See Chap. 3: "Feminisation of policing".

[2] "Full time equivalent".

[3] "Psychs" here refers to young psychologists currently employed by SAPOL.

> the doctor was confident that I could get help. We need to be taught more about what can happen to us so that we can get help sooner.

This is a very clear plea for access to psycho-education, perhaps a central feature in initial academy training with career-long updates.[4]

"Getting on with it" was a regular theme of the interviews, where officers, particularly those with long service in "the job" were crystal clear that acknowledging work-related stress reactions at work was never a good idea. The repercussions were clearly foreseen, and included being sidelined, being overlooked for promotion or more challenging duties, being discriminated against by colleagues, and being the subject of rumour and innuendo.

Another Officer told of a positive return to duty:

> I took two months off work. I had a really good Boss, when I returned to work, he started me with easy tasks, then I was offered a project which built up my confidence. Medication helped, it has been up and down. I had a back injury as well so I couldn't go back on the road. Psych support has been really, really helpful as has been my gym membership and access to the local swimming pool. Seeing a local psych at the beginning was difficult, so I came to Adelaide for treatment, with accommodation at the Academy and a car to travel to the psychologist's rooms. Some cops expect everyone to drop everything, I didn't. Both psychs were different. The first one used Cognitive Behaviour Therapy…set out mantras on a page showing the realities of my obsessional thinking. The second psych focussed on dealing with the stigma I felt about not being involved in "real policing" as I was depressed at that stage. He put things in context.

The "really good boss" in this officer's experience was obviously of crucial importance to this outcome.

Those interviewed confirmed the literature that describes reluctance to seek stress-related help from within police organisations, based on the culture of toughness and a macho emphasis on "being up to the job". There was, however, some evidence from the interviews that officers are often prepared to make their own external arrangements to maintain their mental health and that a minority are prepared to trust the Employee Assistance programme in seeking help with them.[5]

6.3 Asking for Help from the Psychology and Psychiatry Interviews: Themes

In addition to the 50 interviews conducted with police officers, I also interviewed a cohort of psychiatrists and psychologists who have treated officers or assessed them in the context of WorkCover claims relating to duty-related psychological injury. Specifically, three psychiatrists and three psychologists were contacted, some on the recommendation of police officers and some as the result of information given to me

---

[4] See my recommendations in the "Conclusions" section.

[5] See my "Conclusions" section, containing recommendations for change in this area.

by their professional colleagues. All volunteered to participate without hesitation. The intention of these interviews was to offer a degree of triangulation to the fifty officer's views around the attitude of SAPOL to trauma-related injuries, Work-Cover applications, treatment offered, and the perceptions of the helping professionals with regard to factors that contribute to police officers making contact with them.

Prior to the interviews commencing, participants were given a copy of the information sheet for psychiatrists and psychologists,[6] and signed the interview consent form. As with the 50 officer interviews, I set out to identify significant themes that emerged from these conversations. I began by asking the participants to outline their level of involvement with officers and the most common reasons they present.

The responses included, "Officers often present with psychological injury, major depression and PTSD. These can be the result of disciplinary issues, personal chronic exhaustion by what they have seen" said a psychiatrist. A colleague agreed, "They present with adjustment disorders, very low numbers with full PTSD. Usually work related anxiety and depression. It is usually the work environment, discipline culture and procedures. Police culture magnifies organisational issues and makes members more vulnerable".

In terms of the work environment that leads many officers into treatment, one psychologist was clear about police officer perceptions of SAPOL's attitude to work-related stress and injury and quoted officers as frequently expressing the view that, "they don't look after us, we don't expect them to". This clearly reflecting the view of many of the officers I interviewed. A psychiatrist explained that he only saw officers after they had made a Work-Cover claim asking, "Why can't they be referred before such a claim? They are alienated by then. SAPOL makes no effort to dispel this. There is often bullying and un-reasonable actions against them". He went on to give an example of a motorcycle officer after thirty years' service undergoing eight hours of psychological tests before being referred to his practice, surmising from this that, "They wanted him out!" In a clear indication of his frustration he went on, "You would hope that police psychologists are a bridge between us and SAPOL. They are not! Cops only see a psychologist if there is no Work-Cover claim. This is a diversion to keep them off Work-Cover. There is much administrative bullying". He went on, warming to his task, "SAPOL discriminates against coppers on the basis of an injury they have caused". And further stated, "SAPOL is one of the most toxic psychiatric environments!!" A similarly frustrated psychiatrist explained, "In South Australia there is no civil litigation where an employee can sue an employer for negligence". Adding that in his view "The present Work-Cover situation arose out of the 1990s when the Labor Government of the day took over the Work-Cover scheme and tried to work out ways not to be sued". He continued, "These are not malingerers, they are a decent group of people who are injured. Like veterans, they endure levels of discomfort without seeking help. In SAPOL there are substantial disincentives to putting your hand up". He added, in line with a view frequently expressed by officers I interviewed, "SAPOL fears an epidemic". Continuing, the same psychiatrist clearly

[6] See Appendix D.

expressed his view that, "The military have a higher duty of care than the police. Police protect our society from the inside".

One of the psychologists interviewed expressed a similar view, "Much of the officer stress is due to poor management issues. SAPOL is a non-caring system. It's OK if you are functioning OK, otherwise you are a broken biscuit! Once you are wounded, you don't get the support. They don't trust that you will operate well when under attack". Referring to an officer whose mouth was spat into by an offender, he added, "SAPOL brought in lawyers, wouldn't pay for medication. They are afraid of precedent". This is a very clear indicator of why officers are very hesitant to seek help from within.

A former SAPOL psychologist explained that in his view, "I saw a change in culture under ******,[7] it went from a family culture to an organisational one". Reflecting the comments above, he went on, "They don't know who you are". Later in the same interview, he repeated his view that "At the centre it's around the organisation better prioritising the well-being of their staff. SAPOL is a hard place to work because of the unrelenting high expectations. We need to get rid of non-supportive management and bullying and harassment". This concern was clearly expressed in the police officers interviewed for this research and recently in a study of the mental health of Victoria police (Cotton, 2016).

Another psychiatrist interviewed had a more positive view of SAPOL's approach to work stress-related issues, "My perception is that SAPOL are largely fantastic. I have seen some really good outcomes". He went on, "Eighty percent of my patients go back to work. Senior coppers are less likely {to go back to work} they are chronically exhausted by what they have seen". He was aware that camaraderie is important in such matters but explained that, "Support from their mates is common but senior managers don't ask 'what can we do to help?' Internal investigations are often the cause". He went on, "There is a senior management dichotomy around giving support to officers around challenging taskings". He continued in terms of the experience of many female officers he has treated, "Women's response to trauma is different. There needs to be more awareness of the damage done by harassment". With mounting frustration, he added, "The organisation has let its women down with flagrant harassment and sexual assault". Management and leadership issues within SAPOL were seen by all the clinicians interviewed as major contributors to officer stress. Commenting on what he called "the power of feedback" a psychiatrist argued that a simple "how are you guys doing?" from a senior officer after a difficult experience was worth more than a critical incident debrief. Another added, "fault finding is the norm in SAPOL. Praise is important. Good leadership inspires troops". The significance of this issue to those interviewed was further enhanced when a past SAPOL psychologist opined, "They've got to be leaders, we don't have leadership. They have played the game {conformed} to get where they are".

A psychiatrist added in the same vein, "Cops are alienated by a huge vested interest that wants it {SAPOL} not to change. There are many incompetent managers from Senior Sergeants up". Emphasising the need for change in terms of contemporary

[7] Former long-serving commissioner.

management theory around "top down" management, a psychiatrist was clear, "The tone of any school is set by the Principal. SAPOL is no different! The top needs to respond to the new order". He added optimistically, "If they did so upper management would be impressed with the reduction in Work-Cover costs". Identifying effective support for and trust in the competence of its officers as good leadership another psychiatrist added, "SAPOL has a lot of extremely good people who need good leadership and support".

A SAPOL psychologist, now retired, was forthright in his view that "SAPOL needs to put more energy into looking after their employees, there is no support from upstairs. I get stories {from officers} it's all gone to God and the Devil in SAPOL". Referring to his view that micromanagement and risk aversion are real issues, he went on, "Coppers need to be allowed to do their job". He continued, "I've only seen one copper who was crazy. They are really nice people. Poor management is responsible for what has happened to them". "It's always complaints about the bosses!" This comment could not more clearly express those of the officers interviewed. A change in the culture of management in SAPOL is seen as long overdue.

Prevention and early detection of negative responses to critical incidents and ongoing stress were high priorities for the clinicians interviewed. Commenting on present practice one said, "Annual reviews are effective for some, but is there a better way? The concept is good as are debriefs after critical incidents. Compelling people to participate in both is counter-productive. Helping professionals should be highly visible at such times". In line with debriefing best practice he went on, "We should get their names after critical incidents and follow up later. The power of someone being there for them is crucial to resilience". Such an approach, if adopted across SAPOL would inevitably impact positively on the present fear of "putting your hand up" and its inevitable negative consequences.

Recruitment practices were seen by many of the clinicians as being of crucial importance. A former police psychologist pointed out, "Our job was debriefing, training, personal counselling and selection of suitable cadets. In terms of recruitment, we looked for personality and emotional strength, stability in home life, attitudes to the job and responses to previous trauma". Another colleague added, "Preventative actions are crucial in recruitment and selection. How do you scaffold people in the first twenty four months? We need to promote Post Traumatic Growth not PTSD. You need to reward senior cops for prioritising these things. It won't open the floodgates, it's all about training and scaffolding".

Said one very experienced clinician, "The holy grail is early detection, and individual understanding and a lot of resilience training. There needs to be a skills based approach to training", again expressing strong support for the recommendations of much research into the importance of a profound cultural change in the present "command and control" (Cotton, 2016) approaches to management in SAPOL and most "democratic policing" (Manning, 2015) organisations.

6.4 Treatment

All of the clinicians interviewed made reference to their treatment practices and to positive outcomes in terms of officers returning to work. A wider knowledge of such positive outcomes across SAPOL might well encourage officers to acknowledge trauma-related issues with less discomfort than at present. One psychiatrist began his comments in a cautionary mode around the challenges of offering psychological services and support to police officers, "Coppers make terrible patients. There is an absolute denial of discomfort and fear". Another in reference to what he and some of the literature call the "trauma industry" commented that "Because of advances in our understanding of brain chemistry and structure we are better able to understand how social interventions help recovery". As an example of such outcomes, he commented, "Such interventions might include the benefit to operational resilience that comes from looking into the eyes of your dog".

Exposure-based treatment approaches were favoured by the clinicians interviewed, with frequent reference to the effectiveness of cognitive behavioural interventions resulting in high levels of return to operational duties. One psychologist explained in terms of his use of a CBT approach and exposure therapy, "Unresolved trauma is stored in the body. The body keeps the score".

A psychiatrist who has worked with SAPOL officers for 30 years was clear about his treatment approach, which consisted of three components:

1. Geography: remove them from their situation.
2. Stop GP medication and fix sleep disturbance.
3. Back into the workplace.

He added, "I don't use much medication. Most of my patients are on no medication at all". Others advocated a combination of drug and psychotherapy, arguing that prolonged exposure therapy works well for veterans of military conflict and also is effective for police officers. Debriefs conducted by well-trained and respected police peers were considered effective after critical incidents, but several clinicians added that if non-police de-briefers were used, they "need to know about policing". Another added in this vein, "Most professionals have never faced an angry man".

Explaining his approach, a psychologist added, "PTSD is not anxiety, more a dissociative disorder. I look for the dis-association and a safe place to explore. There are many non-specific factors, it's about what they {the officers) bring to it". Approaching treatment in this way, if promoted by SAPOL in police language and avoiding the use of clinical terms, would greatly encourage officers who may be afraid of a PTSD diagnosis. Looking for a "safe place to explore" is a strategy that once effectively employed, would encourage less anxiety about trauma-related reactions and the perils of "putting your hand up" resulting in early interventions where necessary.

A combination of drug and psychotherapy that is evidenced-based, and exposure-based therapies were the staple treatment modalities for one psychologist, who when questioned about the efficacy of Mitchell-based critical incident debriefs commented,

"CISD? The data suggests it doesn't work. I support peer initiated debriefs, camaraderie and moral support, pre-event briefings and debriefs embedded in police teams. These approaches are most effective when they also have professional back-up". He added, agreeing with his colleague quoted above, "Professionals who do this work, need to know about the mission of policing". Sergeants, he opined, given appropriate training, would ideally fill the role of peer-based debriefs and support.[8]

Exposure-based treatments were also preferred by a psychiatrist, who added in reference to removing officers from the front line during treatment, "There are many safe roles within SAPOL for police while they recover. There needs to be more workplace planning in this regard". One psychiatrist with many years of experience in this field was very clear about the efficacy of some forms of medication, "Everyone I see has failed to respond to anti-depressants. They are a splint around the broken brain".

In terms of preventative measures and a more positive approach to trauma within SAPOL one psychiatrist argued, "There is a need for psycho-education around trauma, coping strategies that work, a treatment flow chart that reframes the trauma incident. For example, I worked with an officer who after an operational critical incident was much traumatised. He said 'the girl died in my arms', I responded, I bet her parents would have been pleased you were there!".

In summary, the psychologists and psychiatrists interviewed with one exception were very clear in their criticism of SAPOL's response to officers who "put their hands up" at times of mental health challenge and ask the organisation for help. Most psychological injuries were inflicted by the organisation itself in their view, including "administrative bullying", one describing SAPOL as "one of the most toxic psychiatric environments!" This is a bleak picture of an organisation frozen by its fear of a PTSD epidemic, where no psycho-education around risk and resilience is offered and "much of the officer stress is due to poor management issues". Citing the case (above) where a female officer who contracted an untreatable viral infection after an offender spat into her mouth, a psychologist explained how SAPOL brought in lawyers and refused to pay for medication. This he assumed clearly demonstrated the organisation's fear of what he called "precedent". The clinicians pointed to disengaged senior managers who found giving positive feedback very difficult although said one, "a how are you going?" from a Senior Officer after a critical incident was worth much more than a debrief in terms of the officer's resilience and well-being. Pointing to fault finding and risk management as indicators of "command and control" SAPOL management, several of those interviewed expressed very clear views that such approaches needed to change, with resulting improvements in the mental health of officers and significant savings in WorkCover payments. "The power of someone being there {after critical incidents} is crucial to resilience".

These clinicians see the need for urgent, radical change in management, support, early intervention, psychoeducation and resilience training in SAPOL. They are clearly frustrated by the SAPOL response to stress-related issues among their officers. They, on behalf of their clients, see an urgent need for SAPOL to recognise the need

[8] See my Recommendations section.

for change. They are in a very good position to hold such a view. Said one, "SAPOL needs to look at the military. They have a deep understanding of these injuries".

6.5 What Have We Learnt?

It is clear from both the interview data and the international literature that police officers largely look after themselves as far as their mental health and well-being are concerned. SAPOL officers are no exception, with the officers interviewed expressing a clear view that self-care is their only realistic option. "They don't look after us, we don't expect them to", was the most common response, in this case, quoted by a psychologist offering treatment and support. There were some exceptions, with officers fortunate enough to have sympathetic managers giving them access to services and alternative, lighter duties to aid recovery.

The literature tends to underestimate individual police officers capacity to look after themselves even while "embracing a culture of toughness" (Hesketh et al., 2014). However, when an officer is struggling with mental health issues relating to duty-related traumatic events or more likely management-related stressors, there are very good reasons to remain silent.

There is no evidence of early intervention approaches to well-being in SAPOL, nor any relating to basic psycho-education that may identify and deal with early indicators of more serious challenges to well-being. Resilience training is absent from the police academy curriculum and is only rarely discussed in in-service training. This silence clearly discourages individuals from acknowledging exhaustion or early indicators of trauma-related problems. It is clear that SAPOL has no discernible mental health strategy.

The officers interviewed, as well as the clinicians who treat them were agreed on these issues. The latter showing signs of significant anger and frustration at the way SAPOL treats members who are facing mental health issues. It is "a non-caring system" they said, where "SAPOL discriminates against coppers on the basis of an injury they have caused", and further, "SAPOL is one of the most toxic psychiatric environments!" The way officers are managed is at the centre of these criticisms. "Command and control" approach to management is the SAPOL norm where senior officers are risk averse and refrain from giving positive feedback even in the face of the most confronting operational tasks. Officers, therefore, suffer in silence or seek help and support outside of the organisation expressing distrust in Employee Assistance programmes that "leak" and police psychologists who have a limited understanding of policing. As many of the clinicians interviewed pointed out a radical change in SAPOL's approach to these issues would result in huge savings in WorkCover and treatment costs rather than an uncontrollable outbreak of PTSD, which senior SAPOL management appears to expect.

6.6 Where Next?

SAPOL and similar police organisations in Australia and around the globe face a major challenge in this area. Officers clearly understand the negative career implications of asking the department for help in the face of trauma-related problems. PTSD among them is rare, despite the fact that most take care of themselves and each other rather than engaging with organisational support. Senior managers who adhere to traditional para–military "command and control" approaches and who subscribe to risk aversity above the well-being of their troops are seen as the centre of the problem by both officers and clinicians who were interviewed for this research. SAPOL must develop a mental health strategy that is based on the fostering and maintenance of resilience, the capacity to bounce back after out of the ordinary duty-related events and to "keep well" over a policing career. Psycho-education around risks and early indicators of mental health issues, easy access to support services, both internal and external to SAPOL without disadvantage or discrimination and an overall level of encouragement for officers to seek help and support when they need it most are at the centre of such essential change. The clinical psychologists and psychiatrists interviewed were very clear about these issues and SAPOL would benefit from open consultation with them.

Female officers are more inclined to acknowledge their need for support services, and this should be acknowledged and encouraged by management. Women police may hold the key to a significant change in their organisation's approach to trauma-related issues. It is acceptable for female officers to be emotionally impacted by duties involving out of the ordinary stressors according to those interviewed. Some female officers see changes in the SAPOL culture, which offer effective support and treatment to those who "put their hand up" although this was not evident in the views of the clinical psychologists and psychiatrists who were interviewed. Surviving or getting out of "the job" is the only option for many at much human and financial cost. This is a state of affairs that cannot continue, particularly in the light of the widespread awareness among police and other first responders of the perils of PTSD.

Often officers make their own support arrangements linking up with helping professionals external to SAPOL to ensure their resilience. Others are referred to such services by general practitioners who are often the first port of call for those experiencing trauma-related issues. If you are fortunate enough to have a senior manager who understands such issues and is able to arrange light duties and access to support services your outcomes will be more positive.

The Police Association that boasts a 98% membership of SAPOL officers could well be at the centre of such changes to management culture. Their open support for this research in the context of SAPOL disapproval is a promising sign. Officers will inevitably encounter challenges to their resilience, particularly if they are long-serving. Exhaustion, more often caused by management culture rather than trauma exposure, is a real issue and should not be confused with PTSD.

This research confirms through interviews with officers and clinicians the depth of the need for change within SAPOL particularly with regard to addressing the stigma surrounding the recognition of mental health issues in policing and the provision of training and information that offer officers opportunities to assess their own need for additional training and information around coping with the traumas of policing. The level of frustration expressed by the clinicians interviewed is significant in its clarity about the nature and importance of such changes in terms of the well-being of SAPOL members. The required changes are cultural and practical. The human benefits and fiscal savings, should such change take place, would be massive. Asking for help should be natural and encouraged, not a career-ending risk.[9]

References

Alexander, D. (2000). Debriefing and body recovery: Police in a civilian disaster. In *Psychological debriefing: Theory, practice and evidence* (pp. 118–130).

Blum, L. E., & Blum, L. N. (2000). *Force under pressure: How cops live and why they die.* Lantern Books.

Chae, M. H., & Boyle, D. J. (2013). Police suicide: Prevalence, risk, and protective factors. *Policing: An International Journal of Police Strategies & Management, 36*(1), 91–118.

Cotton, P. (2016). Victoria Police Mental Health Review. An independent review into the mental health and well-being of Victoria Police employees. Australia.

Donnelly, E., et al. (2015). Law enforcement officers and employee assistance programs. *Policing: An International Journal of Police Strategies & Management, 38*(2), 206–220.

Flannery, R. B. (2015). Treating psychological trauma in first responders: A multi-modal paradigm. *Psychiatric Quarterly, 86*(2), 261–267.

Hesketh, I., et al. (2014). Keeping the Peelian spirit: Resilience and spirituality in policing. *The Police Journal, 87*(3), 154–166.

Malcolm, A. S., et al. (2005). Critical incident stress debriefing and law enforcement: An evaluative review. *Brief Treatment and Crisis Intervention, 5*(3), 261.

Manning, P. K. (2015). *Democratic policing in a changing world.* Routledge.

Marshall, D. (2006). *Killing for pleasure: The definitive story of the snowtown serial murders.* Random House.

Mitchell, J. T. (1988). CISML: A new era in crisis intervention. International Critical Incident Stress Foundation.

Rees, B., & Smith, J. (2008). Breaking the silence: The traumatic circle of policing. *International Journal of Police Science & Management, 10*(3), 267–279.

Volkman, V. R. E. (2007). *Traumatic incident reduction and critical incident stress management.* Loving, Healing press.

[9] These issues will be directly addressed in the recommendations contained in the "Conclusions" section of this thesis.

Chapter 7
Sleep. The Elixir of Resilience

Abstract Shift work is notoriously bad for Police Officer's health. With the added ingredient of trauma, this becomes a significant challenge for individual officers. This chapter examines the relationship between sustaining sleep and resilience in policing, highlighting contemporary sleep research as it applies to policing as well as the lived experience of the officers interviewed as they describe career-long attempts to live with poor sleep patterns and the benefits of maintaining effective ones. Again, police organisations offer little to assist with this intensely practical issue. The New South Wales police autobiographies provide stark insight into deteriorating sleep patterns as a precursor to the onset of debilitating trauma reactions. This chapter concludes with suggestions as to how sleep research might better inform rostering and the management of operational, shift working officers.

Well-being for many South Australian Police Officers depends on a range of factors including their individual resilience,[1] the steps they have taken in their personal and professional lives to keep well,[2] the extent of SAPOL's capacity to offer assistance when needed[3] and a range of health-related issues including sustaining, reinvigorating, regular sleep. When consideration was given to the "shape" of the interviews, it was clear that sleep patterns were of central interest in that disturbed sleep and nightmares are indicators of stress both at the level of the DSM diagnostic criteria and at the "sub threshold" levels. Good career-long sleep patterns would, it was thought, indicate effective coping mechanisms and self-care strategies contributing to resilience and general well-being. As well, the ability to accommodate shift work is of significant importance. There is little doubt that consistent patterns of sustaining sleep are a significant protective factor against negative and destructive trauma responses (Âkerstedt, 2006; Åkerstedt, 2003; Calhoun et al., 1999; Crary, 2013; Dement & Vaughan, 1999). All of the officers interviewed for this research were very aware of the importance of sleep to their overall health and revealed how they had dealt with sleep-related challenges throughout their careers.

---

[1] See Chap. 8.

[2] See Chap. 5.

[3] See Chap. 2.

A. Paterson, *Trauma and Resilience in Contemporary Australian Policing*,
https://doi.org/10.1007/978-981-16-4416-0_7

The psychologists and psychiatrists interviewed for this study were all very clear that reinstating and maintaining good sleep patterns were a critical factor in the treatment of officers suffering unwelcome responses to stress. Said one, "My first task is in treating a Police Officer referred to me is to stop GP prescribed medication and fix sleep disturbance". Often such referrals resulted in very positive outcomes as reinstated sleep patterns allowed such officers to return to their duties with added energy and enthusiasm.

7.1 Sleep, the Informing Literature

The Diagnostic Statistics Manual of Mental Disorders 5 (American Psychiatric Association, 2013) in its summary of PTSD symptoms refers to consistent sleep disturbance, the inability to fall and stay asleep, night sweats and recurrent nightmares as indicators of a likely PTSD diagnosis. I asked all of the officers interviewed about the quality of their sleep over their careers with a view to the impact of traumatic duty-related events and shift work. All responded with little hesitation, making a clear distinction between the impact on their sleep patterns of traumatic events and that of shift work. Judith Herman (1997:36) is very clear about the impact of PTSD on sleep patterns, "People with posttraumatic stress disorder take longer to fall asleep, are more sensitive to noise and awaken more frequently than ordinary people". The policing literature abounds with references to sleep disturbance as a central component and indicator of unwanted trauma responses (Amaranto et al., 2003; Blandford, 2014; Blum, 2000; Burke, 2016; Carroll, 2017/2018).

The autobiographical accounts considered in this research all refer to extremes of insomnia, disturbed sleep and nightmares (Horner, 2011; McKay, 2005; Rogers, 1999; Sparkes, 2013; Neil, 2014). Often the nightmares involved profoundly disturbing images of assault on family members committed by the officer him/herself. All reported high levels of exhaustion brought on by their over-commitment to their duties and the demands of on-call operational responsibilities. Such levels of exhaustion led to a cycle of self-medication with alcohol and prescription drugs and a spiral of depression and suicidal ideation, leading in all these biographical accounts to a PTSD diagnosis.

Pietrzak et al. (2014) in a study of World Trade Centre responders 8 years after the 2001 attacks found that sleep disturbance was a significant factor for those still suffering PTSD symptoms and that in terms of other responses (anxiety, hypervigilance, irritability and problems with concentration), good sleep was an important key to recovery.

Consistent, refreshing, uninterrupted sleep is an obvious component of well-being, but it is rarely listed as a protective factor in the trauma literature related to policing. A psychiatrist interviewed as part of my research was very clear about the importance of sleep to well-being and recovery, "Getting them {he police officers being treated or assessed} to sleep properly is my first priority. I usually stop the sleep medication prescribed by well-meaning general practitioners and then work with them offering strategies to fix their sleep disturbance. Then we move on from there". Such an approach acknowledges the central importance of sleep to resilience and in these cases to treatment and recovery.

In a qualitative study exploring Royal Canadian Mounted Police Officers involved in the investigation of child exploitation pornography, Burns et al. (2008) concluded that the evidentiary images regularly viewed had a direct impact on sleep patterns. Interviewees reported nightmares and flashbacks as well as problems falling asleep even when extremely fatigued after a long confronting day at work. Strategies employed by the RCMP to counter such experiences included, regular debriefs, viewing confronting images in the morning to allow time for them to dissipate before going off shift, limiting time viewing such material and undertaking intense exercise and yoga to aid natural relaxation and sleep. Relaxation strategies are commonly recommended in sleep literature, utilising the practice of breathing regulation, which is often applied to falling and staying asleep (Curran et al., 2013; Emerson, 2015; Follette, 2014; Gilmartin, 2002; Harms, 2015; Schiraldi, 2011). Some officers interviewed for my research were well aware of the benefits to their sleep patterns available through such practices as revealed in the interview data below.

Being on call and the challenges of shift work were referred to by many of the officers interviewed. This too is a common theme in the policing and trauma literature where researchers focus on the impact on well-being of long career periods of interrupted sleep (Littles, 2011; Stone, 1999; Violanti, 2014; Warner, 2005). Gilmartin (2002)and also make the point that officers who go off duty and return home with levels of hypervigilance that are a survival tool when on duty, need to develop skills around relaxation and mindfulness that make their sleep beneficial both professionally and personally. Peters (2009) agrees, arguing, that the capacity to relax and sleep well are crucial ingredients to the development of resilience, particularly for those involved in policing. Peters goes on to state that relaxation, exercise, sleep and diet are the four critically important factors in the effective management of stress.

No officer interviewed reported any departmental intervention in this important area by way of the provision of sleep-related training, support or information. Most officers clearly had learned strategies, effective or otherwise from their own experience or that of colleagues. This could well represent an opportunity for academic sleep researchers to make a significant contribution to police well-being and the prevention of stress-related illness and burnout.[4]

William Dement, described by reviewers as a pioneer in sleep medicine in his "The promise of sleep" (1999), draws attention to research outcomes that indicate the critical importance of restful sleep in predicting a long, healthy life. Such sleep he argues, outweighs the importance of diet, regular exercise and heredity. The reasons for our need of regular sleep are less than clear (Krueger, Obál, & Fang, 1999) but include the obvious benefits that accrue to our sense of well-being and cognitive function. Shift work (Âkerstedt, 2006; Åkerstedt, 2003; Sack et al., 2007; Sack et al., 2007) creates significant problems in terms of consistent effective sleep patterns, thus having the potential to be a threat to the well-being of Police Officers who work

[4] See recommendations in my "Conclusions" section.

regular shifts. Impact on alertness, mood, the propensity to be involved in accidents as a result of poor sleep, are all factors considered by sleep researchers. Åkerstedt (2003, 2006) goes further, arguing that long-term shift work may result in chronic insomnia as well as increased levels of vulnerability to stress reactions beyond the normal range. Many of the officers interviewed referred to difficulties accommodating night shifts. Female officers, in line with research outcomes (Åkerstedt, 2003; Sack et al., 2007) may experience more such discomfort related to shift work than their male colleagues, in part because of their domestic responsibilities. Increasing age is also seen as a negative factor in dealing with shift-affected sleep issues, due partly it seems, to accrued health-related issues among shift workers (Krueger et al., 1999; Sack et al., 2007).

Significant levels of physical fitness, abstaining from alcohol and stimulants such as caffeine close to bed time, creating a quiet environment for sleep, the use of short naps and sympathetic rosters where, for example, night shifts are placed at the end of morning /afternoon/night shift rotations are all seen as positive factors in the maintenance of healthy lifestyles in the context of shift work. Tilley and Empson (1978) add another dimension relevant to my research, suggesting that REM (rapid eye movement) sleep has a role in consolidating memory, which may have relevance in terms of PTSD theory that suggests intrusive, uncontrolled memory (flashbacks) is a significant symptom of a trauma diagnosis (Brewin, 2003; Morris, 2015; Young, 1997). If consolidation of memory also has a controlling function, then sleep is of great significance in preventing as well as treating trauma-related disorders.

Crary (2013) mounts a complex argument, pointing out that in his view the concept of sleep is under threat from "late capitalism". In what might be good news for shift workers he predicts that present military research into the need for sleep among combat soldiers may result in prolonged periods of activity that might be sleep free without the assistance of drugs. Crary also offers hope for those such as police in stressful occupations opining that, "Sleep is a remission, a release from the constant continuity of all the threads in which one is enmeshed while waking" (P. 126). The officers I interviewed agreed.

7.2 Sleep Problems and Exhaustion: The Autobiographies

Alan Sparkes (Sparkes, 2013:140) clearly describes his confronting dreams and his inability to sleep. As his post-traumatic stress symptoms increased, he had nightmares in which he had stabbed to death his wife and daughter. These were the source of profound anxiety and fear for him, prompting thoughts of suicide to protect his loved ones from the possibility that his dreams might become reality.

Esther Mckay (2005:265/227) gives an account of nightmares describing a particularly disturbing one where she was "lying naked on the morgue table". Belinda Neil (2014:2) describes "the long working hours with no time to recover from one traumatic incident to the next" and continues, "I was falling apart, exhausted and forgetful".

Geoff Bernasconi (Mckay, 2010:58/59) is "mentally and physically exhausted" and "fatigue was ever-present, especially on long road trips when Geoff would struggle to stay alert". These were officers nearing the limit of their resilience, unsupported by their organisation, isolated and nearing the end of their police careers.

7.3 Sleep: The Data from the Interviews

The majority of officers interviewed had a clear view of the importance of consistent, sustaining sleep in the context of their sometimes challenging duties and the need to maintain their physical health. Most had experienced sleep adjustment problems in early career, often involving difficulty in going to sleep directly related to confronting experiences and directly related to their duties. For most, such issues did not persist as they became accustomed to such challenges and developed strategies to counter them. This is well expressed by a Detective Senior Constable who commented, "I sleep well, I can sleep anywhere. I've dealt with a hell of a lot of disfigurement, it doesn't affect me. I remember every single one. I had nightmares for the first eighteen months, then they stopped and haven't come back". Adjustments in early career such as this were reported frequently as officers made the transition from civilian life into policing. The skills developed were obviously effective, in this case, creating a foundation for career-long resilience is evidenced by sustaining patterns of sleep.

The ability to learn how to deal with confronting images to facilitate sleep was frequently mentioned although detail as to how that was achieved was often lacking. "I'm not predisposed to that kind of reaction" was typical. Some reported diminishing thoughts about confronting cases as time passed, which involved strategies that prevented dwelling on such events.[5] A Detective Senior Sergeant, recently retired from the Major Crime Squad, was also clear about the impact of crime scenes and confronting images as well as his capacity to deal effectively with such images, "I've never had a real issue with going to sleep, although the first few nights after a bad homicide I had trouble going to sleep. I still remember a lot of these things, but I don't think about it too often". Such a response, categorised in the DSM 5 (2013:280) as "Acute stress disorder", was often described in this way by the officers interviewed for this study. A few days were usually enough for officers to deal with the "intrusive symptoms" that impacted on their ability to sleep without interruption. Such temporary disturbance was also reported, thus "I have had periods when it's been difficult due to the impact of situations that stick in your head for a while. You think about them a lot for a week or so, then less following week and so on". In this sense, these officers had learned that this process is "normal" and had accepted it as part of their capacity to deal with such situations testifying for them to their resilience.

A retired Chief Superintendent referred to the early stages of his career and its experiences, thus "During the first five days of my career in traffic, on my first evening

[5] I address this in detail in Chap. 5, "Coping.".

shift I was ordered to go down to the morgue with two bodies, one in a coffin, other young child killed by Mr Whippy van.[6] I stripped the body. I had never touched a body before. I had lots of sleepless nights at that time…somehow you did it!" This confirms the view shared by his colleagues (above) that such issues are a phase that most officers pass through as they gain experience in their chosen profession and is evidence of developing resilience through such experiences. There was also clear evidence that long-serving officers had become accomplished at "sleeping well, sleeping anywhere". This classifies positive sleep as a "protective factor", a learned and developing skill that enhances a policing career. Another Commissioned Officer, after describing a shooting incident early in his career, in response to the question, "do you sleep well?" responded, "Not back then, but sleep is always something I've been good at", suggesting again that the ability to sleep well is a skill that came with career experience of trauma and a developing capacity over time to deal effectively with such incidents. A recently promoted Inspector has similarly developed the capacity to create distance between himself and such experiences, "I have always been able to sleep after dealing with dead bodies. I am able to separate myself. I get over things quickly. I remember dealing with the death of a fifteen year old girl who had tripped over. I took a statement from the family. A whole host of things like that". This is not the testimony of an officer under siege from the ongoing stressors of the job, but rather evidence of the ongoing development of coping skills over the length of a police career.

References to practising meditation skills such as yoga, engaging in a healthy lifestyle where exercise and good food are central ingredients are also common, along with suggestions that such issues should be central to recruit and ongoing in-service police training. "I sleep like a log and do yoga two to three times a week" said a Senior Constable of over 30 years in SAPOL. She went on, "if you wanted to teach resilience, yoga and such like in SAPOL the trainers would have to be from within SAPOL", referring to the need for such trainers to be able to "sell" such approaches in the context of a notoriously cynical police culture around similar strategies.[7] The inclusion of sleep-related topics in initial training and on-going in service courses in the context of SAPOL's present approach mental health policy would indeed constitute a significant challenge.

Being "easy going" and similar personality traits was also seen by those interviewed as an explanation for sustaining, consistent sleep patterns. A Senior Constable with 8 years of patrol experience also reported healthy patterns of sleep offering no insight into such an achievement apart from his laid back approach to his duties, "I have no sleeping problems on the whole. I sometimes think about what's happened but am pretty OK with this area. I guess I am pretty easy going". This officer typically refers to his capacity to deal with confronting duty-related experiences but supplies little detail as to how such skills were developed and sustained. A recovery diver with STAR group also reported a similar attribute, "I've never had a dream about floating bodies. I'm not predisposed to those kinds of reactions".

[6] A mobile ice cream shop, prolific in the 1970s in Australia.

[7] See my recommendations in the "Conclusions" section.

Working in the challenging field of child exploitation investigation, a Detective Sergeant reported sleep problems related not to her duties in that area but to her apprehension about giving evidence in Court. I asked her, "Do you sleep well?" She replied, "Yes I do, except the night before trials". A colleague reported frequent interrupted sleep, linked to organisational frustrations. "I have trouble sleeping from three to four am sometimes. I am frustrated with the organization". Such frustrations are commonly reported as a frequent source of stress (Stinchcomb, 2004; Violanti, 2014).

Some Sergeants, with an awareness of the need to sustain the well-being of their teams, conducted debriefs, including advice about possible temporary sleep disruption, after suicides and other challenging incidents. Preventative approaches such as these were routine for a patrol Senior Sergeant who out of concern for the well-being of his team had adopted a self-taught debriefing strategy, "I always debrief staff after difficult jobs, after a suicide or other distressing incident. I talk about what might happen to them with sleeping patterns and emotions. I notice when team members go quiet and follow up with them then. The Sergeant's position is very important in this area". This is a clue to the way in which less experienced officers develop resilience in their career trajectories. Middle managers undertake these strategies without training, basing what they do on "common sense". Basic training for SAPOL managers at this level would contribute significantly to their confidence in offering such support.[8]

A long-serving Detective Senior Sergeant was very clear about his overall approach to maintaining his fitness and well-being, "My healthy existence has helped, and I've always had good support from my family. My life and career have not been without its ups and downs, but I have come out a much wiser person and could evaluate situations more easily. I always slept well after difficult experiences". The contributing factors to levels of resilience such as this are described here in terms of social support and a consistent regime of exercise and sensible diet. Challenges have been met and the result is growth, increased skill and a sense of achievement. Another officer was similarly clear about his capacity to sleep indicating his lack of reliance on self-medication over a long career, "I don't have a problem with sleeping, even after night shift. I don't know why that is…I don't drink or smoke, take no medication…I know some colleagues hit the bottle, I never have". Similarly skilled in sleep, a retired Superintendent with a broad experience of operational duties including STAR group, in answer to the question, "Have you ever had sleeping problems?" Responded, "I never had trouble sleeping" suggesting significant levels of resilience and coping skills that may well be innate. A retired Detective Chief Inspector was similarly positive about his sleeping patterns, again referring to shift work responding, "It never burdened me, I slept as well as you can when you are involved in shift work". A senior officer who spent many operational years on call responded similarly, "I was lucky, I had no major sleep problems, being on call was OK, I could wake up, make a decision and go straight back to sleep, although seven nightshifts straight was always difficult. My wife was a nurse". The latter comment suggests that this officer had benefitted from his wife's shared experience of shift

[8] See my recommendations in the "Conclusions" section.

work, even though the experience of night shift, as with all officers interviewed, was a consistent challenge.

Those interviewed who had ongoing sleep problems accepted them and got on with their careers. Shift work was a part of such acceptance, "I hated night shift with a passion. I always had a bad week before" and "I catch up (with sleep) on RDO's" {rostered days off} and "I didn't realise how bad nightshift was until I stopped" being typical. Such difficulties are described with levels of acceptance. They are not career challenging, rather accepted as part of "the job". Another officer describing a long career in policing in Australia and the UK was similarly resigned, "I have always had poor sleep". Others who also had less than acceptable experiences of healthy sleep patterns including the perils of shift work, reporting, "I have the odd nightmare about a guy with a mobile phone who starts shooting. I usually got enough sleep although I didn't realise how bad nightshift was until I stopped". Some reported a career-long struggle with sleep issues, responding to the question, "How do you sleep?" directly, "Pretty shit! At most six hours a night, I catch up on rostered days off". Similarly accepting of sleep issues, a Senior Constable said, "I'm an insomniac, I try to get eight hours sleep, I had nightmares as a kid "adding with reference to a nightmare commonly reported in the literature, "I have the rubber gun nightmare occasionally now". The classic "rubber gun" nightmare, where, under threat, an officer's firearm becomes rubbery and useless, was mentioned by only two officers, frequent experiences of such disturbances to sleep were not reported by the majority of the 50 officers interviewed.

7.4 What This Research Reveals

Consistent, sustaining sleep is recognised as of critical importance to well-being, particularly in the context of shift work and first responder experiences. Officers interviewed for this study revealed a range of strategies they employed to stay well as well as the absence of sleep disruption that may qualify them for a trauma-related diagnosis. This was achieved in the absence of organisational input into their well-being and was more likely the result of experience and cultural input from colleagues. Even those who acknowledged ongoing poor sleep were able to compensate and remain resilient.

7.5 Where Next?

There is an opportunity here for SAPOL to make a direct and inexpensive contribution to the well-being of its troops by gathering and making available information and assistance around good sustaining sleep from recruitment to retirement and beyond. Sleep researchers have much to offer, all that SAPOL needs to do is seek their involvement.

Sustaining sleep is a skill that those interviewed either acquired through experience or through genetic inheritance. Those who lacked such an advantage accepted troubled sleep as a price they paid for being in "the job" devising strategies such as sleeping on RDO's or simply putting up with their lot. The majority had learned to sleep well, again in the absence of input from SAPOL, this is being a significant indicator of their resilience.

References

Âkerstedt, T. (2006). Psychosocial stress and impaired sleep. *Scandinavian Journal of Work, Environment & Health* 493–501.

Åkerstedt, T. (2003). Shift work and disturbed sleep/wakefulness. *Occupational Medicine, 53*(2), 89–94.

Amaranto, E., et al. (2003). Police stress interventions. *Brief Treatment and Crisis Intervention, 3*(1), 47.

American Psychiatric Association. (2013). *Diagnostic and statistical manual of mental disorders (DSM-5®)*. American Psychiatric Pub.

Blandford, T. (2014). *A dented badge: Tales from the street*. self-published.

Blum, L. E., & Blum, L. N. (2000). *Force under pressure: How cops live and why they die*. Lantern Books.

Burke, R. J. (2016). *Stress in Policing: Sources*. Routledge.

Burns, C. M., et al. (2008). The emotional impact on and coping strategies employed by police teams investigating internet child exploitation. *Traumatology, 14*(2), 20.

Brewin, C. (2003). *Posttraumatic stress disorder: Malady or myth?* Yale University Press.

Calhoun, L. G., et al. (1999). *Facilitating posttraumatic growth: A clinician's guide*. Routledge.

Calhoun, L. G., & Tedeschi, R.G.*Posttraumatic growth in clinical practice* 1–22.

Carroll, M. (2017). "Head notes" A social and emotional well- being/mental health initiative for South Australian police officers. Police Association of South Australia. Adelaide, SA Government and SAPOL.

Carroll, M. (2018) "A cop in the family" Police Association of South Australia. Adelaide, SA Government and SAPOL.

Crary, J. (2013). *24/7: Late capitalism and the ends of sleep*. Verso Books.

Curran, L. A., et al. (2013). *101 trauma-informed interventions: Activities, exercises and assignments to move the client and therapy forward*. PESI Publishing & Media.

Dement, W. C., & Vaughan, C. (1999). *The promise of sleep: A pioneer in sleep medicine explores the vital connection between health, happiness, and a good night's sleep*. Delacorte.

Emerson, D. (2015). *Trauma-sensitive yoga in therapy: Bringing the body into treatment*. WW Norton & Company.

Follette, V. M. (2014). *Mindfulness-oriented interventions for trauma: Integrating contemplative practices*. Guilford Publications.

Gilmartin, K. M. (2002). Emotional survival for law enforcement. *ES Press, PMB, 233*, 2968.

Harms, L. (2015). *Understanding trauma and resilience*. Palgrave Macmillan.

Herman, J. L. (1997). *Trauma and recovery*. Basic books.

Horner, P. (2011). *Jack Knife: The crashing of a policeman—NSW police and PTSD*. Australia, Zeus Publications.

Krueger, J. M., et al. (1999). Why we sleep: A theoretical view of sleep function. *Sleep Medicine Reviews, 3*(2), 119–129.

Littles, M. (2011). *The Police Wife: Bullets in the washing machine*. USA: Self.

Mckay, E. (2005). *Crime Scene-True stories from the life of a crime scene investigator.* Viking (Penguin) Australia.

Mckay, E. (2010). *Forensic investigator.* Viking (Penguin) Australia.

Morris, D. J. (2015). *The evil hours: A biography of post-traumatic stress disorder.* Health Affairs.

Neil, B. (2014). *Under siege.* Harlequin Mira.

Peters, R. F. (2009). *Police under pressure. (A donkey on the edge).* HEAS Publications.

Pietrzak, R., et al. (2014). Dimensional structure and course of post-traumatic stress symptomatology in World Trade Center responders. *Psychological Medicine, 44*(10), 2085–2098.

Rogers, L. K. (1999). *PostTraumatic Stress Disorder: A police officer's report.* Proctor Publications.

Sack, R. L., et al. (2007). Circadian rhythm sleep disorders: Part II, advanced sleep phase disorder, delayed sleep phase disorder, free-running disorder, and irregular sleep-wake rhythm. *Sleep, 30*(11), 1484–1501.

Schiraldi, G. R. (2011). *The complete guide to resilience: Why it matters how to build it and maintain it.* Resilience Training International.

Stinchcomb, J. B. (2004). Searching for stress in all the wrong places: Combating chronic organizational stressors in policing. *Police Practice and Research, 5*(3), 259–277.

Stone, V. (1999). *Cops don't cry: A book of help and hope for police families.* Creative Bound.

Sparkes, A. (2013). *The cost of bravery.* Penguin Group, Australia

Tilley, A., & Empson, J. (1978). REM sleep and memory consolidation. *Biological Psychology, 6*(4), 293–300.

Violanti, J. M. (2014). *Dying for the job: Police work exposure and health.* Charles C Thomas Publisher.

Warner, J. (2005). *101 reasons why you should not become a cop.* iUniverse.

Young, A. (1997). *The harmony of illusions: Inventing post-traumatic stress disorder.* Princeton University Press.

Chapter 8
Resilience in Policing

Abstract **Resilience. What does this mean to a Police Officer?** There is much literature around resilience and first responders, mostly negative, with a focus on vicarious trauma and the dangers it poses. Here, the focus is on those officers who are optimistic who use their professional culture to build resilience and stay well. Contemporary research around the creation and maintenance of resilience is reviewed, with particular reference to US military systems that promote and monitor "Comprehensive Soldier Fitness" and how these might apply to policing. Officers interviewed reflect on their experiences of "bouncing back" after particularly challenging experiences and on the inevitability or otherwise on cumulative trauma. Most reveal practical strategies they use to stay well and optimistic about "the job". The central importance of policing culture, of "watching each other's backs", of the policing "family" is also evident in the wisdom and experience of those interviewed.

Resilience is the major focus of my study. In this context, it refers to the capacity of officers throughout their careers to "bounce back" from each critical incident that might otherwise lead to unwanted mental health outcomes. Before commencing the 50 interviews with SAPOL operational and retired members and the six clinicians, I had studied the autobiographies of the New South Wales and American officers (Horner, 2011; Mckay, 2005, 2010; Neil, 2014; Rogers, 1999; Sparkes, 2013), whose duties had led them to a PTSD diagnosis in the absence of any mental health-related interventions from their police departments. I noted with dismay how they had then been forced to engage in legal dispute with their organisations after being discharged "hurt on duty" to receive recognition and compensation. These were resilient individuals whose ability to "bounce back" slowly reduced after constant duty-related challenges. I approached my interviews wondering how their South Australian colleagues had fared with the same exposures and a similar lack of departmental interventions in their welfare. The literature around policing and trauma offered me little by way of encouragement that the SAPOL interview cohort would be in any way different. A telephone conversation with Professor Beverly Raphael with whom I had worked in a bushfire disaster in the 1980s was more encouraging (Raphael, 2014). Telephone conversation. A. Paterson. Adelaide, South Australia). The Professor reminded me of Posttraumatic Growth theory and clinical practice (Calhoun, 2014; Calhoun et al.,

A. Paterson, *Trauma and Resilience in Contemporary Australian Policing*,
https://doi.org/10.1007/978-981-16-4416-0_8

1999; Tedeschi & Calhoun, 1995) and its relevance to the development and maintenance of resilience among first responders including Police Officers. Having read their work, I approached the interviews with a more hopeful expectation about the career stories I would hear.

I discovered that the majority of those interviewed had been challenged by their operational duties and in many cases more so by the management and leadership under which they served, but most were resilient and thoughtful around maintaining their well-being while realising that SAPOL had little to contribute to it.[1] Their strategies and insights are discussed below in the data section and in the embedded literature around policing and resilience.

8.1 Resilience: The Informing Literature

The concept of challenged people overcoming adversity, bouncing back and moving on originated in terms of scientific study in the 1960s and 1970s, focussing on children growing up in difficult circumstances (Masten et al., 2009). At the centre of such research was the intention of promoting competence, stress resistance and strength in the face of adversity. Such an approach, it was claimed, resulted in resilience. In the context of contemporary trauma studies, developing resilience in the face of war, disaster, personal challenge or stressful employment is seen as a key to survival (Gilmartin, 2002; Seligman, 2011).

There is no lack of definitions of resilience in the literature referenced in this study. Burke, (2016:20) defines resilience as "The capacity to prepare for, recover from, and adapt in the face of stress, adversity, trauma or tragedy". This is of critical importance to my study in that Burke refers to preparing individuals for traumas to come to ensure that the impact of such events is minimised. Offering operational police such opportunities where possible before critical events as a form of prevention and early intervention should promote the capacity to "bounce back". Critical incident debriefs, properly conducted,[2] could also have significance in terms of recovery and adaptation. Violanti and Paton describe resilient individuals as, "Persons who survive traumatic experiences without pathological outcomes". Clearly such a definition applies to many first responders including police whose "assumptive world" (Janoff-Bulman, 1989) includes an expectation that they will encounter levels of death, mayhem and violence rarely experienced by their civilian fellow citizens. Pole et al., (2006:208) opine that resilience is, "a function not only of the individual, but also of the circumstances and environment in which he or she finds himself/herself", this being an extension of resilient qualities beyond the personal to encompass the impact on individual officers of culture, camaraderie and management structures. Officers interviewed often located stressors and challenges to their coping capacity in "command and control" management and an apparent organisational lack of concern

[1] See Chap. 2 "Power, organisation and police culture, 'the job'".

[2] See "Coping" Chap. 5.

for the well-being. Pole et al. (2006) also see the strategy of avoiding "passive coping" as critically important. Typically expressed as "I didn't let it get to me" and escape/avoidance using drugs and alcohol, as negative responses to stress and trauma and instead favours supportive relationships both in and outside of the work environment as keys to resilience and job satisfaction in the longer term.

Avraham et al. (2014: 12) add that resilience is the product of, "striking a balance between emotional connection and detachment", this is being reinforced by my interviews where officers frequently referred to their capacity to create emotional distance between themselves and the most confronting of duty-related events and is further evidenced in Henry's (2004) study of New York Police Officers who were skilled at "partial professional numbing" as a facilitator of resilience. Burns et al., (2008:22) consider that resilience in a policing context involves the implementation of effective coping strategies employed in this case by police investigating child exploitation through watching evidentiary videos as "hardiness and personal self-efficacy, team support, humour, training and education, physical fitness, having a sense of meaning in their work". The importance of team support in such areas of policing is well attested by my interview cohort as is humour, training and physical exercise. Many officers also spoke very clearly about the importance of "a result" in their investigations and patrol activities in terms of their resilience and positive professional and personal self-image.

Resilience or "bouncing back" says Hesketh et al., (2014: 155) can be learned and add that "resilience is about more than emotions, a spiritual dimension is equally important". Also referring to the possibility that resilience can be learned Brimm (2015) asserts that effective resilience training is very similar to Cognitive Behaviour Therapy and has at its centre increasing the individual's capacity to break down negative thoughts and focus on positive outcomes.

Seligman (2011:128) gave this advice to the US Army, "Focusing on the pathologies of depression, anxiety, suicide and PTSD was the tail wagging the dog. What the Army could do was to move the entire distribution of the reaction to adversity in the direction of resilience and growth". The same advice sits well with the present situation facing police organisations that appear to be frozen into organisational torpor by their fear of a PTSD epidemic (Amaranto et al., 2003; Bannink, 2014; Blum &Blum, 2000; Burns et al., 2008; Cotton, 2016; Mc Farlane, 2016). Resilience for Seligman (2011:90) is closely related to what Seligman calls "flourishing" and encompasses his ABC model "how beliefs about adversity (B) and not the adversity itself (A) cause the consequent feelings (C)".

In his reassuringly "Complete Guide" to resilience, Schiraldi (2011:3/13) suggests that "resilient individuals have the knack of surviving and thriving" and "resilience is the capacity to bounce back and recover from setbacks, to be buoyant and elastic about life and its challenges. It includes the ability to adapt well to stressful circumstances, maintain internal balance … in short, the ability to bounce back and thrive". According to Schiraldi, "PTSD is sometimes described as the exhaustion of resilience" (p. 15). This is an important insight, particularly in view of the opinions of the clinicians interviewed for this research. Most felt that the officers they assessed or treated were not suffering from PTSD but various forms of exhaustion that might bring on a depressive state. Essential components of resilience in Schiraldi's view include a strong sense of autonomy and self-reliance, the ability to remain calm under pressure, the capacity to engage in rational thought processes and maintaining high self-esteem, happiness and emotional intelligence, optimism as well as recognising meaning and purpose in the task at hand. As well he argues that humour, altruism (as in, "I joined up to help people"), character and integrity, curiosity (Seligman, 2011) life/work balance, sociability, adaptability, religious faith, a long view of suffering, good health habits including regular effective re-energising sleep, diet and regular exercise all contribute to a long and healthy police career. Many of these qualities are clearly evidenced in the police interview data central to my research.

Reich et al. (2010) focus on the possibility of building resilient organisations in terms of change, responsiveness, innovation and flexibility. They argue that, "if organisational resilience is defined as the ability to bounce back or to recover from challenges in a manner that leaves the organisation more flexible and better able to adapt to future challenges…then organisational resilience is a quality that leaders and managers in all organisations should foster at all times" (Denhardt &Denhardt, 2010:333). This is of particular relevance to police organisations who are notoriously change resistant (Chapin et al., 2008; DeCarlo & Jenkins, 2015; Huddleston et al., 2006; Loftus, 2009; Parsons et al., 2011; Stinchcomb, 2004; Sparrow, 2016; Cotton, 2016; Manning, 2015). Such resistance often involves police organisations facing challenges around responding to public criticisms of responses to critical incidents, gender-related issues and consequent harassment and bullying and assessments such as the recent Cotton (2016) review of Victoria Police in Australia.

In terms of individual resilience, the Denharts cite Couto (2002:52) who argues that it includes, "the skill and capacity to be robust under conditions of enormous stress and change". In their view, resilience (organisational or individual) is not merely the ability to bounce back after challenge, but more about the capacity to learn, adapt and change as new realities demand a response. There was much individual evidence of such responses in my SAPOL interviews but little in terms of such capacities within the organisation. A resilient organisation focuses on adaptive capacity, not only of individuals but also of the systems that surround them, moving away from placing a priority on defending its past to "making its future" (Denhart & Denhart, 2010; Marin, 2012; Paterson, 2014). Police organisations in Australia and elsewhere, particularly in the western world, are facing such challenges in regard to the well-being of their officers.[3] Building resilience is a challenge they must face, and one that they will continue to avoid at enormous organisational and societal cost (Cotton, 2016; Hesketh et al., 2014; Killmier, 1988; Marin, 2012; Nixon, 2012; Peters, 2009).[4]

Widera Wysoczanska takes a longer view describing personal resilience in terms of its origins, which include the importance of upbringing and family connections (attachment) a sense of autonomy, self-esteem, self-confidence, high levels

---

[3] See also my Chap. 1 "Policing theory, police and trauma".

[4] For a further discussion of such issues related to resilience building among police, see Chap. 6, "Asking for help".

of personal discipline, as well as a sense of humour, a tolerance of uncertainty and distress (in others as well as self) and the ability to transform unpleasant circumstances into learning experiences. Resilient individuals, says Wysoczanska, are optimistic and socially competent. She argues that resilience can be learned and increased, this being a high priority for those interviewed for this research, particularly officers involved in cadet selection and training. Operational Sergeants in my interview cohort had a similar view, pointing out that such issues were part of their responsibilities to their teams, duties they performed at a "common sense" level without the benefit of SAPOL provided training.

"Police under pressure: A donkey on the edge" (Peters, 2009) is the provocative title of a self-help booklet written by Roger Peters, a psychologist of 20 years experience in treating Police Officers employed by the New South Wales police service. Describing resilience as "bouncebackability" (p. 154). Peters is deeply critical of the NSW Police service's lack of policies and practices around the psychological well-being of its employees. Peters highlights "learned optimism" as an essential aspect of developing resilience for Police Officers and referencing Martin Seligman, further argues that such optimism is the opposite to "learned helplessness". Peters identifies "five core elements to coping better", self-esteem (see above), social networks and support (this including family networks and the camaraderie of policing), emotional well-being, spiritual well-being (broadly defined, not just in terms of religious affiliation) and physical well-being. Peters (p. 156) asserts that childlike curiosity, learning from experience, adapting quickly to change, "a talent for serendipity" (the capacity to learn "good lessons from bad experiences"), self-esteem and confidence, good friendships and involvement in loving relationships, the ability to express feelings, optimism, empathy and intuition or "creative hunches" are significant components of resilience.

Kirschman (Kirschman et al. 2015) is a clinical psychologist in the US State of California and has specialised for many years in working with operational and retired Police Officers who are dealing with stress and the other factors central to their careers in Policing. She is married to a Police Officer, hence, the title of her book is "I love a cop"(Kirschman, 2006:106) where she defines resilience as, "How people are self-righting and can use social and psychological resources to bounce back from adversity… it means more than merely surviving". This is a direct reference to "social support" often quoted in the literature but rarely defined as clearly as in this context. In terms of "protective factors" to encourage resilience, Kirschman includes "caring, competent managers, a job with purpose, family support systems, the ability to manage strong emotions and impulses, the ability to reframe thoughts and perceptions, the ability to be an active problem solver and communicator and the ability to distance one-self when appropriate and the ability to find challenge in adversity" (pp. 107–109). Armed with these qualities and resources, as many of my interview cohorts clearly were the expectations surrounding a police career should be wellness and resilience not psychological disorder.

Bannink (2014:15) takes this theme further, arguing from a positive psychology framework and promoting the term "posttraumatic success", suggests that psychotherapists focus on "what is right with your clients, instead of what is wrong with them". Resilience, in this context, is drawing on one's strengths to cope with challenges in life and to adapt in creative ways to them, maintaining thereby, a "stable equilibrium". Bannink suggests ten ways to build resilience, among them making connections with others, seeing crisis as opportunity, accepting and acknowledging that change is an inevitable part of life, having realistic goals and moving in their direction as well as having the courage to take decisive actions in the face of adversity. This relates very closely to foundational social work "strength-based" approaches that have made their way into the emerging positive psychology literature. Saleebey (1996) describes how social work practice, like positive clinical psychology has transitioned to a more positive focus on life's challenges rather than its previous problem focus. This has clear implications for those who have chosen to commit themselves to long careers in stress-laden environments such as policing where they might be encouraged by supportive leadership and management to shift their focus from the negatives of their work to the positive outcomes they achieve.

Others seek to develop resilience through offering training to those most in need of that quality, including police. Shochet et al. (2011) in their "Promoting Resilient Officers Programme" (PRO), a Queensland Australia police initiative, involved surveying police cadets in training and 12 months after graduation. The programme featured input identifying individual strengths, such as keeping cool and calm when provoked, positive self-talk and learning to challenge thoughts that limit resilience and personal growth. As well, the programme encourages developing and maintaining positive relationships in the workplace and holding positive views of career futures. The course consisted of seven face to face training sessions followed by online "refreshers" who remind participants of the central facets of resilience and encourage their continued development. Such "protective factors" are also closely linked to resilience in that they, when developed effectively, contribute to the prevention of trauma reactions among Police Officers.

Yuan et al. point out that in their view, most Police Officers are resilient, having chosen a stressful occupation and passed a stringent selection process. They go on to recommend that we focus, therefore, on positives around the individual officer's temperament, personality, positive world view as well as personality factors such as extraversion, openness and "agreeableness". Such a focus, argues Yuan, leads a more resilient policing approach both organisationally and individually.

Burke and Shakespeare-Finch (2011) describe the resilient officer as highly extraverted, capable of interpreting career events in a positive light but are equivocal about the impact of prior traumatic experience on the development of resilience as a police career unfolds, showing that those police cadets surveyed in their study, who had faced major trauma prior to acceptance into police training showed simultaneous levels of high distress and post-traumatic growth. Violanti and Paton offer another perspective, arguing that "persons who survive traumatic experiences without pathological outcomes can provide important clues to the intervention and treatment of those with PTSD". My interview cohort provided such clues in abundance.

8.2 Resilience and the US Military

Brigadier General Rhonda Cornum (United States Army, Retired) and Martin Seligman (Seligman, 2011) were responsible for the creation and implementation of the "Comprehensive Soldier Fitness Programme" in the US-Armed Forces in 2008. Cornum (1993), serving as a flight surgeon, was shot down by Iraqi soldiers as her helicopter sought to rescue a downed US air-force pilot in 1991. Badly injured with both arms broken, she was taken prisoner, physically and sexually abused, held for 8 days and then released. The account of her ordeal reveals extraordinary levels of resilience that transformed into Post-Traumatic Growth (Tedeschi & Calhoun, 1995). The then Major Cornum, more than survived her ordeal. She grew as a surgeon, "the concerns of my patients were no longer academic", a person, "I felt better equipped to be a leader and commander", a family member, "I became a better, more attentive parent and spouse". As well she described spiritual growth, thus "I was now open to at least the possibility of a spiritual life versus a physical life" and changed her basic priorities (cited in Seligman, 2011:160).

Colonel Jill Chambers, then heading up a Pentagon-based programme for returning veterans, visited Seligman in 2008 issuing a challenge that many academic researchers would simultaneously relish and recoil from:

> We do not want our legacy to be the streets of Washington full of begging veterans, post traumatic stress disorder, depression, addiction, divorce and suicide. We have read your books, and we want to know what you suggest for the army (Seligman, 2011:127).

Seligman and Cornum worked together with a carefully recruited group of psychologists and army personnel to create a programme that would be used to train the entire US army in resilience strategies and to monitor their progress through an online "Global assessment tool". The aim was to create service-wide models of psychological fitness to match the levels of physical fitness required within the military. Using Sergeants, trained in the delivery of resilience topics to offer Comprehensive Soldier Fitness modules to the troops, the "Master Resilience Training Programme" to underpin Comprehensive Soldier Fitness (Seligman, 2011) was born. The content is divided into three parts: Building mental toughness, strengths and strong relationships. Seligman and Cornum paid close attention the effectiveness of the training offered to the Sergeants, ensuring that they developed the skills to engage with their charges and effectively build their capacity in the context of the ABC model: "the emotional consequences (C) do not stem directly from the adversity (A) but from your beliefs (B) about the adversity" (Seligman, 2011:167).

The Comprehensive Soldier Fitness Project is intended to offer US soldiers the opportunity to develop resilience through the development of "healthy" approaches to the adversities of battle and army life as well as their personal lives and relationships. Much of this would directly apply to a policing context. This, I will discuss in much detail, later.[5]

---

[5] See my "Conclusions" section.

8.3 Optimism and Its Impact

Being optimistic and positive about challenging situations is seen by many researchers into resilience and post-traumatic growth as a critically important factor in maintaining individual and organisational well-being (Calhoun & Tedeschi, 2014; Joseph, 2012; Reich et al., 2010; Schiraldi, 2011). It was, therefore, important that the interviews central to this research allowed such a positive focus from the officers interviewed with regard to their view of their careers. At the end of each interview, I asked the following question:

> On a scale of 1-10, one being, "I have just wasted my life on a career in an ineffective organisation, constantly dealing with the dregs of society, with no useful outcomes, and ten being: It's been great. I have achieved a great deal of good outcomes and worked with some wonderful people. What would you score?

The responses were positive, with a very few exceptions. Officers interviewed for my research, regularly expressed such high levels of optimism and enjoyment around their chosen career and in doing so referred, often unintentionally to the issues that abound in the academic and research literature addressing the concept of optimism. Themes emerging from the many conversations within my research, included that of "optimism", defined here as an "attribution or a dispositional style" (Peterson & Seligman, 1987). An optimistic Police Officer is, therefore, likely to have good levels of physical and mental well-being and have the ability to consistently overcome obstacles that lie between her/his professional and other life goals. Such officers have (realistically) positive expectations in situations that may have the potential to produce extremely negative outcomes. This is described by Sharot as "the irrationally positive brain". Many of the Officers I interviewed were clearly optimistic in that sense to the benefits of their long careers in policing both to themselves and the society they serve.

As outlined in my chapter on leadership and management,[6] Sergeants are of critical importance to the process of patrol officers recognising the aspects of their duties that make positive contributions to society's good order. Having the capacity to balance out the "good from the bad" in experiences is critical to their well-being and to stave off the perils of cynicism, warned against by Warner in his "101 reason why you should not become a cop". Kitaeff (2011) references this as "the power of purpose", where the achievements of Police Officers in their everyday duties are recognised and used to build a positive optimism. Clearly such optimism and positivity in a leader such as a Sergeant would have an impact in terms of the "satisfiers" referred to by Paton (2009). It is such "satisfiers" that negate the impact of the 90/10 rule of policing. Plantinga (2014:183) points out that "90% of people are decent. 10% are not. You deal with the 10, 90% of the time". Plantinga identifies optimism as a means of encouraging officers to resist cynicism and to approach their duties with realistic expectations and a degree of hope around positive outcomes.

---

[6] See Chap. 2: "Power, organisations and police culture, 'the job'".

Padhy et al. define optimism as "a generalised expectancy that one will experience good outcomes in life, and interpret past or present events in a positive manner". They go on to establish in their research a relationship between optimism and psychological well-being, concluding that the latter state included six dimensions that comprised, autonomy, personal growth, an acceptance of self, life purpose, mastery or control over one's environment and "positive relatedness", the latter describing among other experiences that of the police "family" culture. Interestingly, this study revealed that officers having more than 10 years of policing experience were more optimistic than their colleagues who had been in "the job" for a shorter period (Balmer et al., 2014). This last outcome was also clearly reflected in my interview data. Padhy et al. also concluded that organisational demands and "hassles" can be as harmful to well-being as confronting operational experiences.

Much of the policing and trauma research literature focuses on risk and protective factors in officer's careers in terms of the likelihood that they will be afflicted with PTSD (Joseph, 2012; Peters, 2009; Sanford, 2003; Toch, 2002; Violanti, 2014; Weiss, 2010). My research identifies the strategies and attitudes SAPOL officers employ to remain healthy. This inevitably addresses issues around optimism, resilience and post-traumatic growth and how such concepts interact with and are impacted upon by other more operational experiences such as regular confronting experiences involving death, violence and injury. Personality factors such as gregariousness, the capacity to see positive outcomes in challenging situations, having clearly defined life and professional goals, accepting and appreciating social and peer support, possessing sense of self-actualisation and control, maintaining physical health and fitness, spiritual awareness, humour, organisational support and recognition are all factors that contribute to optimism and resilience.

Paton et al. reinforce this by describing the process of "finding meaning and insight" as a central indicator of Tedeschi and Calhoun's (2006) "placing meaning, structure and perspective" on confronting duty-related experiences, thus aiding effective coping with the issues raised. This has interesting implications for the process of Critical Incident Stress Debriefing in relation to the well-being of officers after such experiences, as such an approach may offer the opportunity to effectively process critical events. It also reflects the importance of positive leadership[7] and the potential to contribute through appropriate feedback and encouragement to the well-being of those in "the job" (Tedeschi and Calhoun, 2006).[8]

8.4 The Data from the Interviews: Optimism and Resilience

How did the officers who were interviewed maintain their resilience? Some reported active involvement in sport throughout their careers. Many talked about the annual psychological reviews that are supposed to be regularly offered (but rarely are) to

[7] See Chap. 2 "Power, organisational and police culture, 'the job'"..

[8] See also "Coping" Chap. 5.

those Officers undertaking particularly stressful roles within SAPOL. Some Officers had made private arrangements to debrief when necessary with social workers, psychologists and other health professionals. Others had created and maintained a clear demarcation between off-duty and work evidenced by one who always arrived at work in civilian clothes, changed into uniform and back into civvies again to cycle home often having taken a shower at his police station. Some had developed a habitually optimistic approach to their duties, looking for positive outcomes including those related to bringing offenders to justice and victims of crime their right to justice. The officers interviewed were clearly well aware of the concept of resilience, many were acutely aware of the hazards of their profession and all recognised that keeping well was a personal challenge, usually without input from the higher echelons of the organisation. Optimism was seen to be important and was a "habit" for many of the longer serving Officers.

One commented in the context of police culture, "if you wanted to teach resilience, yoga and such like in SAPOL, the trainers would have to be from within the police organization". This clearly indicates how far ahead of SAPOL management many officers are in terms of their knowledge of and interest in strategies that maintain resilience and well-being. Such knowledge and interest motivated many of those interviewed to participate in my study in the hope that change might result. It also shows evidence that private research into options such as yoga were common among my interview cohort to the extent that they had given thought to the implementation of such strategies.

SAPOL, according to many officers interviewed, often uses internal resources, particularly in the context of training, because it is assumed that a knowledge of policing "from the inside" is essential to the establishment of effective communication. This was reflected in my interviews with psychologists and psychiatrists (see below) and in the literature (Kirschman, 2015; Peters, 2009; Wehr et al., 2017). In my recommendations at the conclusion of this research, particularly in regard to management training, I offer an alternate view.

When asked what SAPOL does about individual officers mental and physical health, the response often was, "they don't do anything they are not interested" and "if you show weakness you are out! There is no loyalty you're just a number!" This last statement is from a more cynical retired Police Officer interviewed. Cynical or not, this officer expressed clearly what many of his colleagues said at interview. SAPOL management clearly keeps such issues at arms—length in terms of developing policies around mental health and well-being for reasons that are not always obvious. Individual officers are expected almost by nature to be resilient and to keep well. They are part of a culture that "toughs it out" at times when their "assumptive world" (Janoff-Bulman, 1989) is challenged by unexpected or out of the ordinary duty-related events. SAPOL management shows a consistent reluctance to recognise the impact of such events, including the suicide of officers perhaps for fear of being seen as "soft" by their lower ranked colleagues.[9]

---

[9] See Chap. 4 "Death and bodies".

Others, less cynical officers, made the same point, however, expressing their commitment to wellness in very personal and conservative terms, "I love that I am a police officer, I know that SAPOL won't look after me, so I have to look after myself". Being aware of the need to do so in the context of a job that is enjoyed and seen as significant is at the centre of surviving and thriving in "the job".

Police Sergeants, those with a responsibility for the well-being of their teams within SAPOL, often expressed their awareness of the importance of such issues, referring to "my satisfaction from looking after my troops". At that level, there is clear evidence of more than a duty of care, which recognises and responds at a personal level to such challenges.

Other officers had a clear perception of the ingredients contributing to their resilience, "I can't think of any times of struggle. I always coped. I have never suffered illness. I have been fit and healthy. I always had a fitness regime and never ate rubbish" said a long-serving Detective Senior Sergeant. This is a recognition of the importance of self-care born of the knowledge that "emotional survival" (Gilmartin, 2002) is an individual, not an organisational responsibility. A Sergeant reported challenging aspects related to his career that he thought were not contributing to his well-being, "My eating habits were very bad. I felt compelled to work like that. I then lost twenty kilos started bike riding. I ride by myself a lot. I am much fitter and more relaxed". This is again evidence that such realisations were usually not the result of organisational interventions, but more often self-generated by individual officers as a result of research or feedback from family or colleagues.

Other officers reached a point in their careers where they knew that changes had to be made if they were to survive in policing. One reported, "I thought to myself I can't be doing this for ever. I need to get away from the stresses and strains. I moved into a non- operational role. I had become incredibly tired". "I thought to myself" is significant here in that the comment continues the theme of self-care and career maintenance that flows not from departmental initiatives but from "ruminations" (Tedeschi & Calhoun, 1995) that lead to positive change and post-traumatic growth. Others, similarly planned ahead, "I had clear expectations of the negative possibilities of policing. I thought it's likely to happen to me, so I thought ahead. I'm a realist. I was willing to accept and cause change during my career", said a retired Superintendent, showing evidence of a realistic "assumptive world" (Janoff-Bulman, 1989) that encouraged and motivated effective career-prolonging personal/professional strategies to promote and maintain resilience.

An officer involved in police training reported that she had written a draft proposal for a police academy support officer to assist cadets throughout their training and had suggested a health and well-being section in the course, "we need to implement a few simple tools like breathing and relaxation. The present restructure of SAPOL may help us. Resilience training is also an important target". This is further evidence of efforts to create change from the operational ranks of SAPOL, in this case, at a critically important level. This officer had from her own experience of career challenges and subsequent research made suggestions to her managers that reveal a high degree of motivation toward change. Her suggestion has had no outcome to date.

Another retired Senior Officer reported that it was "important to exercise good judgement when involved in policing. It is a matter of personality, some coppers are angry at management and angry at the world. These people are more susceptible to stress". This reflected much of what policing and resilience literature makes clear, it is not only the operational experiences that induce stress and trauma responses, it is more about the individual officer's interpretation of events and organisational influences. His or her worldview is of critical importance to well-being and resilience.

There was further ample evidence from the interviews of practical strategies that were employed by many to ensure resilient responses to duty-related challenges. Some introduced strict personal regimes that involved drawing a clear line of demarcation between their on and off duty lives: "I go to work in shorts and a t-shirt and as I undress at the end of a shift I peel away the day. I shower and shave at work. You leave your job back there, I walk away feeling refreshed". As well this Detective Senior Constable added, "I go to the gym regularly for physical training, I keep it simple. I prepare myself for the job. I served three years as a child abuse investigator in the mid-2000s I needed to get out. Every two or three years I move to break away and freshen up". This is a comprehensive approach with a rich vein of clarity around duty/personal boundaries as well as the capacity to plan duty changes when weariness threatens. "Walking away refreshed" is the antithesis of the outcomes some researchers (McFarlane, 2011; Nievas, 2015; Paton, 2009) predict as the inevitable outcome of a police career. Police Officers are clearly not hapless, thoughtless, slow moving targets for traumatic responses. Many in the almost total absence of organisational inputs take very good care of themselves.

A Sergeant, approaching middle-age responded in answer to the question, "Is fitness important to you?" "I'm starting to struggle as I get older with injuries and niggles. I do lots of gym work with younger colleagues. I'm addicted to it. The younger cops get a lot out of my experience and I get a lot out of their perspective on things". Intergenerational cultural exchange as well as a career long commitment to well-being in terms of exercise is evident here. This is clearly a healthy addiction! Another Sergeant reported, "self- care is very important. I exercise, use black humour, have other interests outside the job, football and cricket and I don't take work home, although I can talk to my wife as she understands being an ex- cop herself. The emotional side of things I try to leave at work". This reveals much thought about relationships outside "the job". An Inspector reinforcing his clear demarcation between work and personal life said, "I don't talk about work at home, I have close friends outside of SAPOL, I don't carry my badge around when I am off duty. I am not a cop nuffy![10] It's just a job for me, and my wife's not interested". This is clearly about identity and a determination not to "be" the job. The perils of entirely identifying with police culture are clearly recognised here. The intention not to be a cop "nuffy" is clear and reinforced by an off-duty strategy that is characterised by relationships outside of the job. This officer's wife's disinterest in his police activities is seen by him as a positive, as an opportunity to follow Gilmartin's (2002) advice

[10] According to this officer a "cop nuffy" is an officer who has no identity outside of his/her police role.

to avoid the perils of the off-duty rollercoaster. Another officer, commenting on how "being" the job was hazardous, commented, "At the beginning of my career I *was* the police, now I *work* for the police". This is a clearly re-occurring theme in my research. Maintaining a distance from the police organization in personal and private lives is an important aspect of resilience among operational police. One commented, "In Rotary I am {first name}, they know I am a police officer, but it hardly rates a mention. There were only two Police Officers at my fiftieth birthday party. When I am at work I am full on, when I walk out the door…" Being "full on" and leaving to another life is clearly a recipe for well-being in the profession of policing as indicated by other officers who organize their social lives with a focus on friends outside of SAPOL, "I make it a priority to have friends outside of the job. I exercise very little. You can get into exercise in SAPOL. Those who are into exercise don't drink too much". This again is clear evidence of much thought and insight that leads to action. Much of the research that addresses policing and trauma downplays or fails to address the significance of strategies such as these.

In common with other officers, a Senior Constable after more than 10 years of service commented, "My coping process includes talking with my partner who has been with me right through my career. Taking off my uniform when I leave work is a symbol of leaving work behind. I keep fit, often I go to the gym before night shift and I surf and swim. I have many friends outside the job, ex school mates. I see them most weekends". Again there is a clearly recognised strategy here, practical actions augmented by social support, which is recognised as crucial and carefully maintained contribute to resilience and well-being.

Some officers learned from early experiences while in "the job". One, a Senior Constable of 25 years experience underlined this clearly, "I don't write myself off any more. I meditate, I undertake alternative approaches involving creating a peaceful environment for myself. I have many more tools in the tool box". The perils of alcohol self-medication as a stress reduction measure (Mckay, 2005, 2010; McNeil & Wilson, 1993; Neil, 2014; Sparkes, 2013) have been clearly addressed by this officer who has embraced alternative, effective means of maintaining his resilience, again with no apparent external intervention, departmental or otherwise.

Outcomes of investigations and police work can also have a very positive impact on resilience. Said a Detective Sergeant, "There is usually a result in our investigations, we have a very important role. When I leave work I can feel myself taking one hat off and putting another on, for example when I am at my kid's school. That's very important". Much of the trauma and policing literature ignore this aspect of policing (Nievas, 2015; Paton, 2009). Many officers interviewed were acutely aware of the importance of what they do and took great pride in it. This is reinforced by many aspects of police culture and by the camaraderie that enfolds individuals within it. A "result" is always celebrated and makes a direct contribution to the well-being of those involved. Another similar perspective on maintaining resilience came from a Senior Constable", I have had good people to work with, building relationships and understanding people, that's what I like about the job. I am interested in what we do". Building relationships, growing in "the job", maintaining interest are all factors that contribute to resilience, optimism and growth.

Relationships, marital and otherwise are critically important as well in terms of the way in which Police Officers contemplate their well-being. "Social support" is widely seen in the literature as a protective factor that mitigates against negative trauma responses among police and other first responders (Baker, 2006; Burke & Shakespeare-Finch, 2011; Burke, 2016; Gilmartin, 2002; Kirschman et al., 2015). This was born out by many of the officers interviewed, "I have a great relationship with my husband and plenty of connections outside of work" said a Detective Sergeant, working in child exploitation investigation who had clearly given much thought to the hazards of her investigatory field. Others, like this retired Senior Sergeant, at the end of a long career reported, "I never drank or smoked, I am married to the same wife and I could cope because I had faith". "The same wife" being his reference to the positive factors surrounding a long-term supportive relationship along with a clearly defined faith-based world view.

As a clear indicator of a long and healthy career when asked, "Were there times when in your career you felt on the edge?" A retired Inspector was quick to respond, "No! I've bounced around for most of my career, I was single for the early part. Getting bounced around was part of the job. I've had to adapt throughout my career". "Bouncing around", the ability to deal with trauma and move on and adapt in a healthy fashion as well as the benefits of "social support" are clearly represented here, as is evidence of an officer's flexibility that enabled him to consistently cope with the challenges of his career.

Others had a pragmatic approach to their police careers, "work stays at work but every now and then you need a mental health day. I sometimes wake up and say to myself I can't do police today!" Said a Senior Constable who saw no contradiction in this strategy and her status as a highly committed officer. This for her was self-care in practice, a pragmatic and necessary part of her overall commitment to "the job" and her capacity to do policing well.

There were signs among those interviewed that future generations of senior officers might bring with them a different approach to these issues. A young, recently promoted Inspector expressed his plans in terms of resilience in the organisation, thus:

> I have plans in my head around changes in SAPOL in this area. A footy club monitors its players' welfare. I am sure work performance and levels of wellbeing can be changed and maintained. We need proactive monitoring of staff. We need to offer gym memberships and catch officers before they break. We've got a whole lot of broken coppers we can't put anywhere. People should be rotated {through different police roles} rigorously.

Monitoring individual welfare of officers would constitute a radical change and perhaps overcome the traditional reluctance among police managers to address such issues. This is far beyond the much maligned "annual reviews" presently inconsistently offered by SAPOL to selected operational areas and may well usher in a change in attitudes toward resilience, moving it from an individual to a corporate responsibility. Prevention, the "catching of officers before they break" is presently unheard of. The response is almost exclusively to those "broken" officers after they have "broken". Regular rotations through the most difficult postings including Child

Exploitation and Family Violence could also be mandated and debriefs after critical incidents consistently offered, according to this officer's stated intentions.

There was also evidence of post-traumatic growth closely linked to resilience among those interviewed. One officer reported that he had suffered in terms of his inattention to his health and well-being but had come through it in a positive way. "I had a bout of depression at one stage. I didn't realize what it was, I had a heart attack which was linked to the depression. I went to a psych paid for by SAPOL. I was drinking too much. Having a heart attack was the best thing that happened. I have had some other issues as well, my psych was fantastic".

In terms of organisational care a Senior Constable reported, "I was involved in a domestic violence related murder where two patrol cops gave CPR to the victim. No-one said anything to them until I did. We have firearms training every year but no mental health training". This is an extremely telling comment in terms of organisational priorities. Operational skills are understandably highly valued and maintained. IMOST (Incident Management and Operational Safety Training) training is mandated annually for every operational officer, debriefs, psycho-education and self-care input clearly are not. If such a change of policy and practice occurred, career-long resilience would be greatly enhanced for SAPOL members.

Others are careful of the perils of police culture, "I haven't got into the police culture, it depends who teaches you about the job". This is an important insight into the perils of some aspects of police culture. If you are taught by more experienced, cynical officers that you should focus on the negatives, including the citizens routinely encountered who constitute the 10% of the 90%/10% rule, and the uncaring, unconnected distant management of SAPOL then your negative attitudes may be reflected in your well-being. If optimism is discouraged, then these cultural matters are the opposite of the protective factors described above. Cynicism and negativity are best avoided by officers seeking to stay well. The point about "the job" is that it is and should be, "more than a job!"

Resilience training is on the agenda for a lot of younger Police Officers as well. One commenting "Resilience should be taught on the job. Our local training officer conducts training for us every five weeks and a recent one was on resilience. He did one session on it. His central message was 'embrace change!' If anyone trains us, they need to be police or ex police. Our training officer hasn't been operational for seven years. The messenger is important". Interestingly this comment also reflects the intention behind the resilience training offered to this officer. The message was about accepting change in the context of continual SAPOL restructures. Significantly resilience in this context was seen as an operational skill defined in terms of the training officer talking about resilience from memory, not current field experience. Another senior officer in a management role agreed, expressing the opinion that, "The greatest antidote to stress is training". Becoming more specific outlining what they thought were three discreet areas of training, which should be ongoing throughout a Police Officer's career, she continued, "The priorities should be operational training, organisational training and personal health and domestic relationships training". Keeping well and having healthy relationships outside the job are the priorities here. Such an approach to these areas would pay dividends far beyond the cost of its introduction.

One officer recently diagnosed with Post-traumatic Stress Disorder commented, "Resilience training and resilience building is important. I've kept it secret for too long". This is both evidence of personal research around resilience-related issues as well as an experience of recognising warning signs of mounting stress reactions that cannot be revealed for fear of negative career impacts. The autobiographical accounts of police careers cut short by a PTSD diagnosis (Horner, 2011; Mckay, 2005, 2010; Neil, 2014; Sparkes, 2013) make precisely the same point about the need for secrecy and a lack of capacity to recognise the implications of mounting PTSD symptoms.[11]

Protective measures of another kind were outlined by another officer who reported that his successful strategy for maintaining resilience and wellness was as follows, "As far as trauma goes I have compartmentalized it, maintained a clinical distance, you don't buy into it. I probably taught myself to do that. I have always had other interests outside the job, although sometimes you feel guilty about keeping a clinical distance from suffering". Having a separate zone of consciousness where traumatic experiences are placed is a sophisticated strategy sometimes used in the treatment of PTSD (Kitaeff, 2011; Monson & Shnaider, 2014; Sparkes, 2013; Wilson et al., 2012). By maintaining a "clinical distance", this officer replicates the experience of many colleagues in Australia and elsewhere who self-taught, keep well by developing and refining such a strategy (Henry, 2004). The guilt expressed as a result is probably a small price to pay.

Expressing a similar strategy, another Retired Detective Chief Inspector said, "I never talked about work at home, I walked out of the office and left it there", and went on, "as a senior manager and first on scene at a Police Officer's death it was traumatic, but as the senior person there you divorce yourself from emotion and get on with it". Such a competency relates not only to the "just get on with it" traditional approach to policing but also illustrates the necessity of developing a range of skills that most officers view as necessary for them to do their job when circumstances require appropriate professional responses. In their view, this is not a form of avoidance that may have long-term dire consequences, but rather a thoughtful, intentional strategy born of experience and directly contributing to resilience.

In the face of death and suffering other officers have adopted a similar approach, "when you are dealing with drownings and other deaths, you had to be clinical as well as having empathy with the victims. I always had that. You don't dismiss it from your mind and you don't dwell on it either. You need the ability to realize that it is part of the challenge, you force yourself to be detached". This is confronting language where maintaining distance by strength of will is seen as a necessary, professional skill where a balance between compassion (for victims) and detachment (from tragedy) is also considered a vital ingredient to efficiency as well as resilience.

In terms of the possibilities of benefitting from successfully coping with traumatic experience before becoming a Police Officer others also point to the resilience

---

[11] See Chap. 6, "Asking for help".

building possibilities of prior trauma in their lives. "When you have had other bad experiences, hopefully you can learn from them. I should have been more affected than other coppers. My own experience of family tragedy helped me deal with victims", said a retired Senior Officer. This is clear evidence of resilience and growth and has direct relevance for recruitment processes in police organisations (Burke & Shakespeare-Finch, 2011) where conventional wisdom might focus on precluding those who have had traumatic challenges before applying rather than recognising the possibilities in such situations of posttraumatic growth as described here.

As if agreeing with his long-serving colleague, another retired officer, referring to his long career, responded to the question, "Are you positive about your career?" by saying, "Absolutely! I retired with 432 sick days left unused. Resilience is physical and emotional". He went on, "resilience should be tested at recruitment stage. You've got to learn to bounce". The implication here is that resilience is complex, a combination of physical fitness and emotional strength that can be built through training and experience (Schiraldi, 2011). The development of such "skills" in resilience over many years can lead to a long and healthy career of police service.

An Officer looking back over an eventful 35-year career said, "The drug squad was an interesting experience, I developed a worldly outlook, I got on with it and did what was necessary, there were many deaths, violence and bodies. I never gave myself time to dwell on those things. I was very involved in sport during this period". Being "worldly" included for this officer the capacity to deal with challenges far outside of the ordinary citizen's experience. This is a duty-related coping capacity involving self-discipline as well as physical and emotional fitness.

The clinicians interviewed as a part of the study had similar views around resilience and policing. Said a Psychiatrist, "The holy grail is early detection, and individual understanding and a lot of resilience training. There needs to be a skill-based approach to training". Such an approach is not yet evident in SAPOL.[12]

There was a synchronicity evident between what Officers said about resilience and what the literature identifies as important. Many had obviously done their reading! The clinicians were also of the same mind, agreeing that resilience can be maintained and developed by organisational interventions at all levels of policing. Said one, "There is a need for psycho-education around trauma, coping strategies that work, a treatment flow chart in peer support that reframes the trauma incident". Most of those at the SAPOL "coalface" who I interviewed clearly agree. Others envisaged a career-long emphasis on resilience and the prevention of negative reactions to trauma. One said, "Every time a copper sits an exam for the next promotion level they must study mental challenges and resilience". He added, "Career long fitness is a very important buffer and should be encouraged and supported by management. There should be five yearly rotations through challenging roles such as Child Exploitation and Family Violence. The Academy should place much more emphasis on psycho-education around trauma and resilience building. They do very little of that currently".

A colleague agreed, "The Academy needs to accept the need for resilience workshops. Debriefs are important. There need to be more resources in this area". Debriefs

[12] See my "Conclusions" section for a recommendation with regard to such training.

conducted according to the Mitchell model are highly controversial among academic researchers and some practitioners, (Al-Shahi & Warlow, 2000; Amaranto et al., 2003; Curran et al., 2003; Dyregrov, 1998; Peters, 2009; Raphael & Meldrum, 1995; Raphael & Wilson, 2000) but were frequently referred to as beneficial by this and other officers interviewed. They were seen simultaneously as a sign that SAPOL "cared" and as an opportunity to reframe events beyond the usual experienced by operational police involved in them,[13] thus contributing directly to resilience.

8.5 Mates and Camaraderie. Building Resilience Through Culture: Data from the Interviews

If resilience involves the capacity to "bounce back" after significant trauma-related challenge, then camaraderie is an essential ingredient of that capacity. Often mentioned by the officer's interviewed, but left largely undefined by them, camaraderie is part, but by no means all of that which defines police culture. "Watching each other's back", arranging informal debriefs, "anger, laughing, singing" "getting on with it" in the sure knowledge that your sworn colleagues "are all in the same boat" and "understand what you're going through". Such an understanding, in light of "the police macho approach" was often unspoken, but those at the sharp end of policing, in this case a Major Crash Sergeant went further, "we know each other, and we take care of each other. We ask each other, are you OK?" There is permission and expectation at this level to acknowledge and express challenges that are out of the ordinary for officers by expressing such concern. That is an expression of camaraderie.

The importance of working in teams to allow the natural expression of mutual concern and support was themes that were mentioned frequently in the interviews with officers. A Detective Sergeant working in a Family Violence Section put this issue clearly, "We have very few formal debriefs. We do it every day as a team. There are many manifestations…anger, laughter, singing…my colleagues make it all possible". This appears to be a level of collegiality unique to the military and first responders, particularly police. Their awareness of the importance of what they do, gleaned from their shared experience, not from rare departmental or community feedback, binds them together in levels of mutual concern and support unheard of in most professions. In the absence of departmental interventions, feedback and resourcing, officers take care of each other and themselves in a variety of ways.

Camaraderie derives from the policing task, its complexity, its challenges and its potential cost to the individuals who undertake it. It is enjoyed by those who participate. It is part of career-long achievements and is almost always described with reference to personal closeness and humour. Clearly it involves "bonding" and a shared understanding of the world, an understanding not always replicated in professions outside of the military and "first responders". Camaraderie is seen as essential

[13] See "Keeping well, Coping" Chap. 5.

to resilience and "emotional survival". In Australian policing, it may well be the key to a long and healthy career with your "mates". Another was less specific about the issue, referring to the way stressful events were managed he said, "We just got on with it! Camaraderie was important then, it's stamped out now! ****** {a former long-serving Commissioner} made that clear, ordering that we dob in colleagues". The attempted stamping out of camaraderie appears to be greatly exaggerated by this somewhat disillusioned officer, the task of doing so being far beyond the powers of even the most determined of Police Commissioners.

A long serving now retired Commissioned officer spoke fondly of his training in the 1940s, describing relationships then formed that lasted throughout police careers," they taught us everything, etiquette, horse riding as well as the law. We bonded, developed life-long friendships". The same process under different circumstances is alive and well among SAPOL officers, although many (see above) take care to also maintain close friendships outside of "the job" to keep their lives in some form of balance and to avoid the perils of being a "cop nuffy". Such camaraderie was central to the culture of policing for many, "We were supposed to be stronger and tougher. We coped by having a drink, it was the culture of the time and we were all in the same boat and knew what each other was experiencing". And, "You're with your mates, they know what you're going through". The distinction between actually being "stronger and tougher" and the need to cope was achieved in "the culture of the time" by the use/misuse of alcohol and more appropriately by the realisation (often unspoken) that your experiences were shared even when profoundly challenging. This was (and is) the foundation of real camaraderie contributing to real resilience.

Such caring for fellow officers was a frequent theme in the interviews, "Our team runs on the understanding that *someone does care*…we support each other", said a Detective Senior Constable, this being seen as an antidote both to the verbal abuse routinely suffered by officers at the hands of some members of the general public and the other stresses imposed by SAPOL's seemingly distant management processes and structures. In police sections, such as Major Crash Investigation that deal routinely with death and grotesque injury, such mutual support is seen as even more crucially important than more routine policing. This is well expressed by a Sergeant in that section, "The police macho approach is, I can't be seen to be weak". Major Crash is a small Unit, we know each other, and we take care of each other. We ask each other, are you OK?" Such a question would be less culturally acceptable in other areas of policing. Not being "seen to be weak" is avoided at all costs, but here, "knowing each other" and "taking care of each other" are more than just acceptable, it is culturally crucial. SAPOL could well explore the potential in such attitudes and responses to the challenges of policing. A Detective Senior Sergeant, continued this theme, is referring to the stresses of the job and the importance of his close colleagues, "The stress was mental, physical and emotional, facing your demons is embarrassing because you think you're weaker that your mates. I loved patrol work, shift work and the thrill of the chase, but I was a troublesome uniformed person. My mates kept me healthy". Again, this is a clear indicator of how camaraderie assists with the maintenance of resilience at the raw edge of the police experience. This officer, though presumably "troublesome" to senior management was kept healthy by the intervention of his colleagues, despite his and their acknowledgement that the strength needed to "cope" was not always present even when assisted by adrenaline. The precise nature of the interventions his colleagues undertook was not explained, but they were clearly effective as this officer was very much still in "the job". Another Officer put the same insights very clearly, "Camaraderie is very important. You get to know each other well and that helps" {cope with job stressors}. The importance of this aspect of resilience also goes beyond immediate police colleagues to include other first responders, "the St John Ambulance volunteers were the salt of the earth, we dealt with all sorts of bodies, and there was a great sense of camaraderie. Often we had to dodge the blood and guts if a post-mortem was in progress while we were there", said a Chief Superintendent referring to his early career experiences as a young Constable at the morgue in Adelaide. Delivering bodies to the morgue at this time included washing, stripping and identifying them in the midst of such challenging chaos, especially so for young officers at the beginning of their careers. Such camaraderie was critical to either responding with resilience to such challenges or finding another career.

Looking back on her long, resilient policing career, a Senior Constable expressed her satisfaction with "the job", thus, "I have done some amazing things and enjoyed fantastic camaraderie".

Rural and regional policing was also the subject of another officer's thinking around the importance of close collegiality, "There was a lot of working alone in the country. A few times I was nearly killed with rocks… I was hyper vigilant then. The camaraderie in the country balances that out"; this is from a retired Senior Constable, now an academic.

Another Sergeant was clear about the positive and negative aspects, referring to camaraderie, "I've had some hilarious jobs and worked with some great partners. I would let my son join SAPOL" but she added, with reference to the darker side of bullying and harassment in SAPOL and policing in other jurisdictions, "My daughter? No fucking way!" This clear testimony to a high level of thoughtfulness around the preservation of resilience through humour and camaraderie and the hazards (especially for women in "the job") that cannot be ignored and must be endured to ensure a long policing career. This officer entered a service populated with "dinosaurs" who patronised her and subjected her to harassment and bullying. Younger male members in her early years of service treated her differently, but not to the extent that she considers SAPOL to be a safe place (yet!) for her daughter.

With reference to handling the constant of death and injury a Sergeant commented, "Dead bodies are a given, even when looking at a body without realising it was a body. Dealing with the victim's family was the most difficult part. We had our own debriefs over pizza and beer, camaraderie was and is very important. I have always had close police friends". In the context of dealing with death, I asked another how he dealt with such experiences on the job. The retired Chief Inspector responded, "I grew up on a farm, it was an extension of my farm experience with death. You were paired up with a senior, experienced cop who took you through it. It wasn't a good look if you went outside and vomited. There was a great deal of camaraderie in the teams we worked in". This is a very clear expression of how young, recently graduated officers learn resilience and coping mechanisms from their senior colleagues. Being taken "through it" by such a colleague laid firm foundations for a long and productive career.

A long-retired, now elderly Senior Sergeant reflected on the importance of his colleagues in terms of the positives of his career thus, "I was there to serve and help the public. We took an oath, there was not a mark against my name. I kept my nose clean for thirty five years, I looked after the public at times of stress. Mateship is there. Looking after one-another, protecting one-another". He added, "There was also a girl who died in my arms. I had a very good listener in my wife…she understood, my colleagues were good as well". This officer had more that survived his long career, taking pride in his capacity to respond to its challenges and make a clear contribution with his colleagues to the "public" who he helped and served for many years. There are references here to the importance of support from various sources, the central importance of ethical conduct and an optimistic outlook during and after a career in policing. A retired high Ranking officer reflected on the importance of camaraderie in another way:

> Police Chaplains have been a positive resource. The Welfare Branch was run by a Chaplain originally. People affected by the job can be put into easier jobs, people can be shuffled around. The troops rally around in difficult situations, comradeship comes out. A Pt. Pirie police Officer and his wife were both killed in a vehicle crash. The orphaned children went to live with their Uncle. His house wasn't big enough. There was a 98% response to the police Association appeal to extend the house.

This officer makes reference to the importance of the policing "family" in this circumstance as did a much younger, still operational colleague, a Senior Constable who used a movie reference to express a similar view, "Team bonding is important, the blues family is very much alive". In the context of humour, a Senior Constable also referred to the importance of colleagues, "Gallows humour is important. You have to be there…sadness misery everywhere, there are very few wins on the job. The best thing about Policing is the people you work with. Funny and appropriate dry humour is what works best". Many of those interviewed agreed with this assessment of "the job" and its benefits. A Detective Senior Sergeant who was seriously assaulted early in his career, when asked what kept him in "the Job" responded, "I have always been highly motivated and received many awards, Dux of course, Cadet of the year, Qantas award, topped Detective training, surf life saver. I couldn't see why I would need to change. There was good support from SAPOL and much camaraderie from colleagues". Here are exhibited the central tenets of resilient policing, the capacity to maintain high levels of motivation despite serious challenges in the context of a positive view of the organisation and immediate colleagues.

Further positive aspects of the camaraderie in policing in terms of optimism were well expressed by a STAR[14] group Sergeant, "I look at the guys who haven't coped, they look at the negatives of situations. I pick out the positives. It's also important that others (colleagues) are involved as well in those situations. Going out with them

[14] Special Task and Rescue group are heavily armed elite responders to critical incidents.

and having a beer with them is better than going home and pushing your family. Black humour is very important as well. He went on, "The people there, I like the job and the people…go to work, have a laugh with your mates, go home and do it again the next day". This is resilience at its clearest and evidence of the ability to consider operational challenges positively often in the presence of less than desirable outcomes.

8.6 Gilmartin: Helping Cops to "Bounce Back". the Data from the Interviews

Kevin Gilmartin is an American Psychologist who is the author of a self-help book for Police Officers entitled "Emotional Survival for law enforcement—A guide for Officers and their families" (2002). Gilmartin, who is an ex Police Officer has visited South Australia twice gaving lectures to local Police Officers based on the contents of his book. These lectures were attended by 100 of local police, lasted for 3 hours, without a break and were popular in terms of their content and practical application. At the core of Gilmartin's message was his view that Officers are trained to be hyper-vigilant while on duty as an essential occupational safety measure and that many find that off-duty they fall into an opposite state, one of disengagement and torpor, "tired, detached, isolated, and apathetic". This, says Gilmartin, has a profoundly negative impact on friends and family and is the enemy of resilience. His basic message is "only worry about the things you can control", referring to the stress emanating from police management structures and practices[15] What can be controlled, argues Gilmartin, is an Officer's personal (home) life. He had a significant impact on those who attended his lectures and read his book. "When Gilmartin talked about hyper-vigilance, he was right on the money" said one Senior Constable. Another said, "I attended Gilmartin twice—once by myself and once with partner. SAPOL said, "Read the book". This response illustrates what most officers already know about resilience and emotional survival. Self-reliance, "reading the book" and acting on its good advice, in the absence of departmental input, are familiar territory indeed.

Another put his view succinctly, Gilmartin is right on the money". Speaking of his experience of policing in the far North of South Australia he went on, "Gilmartin was right about the hyper arousal, you're "up" in the Lands dealing with riots and then return to Adelaide". Gilmartin's message was clear, hypervigilance is a necessary component of police duties, assuming the presence of threat until a situation is resolved and is critical to survival on the job. Being able to turn off hypervigilance when off duty and not allow it to be replaced with familial disengagement, disinterest and absence was critically important to emotional survival.

In the context of suicide and policing a Senior Constable saw the Gilmartin approach as full of promise in terms of SAPOL developing appropriate policies, "In the seven years I've been in SAPOL there have been three suicides. That has pushed

[15] See "Management and Leadership" in Power, organisation and police culture. Chapter 2.

the organisation and PASA into thinking about welfare and resilience. Gilmartin was fantastic. They don't know what to do, they don't have a policy". Whether or not Dr. Gilmartin will directly contribute to policy development in this area is open to question. As a "fly in fly out" inspirational guest it remains to be seen whether he will influence the present hands off attitudes of SAPOL executive management to such issues. A now-retired Senior Sergeant commented, "Gilmartin was inspiring and very insightful".

His advice was acted upon by an officer married to another member, "Gilmartin is the best book I've ever read, my partner read it as well, if we start being reclusive we bounce off each other. You need to be careful of the tired, no exercise, eat crap, cycle". The Gilmartin lectures were compelling for many of the officers who attended including this one. Gilmartin is a skilled presenter and had obviously made the presentation many, many times before. SAPOL Officers attended in their 100s, many with husbands, wives and partners. A Senior Sergeant somewhat ruefully commented, "Gilmartin was helpful. Our training person said I have four copies. I lost a marriage along the way, if only someone had given me this book when I was a cadet!" Gilmartin's authority lay in his police career and experience. He spoke the language and put his finger on the issues closest to the professional reality of those present. Taking control when off duty, avoiding becoming a victim of your police organisation by being positive about "being screwed" by it (which Gilmartin argues is inevitable at least once in a police career) is, in his view, the key to well-being and resilience.

"Gilmartin almost moved me to tears", said a Sergeant of 25 years service. Such an emotional reaction may be in part due to the scarcity of experiences like this for most SAPOL officers. Direct input into their situation by an individual who has been there and has a high level of empathy is unique for most officers who attended. This was also a factor in the interviews conducted for this research. Many of those involved commented that the experience of telling their career story was unique, emotional and therapeutic.

For some, Gilmartin's message reinforced strategies already in place. An ex UK recruit to SAPOL, compared policing in the UK with local conditions, thus "I am aufait with the Gilmartin approach, I am into fitness. Police here are healthy, the Met is more cynical and bitter". This is a positive insight, largely supported by this research. A comparison with the metropolitan police in this context, by an officer familiar with both organisations, places SAPOL in a more optimistic, less cynical light. This constitutes some good news in terms of the possibility of resilience and post-traumatic growth among its members.

The interview data show how well this was received by operational Officers, but higher ranks were conspicuous by their absence at the presentation. This may have been partly due to Gilmartin being sponsored by the police Union but more likely reflected higher Command's policy of disengagement from "emotional" issues around policing. Officers interviewed for this research were clearly paying attention to such issues is seen by management as perilous in that it may encourage an outbreak of trauma-related issues.

Although relevant and encouraging to those Officers present, Gilmartin's presentations and his book, will have little long-term impact on the resilience of SAPOL Officers. It is good individual advice that is unlikely to impact on mental health policy and practice within the organisation. Without such policy changes, little will change, leaving officers to continue to take care of themselves.

8.7 What Have We Learnt?

It is very clear that much research into resilience in policing focuses on what resilience is (the capacity to "bounce back" after confronting, out of the ordinary experiences) and what constitutes "protective factors" that foster such resilience. The Officers interviewed had given these issues much thought, many had instituted patterns of behaviour that fostered well-being such as making clear demarcation between work and home, cultivating relationships outside of SAPOL, organising private debriefs when necessary and developing what Henry (2004) calls "a balance between emotional connection and detachment". Moving from challenging postings when the need for a change is recognised, being habitually "irrationally optimistic", and seeing achievements in positive investigatory outcomes were also important, as were engaging with colleagues in levels of camaraderie that transcend a merely individual experience of traumatic challenge ("we know each other and we take care of each other"), enjoying supportive personal relationships outside of "the job" and changing eating and fitness habits when the need was also recognised. It was widely acknowledged that SAPOL has little interest in such measures and that individual officers need to take responsibility for their own resilience and well-being, "I know that SAPOL won't look after me, so I have to look after myself".

The need for resilience training was highlighted clearly by many of those interviewed including the clinicians. Those who offer such training must be credible, experienced and currently operational in SAPOL. Such training should commence at the Academy and continue career long.

Younger Commissioned officers on the way up in SAPOL had very clear plans for change; early intervention, monitoring, encouraging physical fitness and moving officers into less challenging postings to avoid exhaustion.

The 1–10 questions at the end of each interview revealed surprising levels of resilience and job satisfaction among those interviewed. They loved and enjoyed "the job" but not "SAPOL" management who were seen by most as a problem to be dealt with. Gilmartin's presentations illustrated how starved these officers were for input, guidance and encouragement. They turned up in their 100s for his presentations, unaccompanied by their senior managers.

8.8 Where Next?

SAPOL could and should do a great deal more to contribute to officer resilience, particularly in terms of on the job training and changes in approach to the welfare of its Officers. The present lack of acknowledgement of the need to do so seems to be based on tradition ("cope or leave") and a level of fear that any movement in the direction of acknowledging work-related stress might cause an avalanche of WorkCover claims. It is also clear that the organisation finds any alternative to "command and control" approaches to management of staff including positive feedback for a job well done or clear indicators of support after challenging operations ("how are you guys going?") unthinkable.

Officers and clinicians who were interviewed agree that there is a need for broad cultural change that recognises the need for resilience to be nurtured and police members supported in "the job" in what Cotton (2016) calls "people focussed leadership". Gilmartin's advice to members about maintaining the "emotional survival" is just that. SAPOL needs much more than advice from outside, it needs a people focussed revolution from within based on a recognition of the perils of policing and building resilience of its members to do more than just survive.

The Police Officers interviewed in this study were well aware of the need for them to take the initiative to develop and maintain their own resilience. In volunteering to be interviewed, they were acknowledging their view that SAPOL does little for its members in this area, leaving responsibility for their well-being up to them. The qualitative interview structure of this research gave them the opportunity to describe their strategies, their awareness of the perils of policing in a conversation that many acknowledged was both unique for them as well as "therapeutic". Rather than measuring levels of distress as in many quantitative approaches to police research, I set out to uncover levels of coping and resilience.

References

Al-Shahi, R., & Warlow, C. (2000). The current status of psychological debriefing. *BMJ, 321*, 1032–1033.

Amaranto, E., et al. (2003). Police stress interventions. *Brief Treatment and Crisis Intervention, 3*(1), 47.

Avraham, N., et al. (2014). Paramedics' experiences and coping strategies when encountering critical incidents. *Qualitative Health Research, 24*(2), 194–208.

Baker, B. (2006). *Becoming a police Officer: An insider's guide to a career in law enforcement*. iUniverse.

Balmer, G. M., et al. (2014). Psychological resilience of Western Australian police officers: Relationship between resilience, coping style, psychological functioning and demographics. *Police Practice and Research, 15*(4), 270–282.

Bannink, F. (2014). *Post traumatic success: Positive psychology & solution-focused strategies to help clients survive & thrive*. WW Norton & Company.

Blum, L. E., & Blum, L. N. (2000). *Force under pressure: How cops live and why they die*. Lantern Books.

Burns, C. M., et al. (2008). The emotional impact on and coping strategies employed by police teams investigating internet child exploitation. *Traumatology, 14*(2), 20.
Brimm, T. (2015). *Building mental resiliency*. Police magazine.
Burke, R. J. (2016). *Stress in Policing: Sources*. Routledge.
Burke, K. J., & Shakespeare-Finch, J. (2011). Markers of resilience in new police officers: Appraisal of potentially traumatizing events. *Traumatology, 17*(4), 52–60.
Calhoun, L. G., et al. (1999). *Facilitating posttraumatic growth: A clinician's guide*. Routledge.
Calhoun, L. G., & Tedeschi, R. G. (2014). *Handbook of posttraumatic growth: Research and practice*. Routledge.
Chapin, M., et al. (2008). Training police leadership to recognize and address operational stress. *Police Quarterly, 11*(3), 338–352.
Cornum, R. (1993). *She went to war: The Rhonda Cornum story*. Presidio Press.
Cotton, P. (2016). Victoria Police Mental Health Review. An independent review into the mental health and well-being of Victoria Police employees. Australia.
Coutu, D. L. (2002). How resilience works. *Harvard Business Review, 80*(5), 46–56.
Curran, L. A., et al. (2013). *101 trauma-informed interventions: Activities, exercises and assignments to move the client and therapy forward*. PESI Publishing & Media.
DeCarlo, J., & Jenkins, M. J. (2015). *Labour unions, management innovation and organizational change in police departments* (pp. 1–44). Springer.
Denhardt, J., & Denhardt, R. (2010). Building organizational resilience and adaptive management. In *Handbook of adult resilience* (pp. 333–349).
Dyregrov, A. (1998). Psychological debriefing—An effective method? *Traumatology, 4*(2), 3.
Gilmartin, K. M. . (2002). Emotional survival for law enforcement. *ES Press, PMB, 233*, 2968.
Henry, V. E. (2004). *Death work: Police, trauma, and the psychology of survival*. Oxford University Press.
Hesketh, I., et al. (2014). Keeping the Peelian spirit: Resilience and spirituality in policing. *The Police Journal, 87*(3), 154–166.
Horner, P. (2011). *Jack Knife: The crashing of a policeman—NSW police and PTSD*. Australia, Zeus Publications.
Huddleston, L. M., et al. (2006). Conceptualizing traumatic stress in police officers: Preemployment, critical incident, and organizational influences. *Traumatology, 12*(3), 170–177.
Janoff-Bulman, R. (1989). Assumptive worlds and the stress of traumatic events: Applications of the schema construct. *Social Cognition, 7*(2), 113–136.
Joseph, S. (2012). *What Doesn't Kill Us: A guide to overcoming adversity and moving forward*. Hachette UK.
Killmier, R. (1988). Interview with Deputy Commissioner of South Australia Police. Unknown. South Australian Police Association.
Kirschman, E. (2006). *I love a cop* (revised). Guilford Press.
Kirschman, E., et al. (2015). *Counselling cops: What clinicians need to know*. Guilford Publications.
Kitaeff, J. (2011). *Handbook of police psychology*. Routledge.
Loftus, B. (2009). *Police Culture in a changing world*. Clarendon Studies in Criminology.
Manning, P. K. (2015). *Democratic policing in a changing world*. Routledge.
Marin, A. (2012). In the line of Duty. Ombudsman's report. Ontario, Canada.
Masten, A. S., et al. (2009). 12 Resilience in Development. In *The Oxford handbook of positive psychology* (p. 117).
McFarlane, A. C. (2011). *Many paths, one purpose. Expert forum*. Australian Centre for posttraumatic mental health.
Mc Farlane, A. C. (2016). *Occupational Safety*. South Australia, Adelaide University. Centre for Trauma Studies.
Mckay, E. (2005). *Crime Scene-True stories from the life of a crime scene investigator*. Viking (Penguin) Australia.
Mckay, E. (2010). *Forensic investigator*. Viking (Penguin) Australia.

McNeil, M., & Wilson, C. (1993). *Alcohol and the Police workplace.* National Police Research Unit.

Mitchell, J. T. (1988). *CISML: A new era in crisis intervention.* International Critical Incident Stress Foundation.

Monson, C. M., & Shnaider, P. (2014). *Treating PTSD with cognitive-behavioural therapies: Interventions that work.* American Psychological Association.

Nievas, V. (2015). Posttraumatic stress disorder and police officers. *Australian Police Journal, 69*(4).

Neil, B. (2014). *Under siege.* Harlequin Mira.

Nixon, C. (2012). *Fair cop.* Victory Books.

Parsons, A., et al. (2011). Effective policing: Management influence and the commitment of senior police personnel. *Policing & Society, 21*(1), 1–26.

Paterson, K. (2014). Modern, motivated, progressive and professional? Flexible work practices and the retention of female members in SAPOL. *Australasian Policing, 6*(1), 21.

Paton, D. (2009). *Traumatic stress in police officers: A career-length assessment from recruitment to retirement.* Charles C Thomas Publisher.

Peters, R. F. (2009). *Police under pressure. (A donkey on the edge).* HEAS Publications.

Peterson, C., & Seligman, M. E. (1987). Explanatory style and illness. *Journal of Personality, 55*(2), 237–265.

Plantinga, A. (2014). *400 things cops know-Street smart lessons from a veteran patrolman.* Quill Driver Books.

Pole, N., et al. (2006). Resilience in retired police officers. *Traumatology, 12*(3), 207–216.

Raphael, B., & Meldrum, L. (1995). Does debriefing after psychological trauma work? *BMJ: British Medical Journal, 310*(6993), 1479.

Raphael, B., & Wilson, J. (2000). *Psychological debriefing: Theory, practice and evidence.* Cambridge University Press.

Raphael, B. (2014). Telephone conversation. A. Paterson. Adelaide, South Australia.

Reich, J. W., et al. (2010). *Handbook of adult resilience.* Guilford Press.

Rogers, L. K. (1999). *PostTraumatic Stress Disorder: A police officer's report.* Proctor Publications.

Saleebey, D. (1996). The strengths perspective in social work practice: Extensions and cautions. *Social Work, 41*(3), 296–305.

Sanford, L. L. B. (2003). Critical incident stress and the police officer a pro-active approach.

Seligman, M. E. P. (2011). *Flourish: A visionary new understanding of happiness and well-being.* Simon and Schuster.

Schiraldi, G. R. (2011). *The complete guide to resilience: Why it matters how to build it and maintain it.* Resilience Training International.

Shochet, I. M., et al. (2011). The development and implementation of the Promoting Resilient Officers (PRO) program. *Traumatology, 17*(4), 43–51.

Sparkes, A. (2013). *The cost of bravery.* Penguin Group, Australia.

Sparrow, M. (2016). *Handcuffed: What holds policing back, and the keys to reform.* Brookings Institution Press.

Stinchcomb, J. B. (2004). Searching for stress in all the wrong places: Combating chronic organizational stressors in policing. *Police Practice and Research, 5*(3), 259–277.

Tedeschi, R. G., & Calhoun, L. G. (1995). *Trauma and transformation: Growing in the aftermath of suffering.* Sage Publications.

Tedeschi, R. G., & Calhoun, L. G. (2006). Expert companions: Posttraumatic growth in clinical practice. In *Handbook of posttraumatic growth: Research and practice* (pp. 291–310).

Toch, H. (2002). Stress in policing. *American Psychological Association Journal.*

Violanti, J. M. (2006). The police: Perspectives on trauma and resiliency.

Violanti, J. M. (2014). *Dying for the job: Police work exposure and health.* Charles C Thomas Publisher.

Wehr, T. E. M., Priority One, staff support services, Queensland Ambulance Service. (2017). *Priority one, staff support services.* Australian Society for Traumatic Stress Studies.

Weiss, P. A. (2010). *Personality assessment in police psychology: A 21st century perspective.* Charles C Thomas Publisher.

Wilson, J. P., et al. (2012). *Treating psychological trauma and PTSD.* Guilford Press.

Chapter 9
PTSD and Policing

Abstract **Is PTSD inevitable?** My local daily newspaper recently featured an article entitled: "PTSD: The dark cloud that hangs over our police officers". Police are well aware of the dangers of their profession, physical as well as mental. This chapter examines the PTSD phenomenon from its inception as "Post Vietnam syndrome" to its contemporary widespread application to a variety of traumatic experiences from its detractors to the fears and hopes of the officers themselves. Biological perspectives are examined as is the debate among health professionals around the contemporary "epidemic" that is the PTSD phenomenon. Interviews with the cohort of psychiatrists and psychologists included in my research shed light on the actual incidence of PTSD diagnoses in South Australian policing, and the wider national and international research literature is also reviewed in detail. The New South Wales police autobiographies emanating from the twentieth century show how police organisations of the period had no interest in linking police duties with possible trauma. The question is then considered: "How much or how little has changed?" Police officers interviewed show a very clear awareness of these issues and in some cases significant anxiety as to this possible outcome during a long career in "the job".

I was a practising social worker in the 1980s when the first Diagnostic Statistics Manual defining Post-traumatic stress disorder was published (American Psychiatric Association, 1980). I had had significant clinical contact with Vietnam veterans through my crisis intervention work with South Australia Police. My colleagues and I perceived that they were over-represented in our domestic violence caseload. As a result, I became involved with a group of psychologists who established the Vietnam Veteran's counselling service to meet that group's particular psychotherapeutic needs. I became interested in how the PTSD diagnosis had been crafted as I was of the view that to characterise a traumatic reaction such as PTSD as a "disorder" was challenging. It seemed more appropriate to consider the veteran's symptoms to be a "normal" reaction to an "abnormal" set of circumstances in which the young soldiers, many of them conscripts, found themselves. I was not alone in that view as has been recently attested by Professor Beverly Raphael (Douglas, 2016:89).

My interest in the history of the PTSD diagnosis and its development persists, and it is highly relevant to this study as it has now been applied to first responders

A. Paterson, *Trauma and Resilience in Contemporary Australian Policing*,
https://doi.org/10.1007/978-981-16-4416-0_9

as well as veterans of war. I seek in my research to answer this question, "how did our present understanding of the health implications of exposure to trauma originate and how does PTSD as a diagnosis apply to non-military environments?".

9.1 PTSD: An Epistemology

David Morris, a US Marine and war correspondent saw action in two tours of Iraq "embedded" with US forces in the most challenging theatres of that war, and who was wounded in an IED explosion, sums up the recent impact of the "trauma industry" on Western culture, "Over the past four decades PTSD has permeated every corner of our culture" (Morris, 2015:1). I will consider this further as a significant aspect of the assumption that continual engagement in stressful and traumatic situations (as in a typical police career) will inevitably lead to stress-related illness (Gilmartin, 2002; Herman, 1997; Mc Farlane, 2016).

World War One's psychiatric diagnostic descriptors including "disordered action of the heart" "railway spine" and later "shell shock" chart the development of theoretical approaches designed to explain responses to trauma exposure unique to the twentieth century. The mechanised, industrialised nature of trench warfare exposed soldiers to a hitherto unexperienced level of stress where they waited for days and weeks in the midst of chaos, death, mutilation and conflagration for a death that seemed inevitable. The casualty rate was unheard of. In the first 12 months of World War One, the British regular army was almost wiped out as a result of the European campaign (Kelly, 2015) and was reinforced by volunteers and later conscripts to fill the gaps created by the massive casualties. At the war's end, 80,000 veterans had been treated for shell shock (Grogan, 2014). Shell-shocked soldiers were tainted by the condition's association with insanity, cowardice and malingering (Lees, 2014). Kelly states that 40% of all casualties were "nervous disorders" with indicators including, anxiety, fatigue, neuralgia (pain), headache and "low mood". "Hysterical" shell shock included symptoms such as mutism or fugue (memory loss), re-enactment in memories of the event(s), dreams and nightmares, the numbing of emotions, avoidance of situations relating to or reminiscent of combat exposure, jumpiness, anxiety and depression. All this clearly prefigures later twentieth century PTSD diagnoses.

The preferred treatments both at the front and in mental health facilities back in the United Kingdom included "Rest, good food, encouragement" (Jones & Wessely, 2005) and hypnosis, shock treatment, "rest of mind and body", (Kelly, 2015) psychosocial support (from colleagues and health professionals) sport and cold baths. Most veterans recovered quickly, and if hospitalised, were discharged within 2 weeks of admission (Morris, 2015; Young, 1997).

The term "shell shock" is now applied journalistically to a wide range of human experiences from the unexpected outcome of a sporting contest, "the batsmen were shell-shocked by the pace attack" to any experience involving high levels of surprise, "the market was shell-shocked by the sudden fall in shares due to a rush on the Banks" (Kelly, 2015).

When the Second World War loomed in the late 1930s, the attention of some clinicians returned to the provision of services to those suffering from war-related anxiety states (Herman, 1997; Jones & Wessely, 2005). In a presentation to the Royal Army Medical College in 1938, Major H.A. Sandiford (1938) a psychiatrist with experience of World War One "shell-shock" and himself a veteran of that war, expressed the view that:

> There is nothing new, produced by war per se, as regards the causation of these diseases, which are seen equally in civil life. They are important from a military point of view because they occurred in large numbers in the Great War, and may possibly occur in larger numbers in future wars unless steps are taken for their prevention. They render a soldier inefficient...or enable him to avoid his duty with impunity. They are to some degree contagious...The subjects of these disorders may find themselves faced with a charge of malingering, cowardice or desertion (p. 231).

In the context of some present estimates that 40–50% of American military personnel are diagnosed with PTSD on their return from war zones such as Iraq and Afghanistan, (Junger, 2015) Sandiford may well be right with regard to the issue of contagion, and his words are eerily predictive of what was to come in terms of the development in subsequent decades of theories and treatments for war and disaster-related trauma. He had a significant concern around "malingering", giving instruction around methods of detection, advising colleagues to "regard each case {of suspected "war neurosis"} with the utmost suspicion and be forceful" (p. 232). In a more positive vein, Sandiford opined that prevention of such neuroses could be achieved by creating high levels of morale through "leadership, discipline, fighting spirit, mental education" (p. 234), although he also cautioned, "do not give any special training in neurosis, it may cause it" (p. 229). This reflects accurately the same apparent fears of many twenty-first century leaders in military and policing organisations. As well, the Major suggests that, "good officers set a good example. They promote confidence and enthusiasm and take an active and personal interest in the welfare and comfort of the men" (p. 230).[1] His insights into the source of such reactions to exposure in the context of trench warfare are also prescient. He describes physical and mental exhaustion as a major factor, as well as the conflict caused in trench warfare, compared with "open warfare" by the inability while cowering in a trench under fire, to "fight or flee".

World War Two was, therefore, expected by many to offer a more significant role to military psychiatrists, who it was hoped, would reduce psychological casualties and more effectively aid the recovery of those who became affected by "battle exhaustion" as the condition became known (Jones & Wessely, 2005). This was not to be, as many contemporary researchers pointed out (Friedman, 2015; Jones & Wessely, 2005; Morris, 2015; Young, 1997). After the war, veterans came home to a hero's welcome after winning a conflict that took a huge toll on the mental health of many of those who fought. On demobilisation, they were told to "forget your experience and get on with the rest of your life" (Young, 1997: 57). Those who returned remained silent about their experience of that conflict. Karl Shapiro a poet Laureate who fought in

[1] See Chap. 2 "Power, organisation and police culture," The job'".

the Pacific War described his own, and his poetic colleagues experience thus, "We all came out of the same army and joined the same generation of silence" (Cited in Morris, 2015:132).

Herman (1997:26) states that "as long as they could function at a minimum level they were thought to have recovered. With the end of the war, the familiar process of amnesia set in once again. There was little medical or public interest in the psychological condition of returning soldiers". It is estimated (Morris, 2015) that in the US World War Two army, there were three times the number of psychological casualties than in World War One. The British and Allied forces had similar outcomes with "battle exhaustion" and aircrews in the RAF Bomber Command who refused to fly missions were described as "lacking moral fibre" (Jones & Wessely, 2005:97). Psychiatric casualties were of major concern, particularly as many so diagnosed were unfit to return to service in the field of battle.

The Vietnam War (1961–1975) heralded a new era of conflict-related psychological injury and distress. US and allied veterans including Australians, returned to their country having fought in a war that was widely unpopular in its latter years. Unlike their colleagues in World Wars One and Two, they were not feted as heroes of a successful conflict, but rather greeted with anger and disgust by some sections of their societies. Vietnam, according to Morris (2015) and others, laid the foundation for a new way of thinking about trauma and its impact, which quickly spread from an association with war and conflict to a broader way of describing events that overwhelmed and confronted the human psyche with long-lasting and devastating impacts.

Diagnostic Statistics Manual 1, published by the American Psychiatric Association in 1952, aimed to create a consistent nosology of psychiatric terms and diagnostic criteria but failed to deliver that outcome as far as the US psychiatric community was concerned (Young, 1997). It featured the term "gross stress reaction", which described a point on the individual's position on a continuum between mental health and illness, with regard to the impact of external events such as warfare, but took that extrapolation no further. DSM 2, published in 1968, made no mention of that syndrome.

What was first described as "Post Vietnam Syndrome" by sympathetic psychiatrists in the United States including prominent academic clinician, Lifton (1983) became "Post Traumatic Stress Disorder" with the release of the Diagnostic Statistics Manual of Mental Disorders (DSM 3) in 1980. This DSM described for the first time a disorder that was a result of the impact of an external event rather than an internal maladjustment of the individual psyche. Lifton, a Professor of Psychiatry at Yale University, was appalled by the Vietnam conflict and particularly by the My Lai massacre, where American Marines killed hundreds of unarmed village residents including women and children. With his colleague Chaim Shatan, also an academic psychiatrist, he formed a therapeutic relationship with an influential anti-war group, "Vietnam Veterans Against the War" after an approach from them asking him to assist them with "the severe psychological problems of many Vietnam Veterans because of their experiences" (Cited in Morris, 2015:140). This intervention took the form of "rap groups" where veterans were able to openly express their experiences, fears and frustrations and discuss their reactions to their involvement in the war. Both Shatan and Lifton entered into a relationship with the Vietnam veterans "that transcended the hierarchical model of doctor and patient and pushed into a new higher plane of social consciousness" (Morris, 2015:143).

Subsequent DSMs have expanded these insights into a broader definition of trauma-related responses, with the 2013 DSM 5 including examples of the impact of exposure, that of police officers viewing images of child exploitation and abuse when investigating such criminal activity. The Gulf, Iraq and Afghanistan conflicts have resulted in a human flood of post-traumatic diagnoses unprecedented in military history (Bistoen, 2016; Brewin, 2003; Junger, 2015; Seligman, 2012). Estimates of numbers of veterans diagnosed with PTSD in the United States vary, but 600–800 thousand seems likely, supported by data from the Veteran's Affairs and Department of Defence Statistics (Brewin, 2003; Rogers, 1999; Wiederhold, 2013). US veterans who receive a full diagnosis of PTSD are eligible to be paid a pension of $3,000 US dollars per month until recovered or in full-time employment (Junger, 2015; Seligman, 2012, 2015).

9.2 The PTSD Literature: The Developing Diagnosis and Response to the Trauma Phenomenon

An abundance of literature regarding Post-Traumatic Stress Disorder has emerged since the early 1970s, initially as a response to returning veterans of the Vietnam War in the United States, Australia and elsewhere (Raphael & Dobson, 2005). In Australia, Cyclone Tracy in 1974 triggered a range of research projects focused on the after-effects of trauma experienced by survivors of natural and man-made disasters (Raphael, 1986). Such research is built on the evidence gained from the diagnosis and treatment of returned Vietnam veterans. At the centre of this approach is the key concept of "trauma" defined as, "a catastrophic stressor outside the range of usual human experience". Subsequently revised in DSM-III-R (1987), DSM-IV (1994) and DSM-IV-R (2000), PTSD evolved into two separate conditions, PTSD and "Acute Stress Disorder", the latter comprising a short-term traumatic response that resolved naturally within a period of 2–3 weeks.

DSM V, published in May 2013, further refines the diagnostic environment, broadening the conditions under which a diagnosis of either PTSD or Acute Stress Disorder might be made. As well, this DSM further defines the difference between direct experience of an event, now only described as "traumatic" and that of the re-experiencing of such events through repeated exposure through work-related activities. This has greatly encouraged research into the long-term career experiences of "first responders" including police. This section of the DSM, notably, includes a direct reference to police exposure to trauma for the first time in a Diagnostic Statistics Manual (p. 270) stating that PTSD may be diagnosed after:

> Directly experiencing traumatic events, witnessing in person the event(s) as it occurred to others. Learning that the events occurred to a close family member or close friend. In cases of actual or threatened death of a family member or friend the event must have been violent or accidental. And in addition, experiencing repeated or extreme exposure to details of the aversive event (e.g. first responders collecting human remains; police officers repeatedly exposed to details of child abuse). A note is added (p.271) "Criterion A4 does not apply to exposure through electronic media, television, or pictures unless the exposure is work related.

"Intrusion symptoms" in the DSM V diagnostic criteria include,

> Re-current, involuntary, and intrusive distressing memories of the traumatic event, re-current distressing dreams related to the traumatic event, dissociative reactions or "flashbacks" relating to the event, intense and prolonged distress when exposed to internal or external cues that symbolise or resemble the traumatic event, marked physiological reactions to internal or external cues that symbolise or resemble the original event, persistent avoidance of stimuli associated with the traumatic event including attempting to avoid memories of the traumatic event as well as efforts to avoid people, places, conversations that are associated with the traumatic event, dissociative amnesia connected to the traumatic event and irritable behaviour, reckless or self-destructive behaviour, hyper-vigilance, exaggerated startle response, problems with concentration and disturbed sleep patterns. (DSM V 2013:271)

The International Classification of Diseases (World Health Organization, 1993) in its classification of PTSD covers similar ground to the DSM, describing the syndrome as "a delayed or protracted response to a stressful event or situation (of either brief or long duration) of an exceptionally threatening or catastrophic nature which is likely to cause pervasive distress in almost anyone". Flashbacks, nightmares, numbness of effect, detachment from others, avoidance of situations remind the sufferer of the original trauma, suicidal ideation, hypervigilance and anxiety and depression. ICD 11 (World Health Organization, 2012) sets out to be less prescriptive, giving clinicians more room than ICD and DSM 5 to exercise professional judgement as they diagnose the disorder.

9.3 Biological Perspectives on PTSD: Diagnosis Made Easy

The development of neurobiological approaches to trauma has evolved largely in the psychiatric community since the late 1970s. Kandel was awarded a Nobel Prize in 2000 for his work on the physiological basis of the storage of memory in the neurons of the brain, is a pioneer of what he calls the "anti-discipline" in psychiatry that moves away from the pervading psychoanalytic behavioural view of mental illness to a "biologic" perception and understanding.

With the advent of more sophisticated means of imaging the brain such as MRI scans, later researchers (McFarlane, 2011; Shalev & Bremner, 2016) have rigorously applied neurobiology to the study of PTSD. Shalev and Bremner (2016) refer to the current definition of PTSD in DSM 5, which moves away from "trauma out of the range of normal human experience" (DSM 3) to one encompassing road trauma, physical assault and other experiences, which influence changes in cognition and mood thus expanding populations of those exposed to trauma who qualify for a PTSD diagnosis. The authors go on to describe PTSD-related "acute and chronic changes to neurochemical systems and specific brain regions" (p. 11). These regions include the hippocampus and amygdala and medial pre-frontal cortex, which are identified as critically important. The hippocampus, according to imaging employed by the researchers, has a smaller volume in those diagnosed with PTSD (in this case Vietnam veterans) than those who have not been so diagnosed. Low levels of cortisol detected in the adrenal system of road trauma and rape victims are also seen in this study as a predictor of an eventual PTSD diagnosis. Early childhood trauma and a small hippocampus at birth are also thought to be contributors to a later in life diagnosis of trauma-related symptoms, although (Shalev & Bremner, 2016) add, more optimistically that the hippocampus is capable of regeneration when appropriately medicated.

LaRowe (2008) also argues from a biological perspective that cumulative stress, such as that encountered during a police career, constitutes "trauma frozen in memory". He goes on to describe neurochemicals including catecholamines, adrenalin and noradrenalyn as critical factors in the definition of trauma-related injuries and professional burnout. La Rowe identifies the amygdala as the brain area, which houses memories and that traumatic memories including flashbacks and intrusive thoughts occur when neurons take a shortcut from the thalamus region to the amygdala bypassing the more rational neo-cortex.

Peters (2009:24) makes it clear that in his view "PTSD is a real medical condition" and once diagnosed it is possible to observe "substantial physiological and neurological alterations to patients with PTSD". This is further evidenced by lowered levels of hydroxicorticosteroids. Peters argues that such changes are permanent and that PTSD is rarely "cured" by psychotherapy or medication and that as a result police officers so diagnosed should not return to operational duties.

Morris (2015) also contends that MRI imaging is now primarily used to prove the existence of PTSD, suggesting that in some areas of psychiatry, neuroscience has become the only reliable rubric for understanding human experience. From the perspective of a PTSD sufferer, however, he goes on to ask whether such an approach has "reached the point of absurdity" (p. 160). Quoting a somewhat cynical Veterans Affairs psychotherapist, he continues, "So tell me about the war so I can better work on your hippocampal transplant!" Morris expresses his frustration at the lack of human experience in such an approach quoting Kandel "The hard-nosed propositions of neurobiology although scientifically more satisfying, have considerably less existential meaning than the soft-nosed propositions of psychiatry".

Joseph argues similarly that "The trauma industry has enthusiastically adopted the language of medicine. Trauma is not an illness to be cured by a doctor" (xv.). He summarises the neurobiological trauma process in terms of "fight or flight" responses where the brain's automatic defence systems "freeze". He goes on to describe the role of the sympathetic and parasympathetic branches of nervous system in the trauma experience. The latter, he argues, slows us down in the face of threat to a motionless state facilitated by the limbic system, wherein the amygdala ("the brain's gatekeeper for incoming information") and hippocampus are placed under stress. The amygdala, argues Joseph, then takes a shortcut to the hypothalamus, which releases the hormone corticotropin. The adrenal glands then release cortisol, which activates the sympathetic nervous system, making the individual ready to fight or flee. The amygdala, continues Joseph, is like a smoke detector in the brain which through the hippocampus organises memory in time and space and usually transfers memory into long-term storage. Under profound threat during traumatic experiences, the activity of the hippocampus is suppressed because the brain structures concerned with memory storage and language have shut down. Joseph, therefore, defines PTSD as "a disorder of information processing" (p. 58).

Seligman (2015) launched Penn State University's Positive Neuroscience project in 2009, drawing together 15 scholars through a series of research awards in the area. His intention is to promote research and practice in the trauma field that in his view "Has focussed on disease, dysfunction and the harmful effects of stress and trauma" and continues, "Very little is known about the neural mechanisms of human flourishing". (Seligman, 2015:2). The first phase of the project was completed in 2013, with much of the research findings now in the process of publication.

9.4 Critics of the PTSD Diagnosis

The PTSD diagnostic approach is also, however, not without its critics, which is some comfort to those who are focused on the positives of dealing with repeated traumatic exposure and the creation and maintenance of resilience (Calhoun & Tedeschi, 2014; Morris, 2015; Schiraldi, 2011; Tedeschi & Calhoun, 1995; Violanti, 2006; Whybrow et al., 2015). Brewin (2003) mounts a significant argument that PTSD diagnosis evolved as a political strategy at the conclusion of the Vietnam War as a means of deflecting attention from the war itself to the suffering and dislocation of its hapless veterans. Brewin quotes "Saviours and Sceptics" on both sides of the argument which questions PTSD diagnosis in the various DSM's as re-invigorating diagnostic criteria that already existed prior to PTSD being introduced as a standalone disorder. Brewin further explores the differences between "ordinary memory" and traumatic memory, arguing that the "medicalisation" of trauma was nothing more than a political device to change focus from the politicians who triggered the war to its veterans, particularly those who on their return from Vietnam protested against its continuance. PTSD according to Brewin is "a cultural and a political construct rather than the description of a mental disorder" (p. 13).

Young (1997:5), in the context of providing a comprehensive history of the development of the PTSD diagnosis, argues that the widely accepted view of the nature of PTSD is erroneous. It is a concept "glued together by the practices, technologies and narratives with which it is diagnosed, studied, treated and represented by the various interests, institutions and moral arguments that mobilised these efforts and resources". He goes on to describe PTSD as a "disease of time", breaking down the usual boundaries between the present experience of reality and the past. He describes the process of healing PTSD sufferers as "reconciling one's world view to what has happened" (p. 9). Arguing that PTSD is as predictable as was "shell Shock" and "battle fatigue" in World Wars One and Two, Young blames such responses on "timidity and a family history of mental health issues". He does, however, not deny the reality of the suffering that precedes the diagnosis or the reality of the events that bring it about. Young's argument focuses on the question, "are the facts now attached to PTSD true and timeless?" (p. 10) and the impact that question has on diagnosis and the creation and viability of the "trauma industry". It is also of interest that Young refers to research conducted in Australia by McFarlane (1993) that categorised fire fighter's responses to the Ash Wednesday bushfires of 1983 in three ways:

1. Responses that show individuals to be "distressed" by the firefighting risk and trauma but not "syndromal".
2. The second category had pre-existing pathological symptoms that McFarlane argues were triggered by the firefighting experience as part of a "feedback mechanism" that exacerbates previous mental health issues.
3. The third category of responses is those triggered by the trauma of the bushfire and could be diagnosed as PTSD in terms of the then DSMIII. (1983). Young's key argument here is that the second group would, in today's trauma climate, receive a full PTSD diagnosis "with concurrent major depression and anxiety disorders" (P138) and has significance in terms of predicting and preventing PTSD. Young comments that few contemporary PTSD researchers have shown interest in Mc Farlane's work.

Bistoen (2016:121) argues that in the context of Western culture, the trauma-impacted individual is focused upon as the locus of trauma instead of the surrounding social conditions that have caused it. In that sense, Bistoen defines trauma psychiatry as a "covert form of neo-colonialism". Referencing Herman (1997), he goes on to argue that trauma is the product of occurrences that challenge and contradict our fundamental assumptions about the world and that PTSD does not reflect "scientifically gathered, objective knowledge" (p. 21). Agreeing with Young (1997), Bistoen points out that PTSD originated from a point it time (post-Vietnam war) in a particular place (post–Vietnam War America) and in accord with a particular "moral and particular agenda" (The Nixon administration of the early 1970s). At the centre of Bistoen's approach is his view that the DSM's aim at reducing PTSD symptoms through their treatment, with insufficient attention being paid to the conditions responsible for those symptoms and pathology in the first place.

Seligman points out that 20% of Iraq and Afghanistan veterans have now been diagnosed with PTSD. He goes on to make the observation that "every soldier going to Iraq or Afghanistan has heard of PTSD…far and away the most usual response is resilience" (p. 157). Referencing a visit, he made to the West Point (USA) military academy, he continues, "90% of the cadets had heard of PTSD which in reality is relatively uncommon, but less than 10% had heard of post traumatic growth which is not uncommon" (p. 158). Seligman argues that the expectation of a PTSD response in the military after a traumatic event "outside the range of usual human experience"

(DSM 5, 2013) is a predictor that a diagnosis will follow, particularly if the individual was a "catastrophiser" before the event occurred. Comparing British military diagnosis PTSD rates of 5% with those above, Seligman alludes to over-diagnosis of the condition in the context of the US life pension of $3000.00 per month for military veterans, many of whom discontinue treatment immediately after a receiving a full PTSD diagnosis and the subsequent pension.

Joseph (2012) makes clear his trenchant criticism of the "trauma industry" by commenting, "for this army of psychotherapists, psychiatrists, psychologists and social workers, business is booming" (xv Introduction). He argues that the focus in matters relating to trauma is now almost always negative, utilising medical language and placing therapists in a "doctor like position" and predicting an inescapable diagnosis of PTSD for individuals who find themselves in situations of great stress and challenge. There is now he believes, "a culture of expectation" that pervades emergency services, victims of crime and natural and man-made disasters, that is, anyone faced with trauma that is beyond the ordinary life experience. An alternative view, argues Joseph is that profound experiences of trauma should be seen as a normal part of human experience, that lead not only to suffering and challenge but also to possibilities of personal and psychological growth that can be overwhelmingly positive.

Derek Summerfield (2001:95) agrees, referring to "the invention of Posttraumatic stress disorder", locating that process in the aftermath in the United States of the Vietnam War as supporters of traumatised veterans sought effective care and treatment for them. He argues that psychiatric diagnoses of PTSD involved then and now "a telling example of the role of society and politics rather than scientific discovery". Pointing to the growth of the popularity of the diagnosis in 2001, Summerfield despairs at the close identification of normal stress responses with "trauma" arguing that the traumatic responses once seen as a result of extreme experiences now apply to more commonplace, everyday life challenges. He asserts that "once it becomes advantageous to frame distress as a psychiatric condition people will choose to present themselves as medicalised victims rather than feisty survivors" (p. 96). This, Summerfield argues has led to the creation of a "trauma industry" comprising not only Joseph's (2011) psychotherapists, psychiatrists, psychologists and social workers but also "experts, lawyers, claimants, and other interested parties" (p. 96).

With reference to over-diagnosis, Rogers (2008:110) makes a similar point in his discussion of malingering and PTSD. Using the DSM 4 definition of malingering, "The intentional production of false or grossly exaggerated physical or psychological symptoms, motivated by external incentives", Rogers describes the difficult task for clinicians of detecting malingerers because of the subjective nature of PTSD symptoms, which are also well known to the general public through a constant media focus on trauma-related issues. He argues that the broadening of the PTSD definition has been "a boon to plaintiff attorneys" (p. 110) and warns that such attorneys may offer coaching to their clients in order to describe symptoms they may not in fact be experiencing. Rogers refers to the life pension available to US military veterans once "full-blown" PTSD has been diagnosed.

Miller (2015:37) in discussing the elements of malingering in this context opines that "some convince themselves that they have PTSD, others with anti-social personality disorders have no qualms and delight in fooling the authorities". He includes fabrication of symptoms, their exaggeration and the intention to extend their impact after they have subsided as components of PTSD related malingering. Detection of malingerers, says Miller can only occur if they confess to their intention or if they are observed undertaking actions that they claim they are unable to achieve. Again this is confirmed in my interviews by a retired detective senior Sergeant, "I don't have flashbacks, a lot of the PTSD is crap. I have seen coppers manipulate the system. A lot of the present concerns have gone too far. I used to say to my teams, come to see me first in confidence before you go to a psych".

Junger (2015) in a similar vein asks why, when only 10% of American troops deployed to war zones such as Iraq and Afghanistan are exposed to combat, PTSD rates are now approaching 30% among all those who return to the United States, that is around 150,000 claims per year. He compares this to the Israeli defence force who have levels of the diagnosis around 1% in the context of generations of conflict and mandated national service. Junger goes on to argue that PTSD might, therefore, be caused not by exposure to combat but by the process of returning home after the deployment, relinquishing the bonds created with fellow soldiers as they experience the mutual reliance that accompanies combat. The argument here is that those who return from combat miss the "human closeness" that is a part of survival in war and that is not available to them in the same measure as they return to civilian life. At war, argues Junger, soldiers are never alone, when they return they are subject to what he calls "the chronic isolation of modern society" (p. 13). This lack of "social support" leads to isolation, depression and the possible diagnosis of a trauma-related illness. Another factor, Junger argues that if the war is perceived by soldiers as just and necessary, then PTSD rates will be lower when they return home. This raises some important questions around policing in that although SAPOL officers are already "home" they are sustained by camaraderie and culture within their organisation and according to those interviewed, also supported by familial and social engagement when they are off duty. Further, if officers see their duties as "just" as most I interviewed did, which serves as a further protective factor, encouraging optimism, resilience and growth. It would seem that the police experience becomes closer to that of the military when they retire and return "home" literally. Further research is needed into that area of policing.

Police organisations across the globe are also beginning to see numbers of veteran and other police officers similarly affected both as the result of extra-ordinarily traumatic incidents and long-term injuries, the presumed result of career long exposure to the everyday traumas of contemporary policing (Chae & Boyle, 2013; Cotton, 2016; Marin, 2012; Ménard & Arter, 2013; Violanti, 2014). In June 1992, the New South Wales Ombudsman, Irene Moss AO, published a report to the state Parliament entitled "Officers under stress-A special report to Parliament under Section 31 of the Ombudsman's Act". The Report focussed on the lack of support for Officers who had been exposed to "traumatic stress". In the introduction to her investigation, the Ombudsman stated:

> As an organisation whose officers are routinely exposed to stress and trauma, the police service needs adequate systems to enable managers to identify and respond to the needs of staff experiencing difficulties. The police Services own research has also highlighted the need for improvements (p.7).

Moss's survey of police personnel involved in critical incidents over a 6-month period in 1998 found that for every five police officers involved in these incidents, only three were offered professional support. Of those who were offered support, 72% were not offered further assistance after the initial intervention, 18% of those interviewed indicated a clinically significant reaction to the incident and only half of this 18% had received assistance. More experienced officers were more likely to be significantly affected. A third of those interviewed were unaware of the police service's psychology and welfare services. The Report's recommendations were two-fold. Moss recommended the implementation of a system to ensure that appropriate support was offered to all officers exposed to traumatic incidents and as a matter of urgency, develop mechanisms and guidelines for managers to obtain reports about officers who exhibit signs that they are not coping and ensure the information issued to support and assist officers (P.8). The well-intentioned report failed to adequately account for the police culture around "toughing it out" and the deeply ingrained belief among (mostly male) officers that you kept such things to yourself and "never put your hand up" when feeling under pressure (Gilmartin, 2002; Henry, 2004; McKay, 2005; Sparkes, 2013; Violanti, 2006;). New South Wales police took no action in response to the Moss report (McKay, 2005; Sparkes, 2013).[2]

A few years into the twenty-first century, autobiographical accounts of career-related trauma began to emerge from the New South Wales Police Department (Horner, 2011; Mckay, 2005; Sparkes, 2013; Neil, 2014). These were written by officers "hurt on duty" after long struggles with PTSD symptoms that resulted in their usually involuntary retirement. Their careers had been marked by a reluctance to seek timely support in the context of a police department that offered very little. Electronic media began voicing concerns about the plight of such officers, Verity (2014) reported on "Our shameful silence on police Suicide" and Kennedy (2015) announced new hitherto unheard of initiatives, "Posttraumatic stress disorder: Australian researchers develop world first guidelines to support emergency service workers". In 2015, a similar report emanated from another State of Australia, "Victorian police Officer's suicide, casts spotlight on mental health toll in Force" (ABC radio, 2015), which gave that organisation and others, an additional incentive to pay long awaited attention to such issues. In response to the issues raised with him, the New South Wales Commissioner of Police made funding available for a trauma support group and encouraged those organising it, to continue to develop their programme (Mckay, 2005, 2010).

Momentum for similar responses from other Australian police jurisdictions is building in the light of recent reviews (Cotton, 2016; Jenkins, 2015; Vincent, 2016) and continuing media attention (ABC "Four Corners: Insult to Injury…how the system damages cops with PTSD" 1/08/16). Police Associations (Unions) in South

---

[2] See also "Asking for help" Chap. 6.

Australia, Victoria and Western Australia as well as New South Wales have agreed to participate in a nation-wide survey of "first responders" in late 2016 to be co-ordinated by the "Beyond Blue" organisation. Professor Sandy McFarlane of Adelaide University's Centre for Traumatic Stress Studies, in a recent submission to a South Australian Parliamentary Inquiry into "Occupational Safety, Rehabilitation and Compensation" (2016), stated, "The Australian Defence Force provides a model for the provision of occupational health services and compensation that require a broad consideration as possible systems of addressing the workplace issues for emergency services", highlighting the general awareness among trauma researchers that the military has responded more appropriately to war-zone deployment-related trauma than have police organisations to the challenges of everyday police work and management (Seligman, 2012).

9.5 PTSD and Policing

This study sets out to explore mechanisms police officers use to "normalise" their experiences to preserve the delicate professional balance between "coping" that Henry (2004) calls "psychic numbing" and being responsive to victims and survivors in their everyday work environment. Recent advances in post-traumatic growth theory set out to re-interpret exposure in a positive context as well as preventative experience in Australia and internationally.

The examination above, of the present research into PTSD and its development through wars, responses to natural and man-made disasters and application to broader trauma-related experiences is an essential part of my study. Schiraldi (2011:15) defines resilience as "the ability to bounce back after adversity and thrive" and goes on to define PTSD as "the exhaustion of resilience." It follows that resilient police officers will be less likely to succumb to PTSD even after a long career confronting death, injury, violence and mayhem.[3]

9.6 The Autobiographies: Themes from a Police Journey into a PTSD Diagnosis

Resilience in the context of recovery from a full diagnosis of PTSD is rarely present in discussions around the long-term impact of repeated exposure to the traumas of everyday policing. Officers so diagnosed usually do not return to full operational duties due to organisational responses discussed above. Several autobiographical accounts of police officers experiencing severe PTSD reactions have recently been written in Australia (Sparkes, 2013; Mckay, 2005, 2010; Horner, 2011).

[3] See Chap. 8, "Resilience.".

Sparkes (2013) is a 20-year veteran of police service in New South Wales, including 15 years as a CIB Detective. In 1996, Allan received a Cross of Valour bravery award for his rescue of a boy from a stormwater drain. Immediately after the incident, he began his descent into classic PTSD symptoms until his discharge on medical grounds several years later. His torment included periods of severe depression, which culminated in significant bouts of suicidal ideation and nightmares in which Allan committed acts of violence on his wife and children. He finally confided in his wife, commenced successful treatment including counselling and anti-depressant medication as well as a strict, self-imposed fitness regime.

Allan had all the typical duty-related death encounters during his career, which included attending sudden deaths, often involving decomposed and mutilated corpses. He was also involved in an operation where two of his police colleagues were murdered by a gunman. He eventually made a significant recovery and now works as an Ambassador for the Beyond Blue organisation and is in high demand on the lecture circuit as a motivational speaker.

Mckay (2005) served in the NSW Police Department as a Forensic Services (crime scene) examiner. She began her career in this area with little technical training and encountered unimaginable horror and death over the next 17 years of her service. Her experience was similar to that of Allan Sparkes, in that her post-trauma was gradual, profoundly private and involved an escalation of symptoms including sleep disturbance, intrusive thoughts, nightmares, avoidance and profound work-related anxiety. One evening, when Esther was on call at home, her suicidal thoughts became so compelling that she moved her firearm from her bedroom to the police vehicle parked outside. This was against regulations and is an indication of her state of distress. She was discharged from New South Wales Police in 2001 "hurt on duty" with a diagnosis of PTSD. She now coordinates the Police Post-Trauma Support group in New South Wales, which has received recognition and a great deal of support from New South Wales Police at a very high level, including that of the present Chief Commissioner.

Mckay also wrote another book on behalf of a police crime scene colleague entitled "Forensic Investigator True Stories from the life of a country crime scene cop" (2010). This describes the career of Senior Sergeant Jeff Bernasconi who was also a crime scene investigator for 13 years as a Detective Technical Sergeant. He was during his career, a union rep and a peer support officer. He worked for all of his 16 years as a crime scene police officer often unsupported and frequently on call or on duty for long periods of time without a break. Jeff performed all the duties that crime scene investigators are generally called upon to perform including the attendance regularly at murder scenes, road crashes and various forms of human disaster. He was diagnosed with PTSD in February 1999 and left the New South Wales Police organisation in the year 2000. His duties and experience closely parallel those of his colleague Esther Mckay as did his eventual PTSD diagnosis. In both cases, it is clear that New South Wales Police saw neither issue with both officers remaining in their challenging roles for such long periods nor did they offer any form of support to facilitate their well-being.

In both cases, Allan and Esther were unwilling to discuss their problems, an issue clearly explained by Esther in her book "Crime Scene" (2005). Her new "boss" was a Sergeant called Pieter:

> One of Pieter's main concerns was our welfare and he constantly checked on us. Right from the start he touched on the subject of stress, saying that at some stage we might all suffer varying degrees of stress, and even be prepared for a possible nervous breakdown. It was his experience, he said, that after working in the scientific field for two to three years, all sorts of symptoms such as sleeping difficulties, stomach upsets and avoidance of the workplace might occur. It was almost as if Pieter was suggesting it was par for the course, and at the time I was surprised at his frankness-this was a subject that was never discussed. It was part of police culture that emotional problems were kept quiet, because any indication that you weren't coping could mean a transfer and a notation on your service register excluding you from future promotion. This was why stress was usually resolved by a visit to the pub (p.140).

This is entirely congruent with my observations of police culture and is frequently referred to in much of the literature (Henry, 2004; Mckay, 2005, 2010; Neil, 2014; Raphael & Dobson, 2005; Seligman, 2012; Sparkes, 2013). As discussed above, there is classic catch 22 in police organisational culture…if you put your hand up acknowledging developing traumatic responses to your operational tasks, you will be punished. This usually leads to the individual officer saying nothing about their problems until the indicators are so obvious that they are career and/or life threatening.

All of the officers' experiences recounted in these writings, included significant levels of suicidal ideation.[4] Often, media organisations report police officer suicides as a direct consequence of the trauma that officers experience in the exercise of their duties. (Verity, 2014, "Our shameful silence on police suicide", Police Officer's suicide call, I'll be gone before you arrive. Channel 7 Sunday Night.) "Victorian Police Officer's suicide casts spotlight on mental health toll in force" ABC news 2015). Such reports are usually linked with the incidence of PTSD in police organisations and the stresses of the policing environment as the major contributor to the completion of the suicidal act often without justification or evidence (Chae & Boyle, 2013; Henry, 2004; Kroes, 1976; Violanti, 2014). Often the causes are far more complex, reaching into relationships, depressive states and a wide range of contributing factors. In the case of the five officers whose autobiographies/biography are considered throughout this research, there is a consistent theme of the advancing PTSD symptomatology and their subsequent distress and overwhelming sense of failure at several levels being a very significant factor in their intrusive thoughts of suicide.

Neil (2011) rose to the level of Inspector in the New South Wales police, having joined in 1987 as a 19-year-old. Her career spanned 18 years as a police officer and included general patrol duties, undercover work including drug investigations, major crime section, organised crime and homicide investigations. She was 32 years old in 2000 when she was appointed team leader of one of five counter-terrorism negotiator

[4] See also Chap. 4 "Death and Bodies".

units for the Sydney Olympic Games. In 2002, she was commissioned as an Inspector and in 2005 retired from New South Wales Police "hurt on duty" diagnosed with PTSD.

Paul Horner began his working life employed by Woolworths and served for 12 months as a prison officer within Correctional Services in New South Wales, joining New South Wales Police in February 1997. His first appointment was to Mount Druitt in New South Wales, he then spent 3 years in the Western New South Wales town of Bourke, which at the time was a violent community, with significant crime and disorder issues. During his appointment, where he was seriously injured while making an arrest in the midst of a violent melee after being hit in the face with a bottle. He then transferred to Byron Bay and was medically discharged in 2007 diagnosed with PTSD.

Ken Rogers worked within Pleasant Ridge Police Department in the State of Michigan in the United States and was for 21 years a sworn officer in that small police organisation. One evening while on duty, he fired upon and wounded an armed offender. As a result of that experience, his life changed as he began the process of confronting and working through developing PTSD symptoms. He wrote of his experiences in a book entitled "PTSD: A police officer's story" (1999).

The absence of debriefing after critical events, the constant exhaustion due to over-commitment and organisational demands, the lack of opportunity to move from ultra-stressful roles into less demanding ones, the cultural underpinning of "shape up or get out", the prevalent use of alcohol as self-medication and the lack of input to police officers around self-care and early detection of PTSD symptoms. All this, along with the reluctance of police organisations to confront these issues, leads directly to the outcomes for the five officers who have written of their experiences so compellingly.

It was clear from the outset that while reading these autobiographical accounts, one could predict the eventual outcome. Indicators of increasing dysfunction and despair emerged that went unnoticed by senior officers and colleagues. Those officers in my interview cohort had a different story, one of resilience and growth not a gradual descent into mental illness brought on by policing duty-related trauma. This is connected to the question asked. In the police autobiographies, the question was, "How did I get to the point of a PTSD diagnosis?" I asked my interviewees, "How have you remained healthy?"

9.7 PTSD from the SAPOL Interviews: The Data and Discussion

Many of the officers interviewed spoke of PTSD in a wide variety of contexts. It was obvious that for some it was a source of anxiety, a threat to their well-being that they considered beyond their control. Others had experienced reactions to confronting events that had caused them concern. None reported any attempt by SAPOL to allay their concerns. The common view was that it was hazardous to seek support when under trauma-related pressure and that departmental interventions such as annual psychological reviews offered in some SAPOL units were haphazard and of little value in terms of long term well-being. Many had thought deeply about their mental health, often at the behest of life partners and had taken practical steps to stay well. Two officers who had been diagnosed with PTSD revealed that their descent towards that diagnosis had gone un-noticed by managers and colleagues, as in this comment, "People on the ground can't see how deep in it you are". "You grow in confidence, you don't like to think anything can shatter that, you always just push it down".

A retired Sergeant who had a specific and well-researched knowledge of the condition was clear about his approach to the issue, saying "I didn't give myself time to get PTSD". This is more than avoidance behaviour (Amaranto et al., 2003; Burke, 2016) with this officer very clear that his long career would have been threatened if he had focussed inappropriately on possible negative outcomes. Instead, like many of his colleagues, he developed the ability to create distance from tragedy, not giving emotional reactions "time".

Others spoke of their reaction to PTSD diagnoses among colleagues, "I am aware that some colleagues have questionable PTSD symptoms and been diagnosed with it". This Detective Senior Sergeant went on, "I know that I could have probably qualified with PTSD if I had wanted to…" There is evidence here of a suspicion that such a diagnosis offers a way out for disgruntled officers (Junger, 2015; Miller, 2015; Rogers, 2008) and that to "qualify" for such an outcome was not culturally or professionally acceptable. A sergeant of over 30 years' experience was similarly aware of PTSD and its impact, "Some of my colleagues have been diagnosed with PTSD. I am sceptical about how genuine some are, but there are more legits than malingerers. One colleague who was a crime scene officer at Snowtown[5] was rooted and left the job". The Snowtown investigation took years to complete and involved investigating the deaths of 12 individuals who were murdered and some of whose decomposed bodies were stored in plastic barrels when discovered by investigating police. The investigating officers were well supported by SAPOL during the prolonged investigation and trial.

Another retired Detective Senior Sergeant commented after describing a career typically full of grotesque death and mayhem, "I don't have flashbacks, a lot of the PTSD is crap. I have seen coppers manipulate the system. A lot of the present concerns have gone too far. I used to say to my teams, come to see me first in confidence before you go to a psych". This officer was well aware of the career cost of submitting to a PTSD diagnosis. Seeing him in confidence before a SAPOL "psych" was recommended. Like much of the literature (Addis & Stephens, 2008; Berger & Weiss, 2009; Bistoen, 2016; Brewin, 2003; Curran, 2003; Janoff-Bulman, 1989; Morris, 2015; Seligman, 2012; Young, 1997), he felt that over-diagnosis of first responders was rife and that his form of early intervention was a preferable alternative. He offered no details of the outcomes of such conversations.

[5] See my reference to these murders in my "Coping" and "Death and bodies" chapters.

A long-serving Major Crime Detective, commenting on his career total of over 200 homicide investigations described the everyday impact on him: "These things you often remember simply by driving past the area where they occurred or someone mentioning a name or place that brings it all back to you. I've never had a real issue with going to sleep, although the first few nights after a bad homicide I had trouble going to sleep. I still remember a lot of these things, but I don't think about it too often". Another Officer with a long career in Major Crime made a similar comment regarding intrusive images of murder crime scenes, "You can't forget anything it's always there, you sometimes think about it even though you don't want to. The images are very vivid at first and they never fade completely. The first few days after one of those incidents are the worst". For these two, after long careers and countless murder scenes, acknowledging the long-term cost of such exposures was matter of fact and indicative of short-term reactions that subsided, followed by permanent, largely controlled memories. There is no evidence in these comments that SAPOL or the Major Crime Squad provided any support or interventions that assisted the natural process, such was the organisational culture of the time.

Some officers saw the need to change career trajectories in the interests of resilience and the expected impact of long-term career exposure to trauma. A Detective Sergeant investigating child sexual abuse over a long period had obviously thought about and researched the possible impact of such exposure, "I have seen and done things that didn't bother me at the time…it must be having an effect, but not to the point that I can't function. But I need to move on". This comment also reveals the expectation, often evidenced in the literature (McFarlane, 2011, 2017; Peters, 2009; Rees & Smith, 2008; Violanti, 2014; Woodberry, 1987) that routine trauma exposure might inevitably lead to dysfunction.

A Brevet Sergeant in Family Violence investigation was similarly philosophical, "I've been told, you probably have PTSD at some level". An Officer of 35 years' experience, when asked, "Have you read much about PTSD?" Responded, "No, I've talked about it with my therapist". The likely positive impact of even basic psychoeducation around PTSD early indicators would prove helpful to officers such as these offering either reassurance or the opportunity to seek support before symptoms progress.

Anxiety around the possibility of a PTSD diagnosis was well expressed by a young Senior Constable after a particularly difficult unsuccessful attempt to save the life of a young woman who had attempted suicide, expressed the uncertainty of such situations clearly, "She died later. My partner on the day struggled afterwards. He was in a liquor store which had the same name as her first name and later burst into tears in a cheese shop. This was worrying for me as he seemed to be solid in the job. I wondered if it would creep up on me the same way. He is OK now". The lack of departmental interventions after such an event, clearly out of the ordinary for even the most experienced officer, adds to the discomfort of those involved and to the expectation that something negative might follow or accumulate. The briefest of interventions, debriefing or Psychological First Aid, might dispel such anxieties and offer a healthy context for post-operational ruminations (Al-Shahi & Warlow, 2000; Alexander, 2000; Australian Red Cross, 2009).

A STAR group recovery diver earlier in his career had the same concerns:

> I hear of people in similar situations who suddenly have a breakdown, I have a different attitude, I don't have nightmares about bodies, when I first started I used to try to tidy up bodies as we took them back in, I don't do that so much anymore. I sometimes worry when I hear stories of people who I believe are seeing and experiencing similar things to me and eventually have a breakdown. I wonder why, and if they have a happy home life or they have other personal issues that contributed to their breakdown.

Not "tidying up bodies" is an indicator of this officer realising that he was getting emotionally too close to victims and that he needed to take steps to re-establish boundaries between the deceased, their loved ones and himself. His clearly expressed concerns about other officers succumbing to "breakdowns" in similar situations to his own could well be lessened by basic psycho-education and debriefing.

A Detective Sergeant who was threatened by an offender with a knife in 1980s commented, "I must have some PTSD around that experience, I still have no memory of what happened. I attended many, many car accidents, fights, pub brawls, domestics". He reflects the view among many officers that there is an inevitable link between such events and an eventual PTSD diagnosis even though his lack of memory of the event conflicts with the nature of a PTSD diagnosis where such memories would be ever present and intrusive rather than completely absent.

An insight into how such thoughts around this issue are dealt with was provided by a retired Detective Chief Superintendent who said, "How you handle stress comes down to personality. I have known people who have had issues with various commands. Early interventions to deal with it are really important. I haven't had a lot to do with PTSD, I'm not sure whether Detectives are over or under represented". An officer at this level in the chain of command is clearly in a similar position to his lower ranked colleagues. An awareness that personality type has a great deal to do with resilience, as well as the importance of early intervention to sustain it indicate that much thought has been given to the issue, again with no reference to helpful Departmental inputs or interventions.

A Senior Constable who was shot while on duty described his experience of post-incident events with regard to PTSD, "I didn't say much to anyone. In saw Employee Assistance and a Psych who explained PTSD curve. My senior partner was very supportive. SAPOL was very good, I can't say anything bad about SAPOL at all". This was, however, a SAPOL response to a visible, physical injury where accompanying emotional responses become acceptable. Invisible, stress-related injury usually provokes a different organisational response. A Sergeant in Major Crash confirmed this, commenting, "There is still a stigma about going to health or welfare sections. If you say I have PTSD forget your career!"

In answer to the question, "Is the UK policing approach around well-being of Officers different?" An ex UK recruit commented, "I don't know, I never sought assistance in the UK or here". He went on, "PTSD can be claimed if you don't have it and many officers who do have it live with it! I don't trust the organisation, I wouldn't go to them if I had problems, I wouldn't go to the EAP…it's a fundamental matter of trust. SAPOL needs to use confidential external services then coppers would use them". The benefit of the experience of a different policing approach is evident in this comment. From observation, this officer is clear that PTSD is subject to both malingering when not present and co-existence when it is. SAPOL has a difficult task in encouraging the levels of trust necessary for officers to come forward when challenged by trauma even at levels below the diagnostic threshold.

Expressing an alternative view, another officer opined, "We deal with contingencies, not our emotions. Depressive periods are normal. PTSD should be accepted as normal!!!" A Detective Senior Sergeant, who was seriously assaulted early in his career, was also aware of such lack of response, "I am sure I had a touch of PTSD after the assault. I had a blandness of affect. I've never had an annual review". Both reflect an awareness of PTSD symptomatology and the readiness to live with their "indifference and blandness" although it may be a coping strategy rather a symptom. Again, a simple departmental intervention around the realities of trauma responses may reassure both officers.

Two officers were interviewed who had been diagnosed with PTSD. One expressed the relief that the diagnosis brought after years of self-concern about his feelings and behaviour, "I had a PTSD diagnosis which was Work Cover approved. I'm better since I've been broken {diagnosed?] but not before, it's the job that does it to you". An officer also diagnosed while stationed in a regional setting and who had experienced a challenging series of events commented, "Before diagnosis I had three fatal MVA's {motor vehicle accidents} in ten days. I didn't know the victims personally. All I got was a phone call from EAP {SAPOL Employee Assistance Programme} asking "are you OK?"

An operational Senior Constable described his experience of the onset of PTSD symptoms after a stabbing injury leading to a diagnosis:

> On the 9th of September 2002 I realised I was not right. I had nightmares, was hyper vigilant. I was always wondering where the next ambush is coming from. On September 11, 2002, I stopped a car the same type as the one where I was stabbed, with four shitheads in it. I panicked, I couldn't breathe. I drove off. I can't do this anymore! I went home and had four months off work. I ticked every box and was diagnosed with PTSD and mild depression".

The Departmental response was less than satisfactory from his point of view, "I was refused WorkCover. SAPOL disagreed with the diagnosis. I took sick leave and PASA (the police Union) sued SAPOL. Management don't care. We are cannon fodder!" The same Officer went on, "My PTSD has gone up and down. From hyper to laconic. There is a solid group who I trust, people know me! I have seen a lot of death and violence, countless suicides, vulnerable and innocent people. It could have been me!" This account illustrates clearly the variety of organisational experiences police officers can have before and after a PTSD diagnosis. This officer had little effective support after a period of intense trauma exposure, although he "ticked every box" had to endure protracted litigation to obtain Workcover benefits.

Another colleague, upon receiving his diagnosis, expressed relief and a clear belief that he recognised the source of his affliction as "the job". These officers expected that after treatment, their careers would continue, which being a possible sign of progress in terms of past organisational responses to PTSD, particularly in Eastern Australian police organisations.

A retired Senior Officer commented briefly, referring to the implications of trauma for senior SAPOL management, "the lid's off PTSD" and added, "retirement is a crucial process with regard to PTSD". How far the lid is actually off, in the sense that it is no longer possible for police leadership in Australia to ignore trauma management is not clear, but pressure from within police organisations (for example, from unions and past members) as well as from without (the media and academic researchers) is mounting and may well be irresistible. This officer's reference to retirement is a case in point. At present, an officer retiring from SAPOL is offered a free physical examination. As one long-serving officer on the brink of retirement commented, "this week I am a Sergeant in Major Crime, next week I will be a golfer!"

As if in summary of this section, a Major Crash Officer was of the view that, "PTSD is rarely discussed. The army has mandatory suicide awareness training. SAPOL thinks that if they focussed on PTSD awareness, half their workforce would disappear". This may well explain the apparent lack of a mental health strategy in SAPOL and the resulting clear need for officers to take care of themselves and each other.

9.8 The Incidence of PTSD Among SAPOL Officers: (Psychologist and Psychiatrist Interviews) the Data

Three psychiatrists and three psychologists were interviewed as a part of this research who all had extensive experience treating and/or assessing SAPOL officers. This was intended to provide some triangulation of the data obtained from the 50 officers who were interviewed with a focus on their coping strategies on "the job" particularly with regard to SAPOL executive management's approaches to officers experiencing challenges to their professional resilience. When asked about their view of the size of the SAPOL operational cohort who are negatively impacted by trauma, there was some disagreement among them. One psychologist commented that among his police clients, "not many have PTSD". A colleague surmised that, "fifteen percent of current SAPOL workforce are impacted, many whom are un-diagnosed with PTSD". Agreeing and commenting on his own view of his psychiatric profession, another confirmed, "PTSD is under recognised. The hypocrisy of psychiatry lies in the fact that the level of functioning of the individual is the critical issue. The diagnosis doesn't matter!" He went on, "I've only seen one copper who was crazy. They are really nice people. Poor management is responsible for what has happened to them. It's always complaints about the bosses!"[6]

A psychiatric colleague, expressing his view of an over-diagnosis of PTSD in this sector was cautious, "They present with adjustment disorders, very low numbers with full PTSD". He added in agreement with his colleague above and much of the

[6] See Chap. 2 "Power, organisational and police culture, 'the job'".

research into the sources of stress, "It usually involves work related anxiety and depression. It is usually the work environment, discipline culture and procedures. Police culture magnifies organisational issues and makes members more vulnerable". A psychologist agreed stating that, "Many officers present with psychological injury, major depression and PTSD due to trauma exposure, disciplinary issues and interpersonal issues". He gave as an example an internal investigation after a police car was involved in a duty-related crash. The officer driving was later diagnosed with PTSD.

In line with the views of many of the police officers interviewed, a psychologist was clear that "A proportion of apparently healthy cops have issues. Individuals don't trust the organisation to seek support". He continued, "The DSM's aren't adequate. We need another diagnostic approach which includes avoidance behaviours, genetic influences and bio-chemical imbalances".

9.9 What Have We Learned?

Post-traumatic stress disorder diagnostic criteria first appeared in the 1980 edition of the American Psychiatric Association's Diagnostic and Statistical Manual of Mental Disorders (DSM 3) (American Psychiatric Association, 1980). It had been developed as a direct response to the experiences of American military personnel who had been deployed as part of the Vietnam conflict (1954–1975). The diagnosis has through subsequent DSM's been applied to civilian experiences of extreme trauma such as natural disaster and criminal victimisation and accident to other "first responder" populations including police. It is now almost an expectation that police officers "when exposed to enough trauma" (McFarlane, 2011) will succumb to a PTSD diagnosis. Such an expectation assumes that even the most resilient of individuals will lose the capacity to "bounce back" (Schiraldi, 2011) after challenging tasks outside of their "normal" operational experience. The "intrusion" (Morris, 2015; Seligman, 2012; Summerfield, 2001; Young, 1997) of the diagnosis into areas such as policing constitutes a challenge to executive police management to dispense with traditional, cultural expectations that their members will tough it out and maintain their well-being without departmental intervention. It is crucially important that police organisations, despite their apparent fears of a PTSD epidemic, respond to these challenges effectively in the face of mounting pressure from unions, individual officers and external reviews and the media in the interests of the well-being of their members.

9.9.1 Where Next?

Direct comparisons in terms of traumatic experiences and organisational responses between para-military and military organisations are often made without acknowledgement of the differences in the experiences of such organisations (McFarlane, 2017; Morris, 2015; Rivard et al., 2002; Sadulski, 2017; Schaffer, 2014; Sutton, 2005). Police officers cannot discriminate between the "battlefield" and home soil. They are potentially never absent from the field of conflict. They cannot return from tours of duty to recover or confront their demons as their military counterparts do. They are challenged to devise and maintain strategies to remain well over long careers, often with little or no meaningful organisational support being provided. The 50 interviews conducted for this research with SAPOL officers and the six clinicians who support and assess them reveal clearly that SAPOL's present "command and control" approaches to management, and reluctance to address trauma-related issues are out of step with more progressive responses such as those of the Australian and US military (McFarlane, 2017; Seligman, 2012; Stinchcomb, 2004).

This study has enabled the voices of the SAPOL officers interviewed to be heard, revealing their optimism and pride in their identity and career achievements, despite their awareness of the hazards of their profession. Their knowledge of PTSD is significant, they are aware of colleagues who have been "broken" and they take steps to remain well in the knowledge that their organisation (SAPOL) will do little to assist them.

References

Addis, N., & Stephens, C. (2008). An evaluation of a police debriefing programme: Outcomes for police officers five years after a police shooting. *International Journal of Police Science & Management, 10*(4), 361–373.

Alexander, D. (2000). Debriefing and body recovery: Police in a civilian disaster. In *Psychological debriefing: Theory, practice and evidence* (pp. 118–130).

Al-Shahi, R., & Warlow, C. (2000). The current status of psychological debriefing. *BMJ, 321*, 1032–1033.

American Psychiatric Association. (1980). *Diagnostic Statistics Manual of Mental Disorders.* American Psychiatric Pub.

American Psychiatric Association. (2013). *Diagnostic and statistical manual of mental disorders (DSM-5®).* American Psychiatric Pub.

Amaranto, E., et al. (2003). Police stress interventions. *Brief Treatment and Crisis Intervention, 3*(1), 47.

Australian Red Cross (2009). Psychological First Aid: An Australian Guide. *Australian Psychological Society.*

Berger, R., & Weiss, T. (2009). The Posttraumatic Growth model: An expansion to the family system. *Traumatology, 15*(1), 63.

Bistoen, G. (2016). *Trauma, ethics and the political beyond PTSD: The dislocations of the real.* Springer.

Brewin, C. (2003). *Posttraumatic stress disorder: Malady or myth?* Yale University Press.

Burke, R. J. (2016). *Stress in Policing: Sources.* Routledge.

Calhoun, L. G., & Tedeschi, R. G. (2014). *Handbook of posttraumatic growth: Research and practice*. Routledge.
Chae, M. H., & Boyle, D. J. (2013). Police suicide: Prevalence, risk, and protective factors. *Policing: An International Journal of Police Strategies & Management, 36*(1), 91–118.
Chopko, B. A., & Schwartz, R. C. (2013). The relation between mindfulness and posttraumatic stress symptoms among police officers. *Journal of Loss and Trauma, 18*(1), 1–9.
Cotton, P. (2016). Victoria Police Mental Health Review. An independent review into the mental health and well-being of Victoria Police employees. Australia.
Douglas, B., & Wodak, J. (Eds.) (2016). *Trauma related stress in Australia: Essays by leading Australian thinkers and researchers*. ACT Australia: Australia 21 LTD.
Friedman, M. (2015). *Posttraumatic and acute stress disorders*. Springer.
Gilmartin, K. M. (2002). Emotional survival for law enforcement. *ES Press, PMB, 233*, 2968.
Grogan, S. (2014). *Shell shocked Britain: The first world war's legacy for Britain's mental health*. Pen and Sword.
Herman, J. L. (1997). *Trauma and recovery*. Basic books.
Henry, V. E. (2004). *Death work: Police, trauma, and the psychology of survival*. Oxford University Press.
Horner, P. (2011). Jack Knife: The crashing of a policeman- NSW police and PTSD. New South Wales, Australia, Zeus Publications.
Janoff-Bulman, R. (1989). Assumptive worlds and the stress of traumatic events: Applications of the schema construct. *Social Cognition, 7*(2), 113–136.
Jenkins, K. (2015). Independent review into sex discrimination and sexual harassment, including predatory behaviour in Victoria Police. Victoria, Australia, Victorian equal opportunity and human rights commission.
Jones, E., & Wessely, S. (2005). *Shell shock to PTSD: Military psychiatry from 1900 to the Gulf War*. Psychology Press.
Joseph, S. (2012). *What doesn't kill us: A guide to overcoming adversity and moving forward*. Hachette UK.
Junger, S. (2015). How PTSD became a problem far beyond the battlefield. *Vanity Fair*.
Kelly, B. D. (2015). Shell shock in Ireland: The Richmond War Hospital, Dublin (1916–19). *History of Psychiatry, 26*(1), 50–63.
Kroes, W. H. (1976). *Society's victim, the policeman: An analysis of job stress in policing*. Thomas Springfield.
La Rowe, K. (2008). *Breath of relief: Transforming compassion fatigue into flow*. Healer–Warrior. INC. Second edition.
Lees, P. (2014). *Shell shock: Traumatic neurosis and the British soldiers of the first world war*. Palgrave Macmillan.
Lifton, R. J. (1983). *The broken connection: On death and the continuity of life*. American Psychiatric Pub.
Marin, A. (2012). In the line of duty. Ombudsman's report. Ontario, Canada.
McFarlane, A. C. (2017). Improving internal practices to support emergency services. In *Mental Health strategy for first responders: Tackle stigma &enhance prevention strategies*. Melbourne Australia: Criterion Conferences.
Mc Farlane, A. C. (2016). *Occupational safety, rehabilitation and compensation*. South Australia: Adelaide University. Centre for Trauma Studies.
McFarlane, A. C. (2011). *Many paths, one purpose. Expert forum*. Australia: Australian Centre for posttraumatic mental health.
Mckay, E. (2005). *Crime Scene-True stories from the life of a crime scene investigator*. Australia: Viking (Penguin) Australia.
Mckay, E. (2010). *Forensic investigator*. Australia: Viking (Penguin) Australia.
Ménard, K. S., & Arter, M. L. (2013). Police officer alcohol use and trauma symptoms: Associations with critical incidents, coping, and social stressors. *International Journal of Stress Management, 20*(1), 37.

Miller, L. (2015). *PTSD and forensic psychology: Applications to civil and criminal law*. Springer.

Morris, D. J. (2015). *The evil hours: A biography of post-traumatic stress disorder*, Health Affairs.

Neil, B. (2014). *Under siege*. Australia: Harlequin Mira.

Peters, R. F. (2009). *Police under pressure. (A donkey on the edge)*. New South Wales, Australia: HEAS Publications

Raphael, B. (1986). *When disaster strikes: How individuals and communities cope with catastrophe*. Basic Books (AZ).

Raphael, B., & Dobson, M. (2005). *Acute posttraumatic interventions: Treating trauma and PTSD*. Cambridge University Press.

Rees, B. & J. Smith (2008). Breaking the silence: the traumatic circle of policing. International Journal of Police Science & Management 10(3): 267–279.

Rogers, L. K. (1999). *PostTraumatic Stress Disorder: A police officer's report*. Proctor Publications.

Rivard, J. M., et al. (2002). Acute dissociative responses in law enforcement officers involved in critical shooting incidents: The clinical and forensic implications. *Journal of Forensic Science* 47(5): 1–8.

Rowe, A., & Regehr, C. (2010). Whatever gets you through today: An examination of cynical humor among emergency service professionals. *Journal of Loss and Trauma, 15*(5), 448–464.

Sadulski, J. (2017). Understanding how police cope with stress to promote resiliency: Multiple case study. Northcentral University.

Sandiford, H. (1938). War neuroses. *Journal of the Royal Army Medical Corps, 71*(4), 222–234.

Shalev, A. Y., & Bremner, J. D. (2016). Posttraumatic stress disorder: from neurobiology to clinical presentation. *Posttraumatic stress disorder: From neurobiology to treatment* (p. 1).

Schaffer, B. (2014). *Way of the Warrior*. Self- published.

Schiraldi, G. R. (2011). *The complete guide to resilience: Why it matters how to build it and maintain it*. Resilience Training International.

Seligman, M. E. P. (2012). *Flourish: A visionary new understanding of happiness and well-being*. Simon and Schuster.

Seligman, M. E. P. (2015). Positive neuro science.

Stinchcomb, J. B. (2004). Searching for stress in all the wrong places: Combating chronic organizational stressors in policing. *Police Practice and Research, 5*(3), 259–277.

Sparkes, A. (2013). *The cost of bravery*. New South Wales, Australia: Penguin Group, Australia.

Sutton, S. R. (2005). *True blue: Police stories by those who have lived them*. Macmillan.

Summerfield, D. (2001). The invention of post-traumatic stress disorder and the social usefulness of a psychiatric category. *Student BMJ, 9*.

Tedeschi, R. G., & Calhoun, L. G. (1995). *Trauma and transformation: Growing in the aftermath of suffering*. Sage Publications.

Verity, W. (2014). Our shameful silence on police Suicide. The Drum, Australian Broadcasting Corporation: 20 minutes.

Violanti, J. M. (2006). The police: Perspectives on trauma and resiliency.

Violanti, J. M. (2014). *Dying for the job: Police work exposure and health*. Charles C Thomas Publisher.

Vincent, N. (2016). Sex discrimination, sexual harassment and predatory behaviour in South Australia Police. Independent review. South Australia: Equal Opportunity Commission.

Whybrow, D., et al. (2015). Promoting organizational well-being: A comprehensive review of Trauma Risk Management. *Occupational Medicine, 65*(4), 331–336.

Wiederhold, B. (2013). *New tools to enhance posttraumatic stress disorder diagnosis and treatment: Invisible wounds of war*. IOS Press.

Woodberry, J. M. (1987). An examination of stress in the police force. South Australia.

Young, A. (1997). *The harmony of illusions: Inventing post-traumatic stress disorder*. Princeton University Press.

Chapter 10
Post-traumatic Growth in Policing

Abstract Post-traumatic growth in policing: How officers grow in many important ways through a long career. This is a far more positive and optimistic approach to mental health and policing framed by post-traumatic growth theory and confirmed by the officers' interviews, the majority of whom had enjoyed their careers and who would "do it all again in a heartbeat". This chapter has a clear focus on the benefits that flow from a career in policing, the significant increases in self-awareness and the long term satisfaction that comes from such service. The qualitative interviews allowed officers to express positive perspectives on "the job" and its significance to the society they serve. Clear linkages are made here with the theory of post-traumatic growth and how participants described its importance to their professional and personal growth. At the end of each interview, I asked participants, "on a scale of 1–10, 1 being, I have just wasted my life working in a dysfunctional organization, with little achieved and few positive outcomes and 10 being I loved every minute of my career and would do it all again" most answered above 7 or 8.

Post-traumatic growth theory (Tedeschi & Calhoun, 2006) offers an alternative model to encourage and promote resilience among police officers and others who routinely confront trauma as they perform their duties. According to some researchers (Bistoen, 2016; Brewin, 2003; Douglas & Wodak, 2016; Huddleston et al., 2006; Kates, 2008; McFarlane, 2011; Rees & Smith, 2008; Seligman, 2012; Young, 1997), frequent encounters with traumatic incidents are now seen as an almost inevitable precursor to a post-traumatic stress disorder diagnosis particularly for first responders, including police officers. Professor Alexander McFarlane put this very clearly as quoted by Belinda Neil (2014) in the opening page of her autobiography, "Even the healthiest individuals will become unwell when exposed to enough trauma" (McFarlane, 2011; Neil, 2014). What constitutes "enough trauma" is not clearly defined but almost all of the 50 officers interviewed for this research were aware of the perils of PTSD but also described an awareness of the possible benefits of their chosen career. Most were well and enjoyed their duties. Most had learned to distance themselves appropriately from scenes of death and carnage. Most recognised that their careers had changed them in positive ways, and most recognised positive outcomes, professional development and an overall sense of achievement. What would constitute a critical traumatic incident

A. Paterson, *Trauma and Resilience in Contemporary Australian Policing*,
https://doi.org/10.1007/978-981-16-4416-0_10

for civilians had little long-term impact on them. Their "assumptive world" (Janoff-Bulman, 1989) included an acceptance of the need to process other people's trauma as being external to them and allowed them to remain "well" even when exposed to "enough" trauma. This is post-traumatic growth, not disorder. This, in the context of my interviews the literature review and discussion, is a more positive contribution to knowledge in the field of policing and post-traumatic growth.

Post-traumatic growth is defined as, "The experience of positive psychological change, reported by an individual as a result of the struggle with trauma or any extremely stressful event" (Calhoun et al., 1999:22). This theory is central to US Military "wellness and resilience" programmes (Seligman, 2012) and has been explored in this study in terms of its potential to encourage cultural change in police training and operational management.

Police Officers in Australia and elsewhere serve in a wide variety of functions including patrol duties, traffic enforcement, special task groups who respond to armed offenders and critical incidents, court prosecutors, criminal investigation (Detective) duties, family violence and child protection investigations, prosecutions and the administration of restraining orders, crime prevention, community policing, youth justice, crime scene investigation, responding to sudden deaths in the community and many other activities that could be described as welfare work and information giving. As Gilmartin (2002) notes, police are trained to be hyper-vigilant and are armed with hand-guns and an array of other equipment to immobilise and restrain offenders. They have the power of life and death over their fellow citizens should situations arise where they have to protect the safety of themselves or members of society. Their shift rosters operate in 4- and 7-day blocks, requiring constant alterations of their body clocks. Most police officers are to varying degrees socially isolated due to their police role, many socialising with colleagues when rosters permit rather than civilian friends and relatives. Police culture and the nature and pace of their work impact negatively and positively on the well-being of police officers. These are structural and cultural factors that simply go with "the job". Officers interviewed for this research were all aware of the stressors of their chosen profession and were particularly cognisant of post-traumatic stress disorder that is a possible outcome of their constant exposure to trauma. A Detective Brevet Sergeant described how she and her partner, a civilian, attended a party where, as part of a game he was asked, "What is your partner's greatest fear?" He answered without hesitation, "PTSD". She commented, "He was absolutely right, although we had never discussed it". Most officers interviewed were very aware of PTSD, very few had heard of post-traumatic growth. In order to understand this, it has been necessary to explore the history of PTSD[1] and the way in which the condition has come to dominate the awareness of soldiers and "first responders" including police.

Post-traumatic growth theory is closely related in the literature to resilience research in the context of continual exposure to trauma. Resilience is the ability to deal with adversity and "bounce back", post-traumatic growth theory goes further arguing that exposure to significant trauma, be it the result of illness, natural disaster

[1] See Chap. 9 "PTSD and policing".

or man-made misfortune can result in personal growth. Post-traumatic growth theory (PTG) has evolved from the pioneering work in this field of Richard Tedeschi and Lawrence Calhoun (Tedeschi & Calhoun, 1995). At the heart of PTG is the assumption that there are possibilities for human growth and positive change as a result of traumatic experiences. Religions including Buddhism, Christianity and Islam feature the theme of suffering being ennobling and character building at the very least. Researchers within the fields of psychology, social work, counselling and psychiatry have in the last 50 years conducted qualitative and quantitative research, including Caplan (1964), and Frankl (1968) seeking to establish the "possibility of positive outcomes arising from the encounter with negative events" (Tedeschi and Calhoun 2006). This is seen by these theorists and others as a direct contrast to the gloomy and foreboding predictability of much of the PTSD literature (McFarlane, 2011; Morris, 2015; Rivard et al., 2002; Violanti, 2014; Violanti & Paton, 2006; Young, 1997). This was well represented for me after the 1983 Ash Wednesday Bushfires when Dr Sandy McFarlane, a then fledgling psychiatrist, predicted a rise in child abuse and domestic violence in communities directly affected by the disaster (Unknown: "Border Watch" September 1983). In addition, many of those diagnosed with PTSD, identify with the diagnosis as a life-long condition (Endersby, 2004).

Tedeschi and Calhoun (2006) go to great lengths to explain that their post-traumatic growth approach does not ignore the pain and loss associated with trauma encounters and that from their perspective, traumatic responses and PTG can and do co-exist simultaneously (Shakespeare-Finch & Lurie-Beck, 2014). The "Post-Traumatic Growth Inventory", an instrument developed by Tedeschi and Calhoun (1996) sets out to measure and quantify positive as well as negative outcomes in areas including a changed perception of self, relating to others, (greater intimacy and compassion) changed philosophy of life, (spiritual change) new possibilities, (a deeper appreciation of life) and an observed increase in personal strength (feeling personally stronger and more resilient). At the centre of this discussion is the assumption that a particular cognitive engagement with the traumatic event may enable an individual to "reframe or normalise" what has happened in terms of a different world view compared with that held before the challenge of the crisis. "Rumination" is essential to this process, this being defined as "persistent thoughts about one's symptoms of distress and the possible causes and consequences of those symptoms" (Tedeschi & Calhoun, 1996).

Nolen-Hoeksema cited in Calhoun and Tedeschi (2006:10) further defines this concept as "thinking that revolves around resolving discrepancies of thinking and making sense of one's previous goals and self and one's current reality". PTG encourages a different view of the impact of trauma, which is a far cry from much PTSD-related literature, which focuses on damage and the negative impact of a diagnosis (Wastell, 2005). This fits as well with the similarities between the positive psychology movement and PTG as well as the strengths perspective of contemporary social work described above. This is particularly relevant to a study of those whose profession inevitably leads to traumatic exposure and promises to cast a more positive and encouraging light on their experiences in terms of long-term health and career satisfaction.

Chopko and Schwartz (2013:10) explored this possibility in a quantitative study concluding that the 183 police officers who filled out a questionnaire at roll call before commencing their duties recognised, "a greater appreciation of their lives, a positive contribution to their close relationships, an increased sense of personal strength in accomplishment and in some, enhanced spiritual beliefs" as a result of their law enforcement activities.

Padhy et al. (2015) in another quantitative study surveyed two groups of police officers the first having less than 10 years' experience in "the job" and the other more than 10 years. Using the term "psychological well-being" as an alternative to PTG, the researchers concluded that optimism about life and police work was a feature more often found in those having longer years of service. They noted as well, that qualities including acceptance, (of change and challenge) a sense of contribution to society through policing, coherence and integration (with colleagues) personal growth (PTG?) self-acceptance and the ability to accept and deal with the trauma inflicted by the organisational aspect of policing, were positive outcomes resulting from dealing daily with societal and individual trauma.

Middleton (2016:134) defines PTG or "flourishing" (Seligman, 2012) in terms of "an individual as an essentially creative entity, moving toward self-actualisation". Middleton refers to his study of survivors of the Herald of Free Enterprise Ferry disaster of 1987 where 47% of those who had lived through the disaster acknowledged that their lives "had changed for the better" as a result of the trauma they had suffered. "PTG" claims Middleton, "is an independent, valid and measurable phenomenon" (p. 135).

Tedeschi and Calhoun have refined their post-traumatic growth theoretical approach since their first publication in 1995 which dealt with "Trauma and Transformation". Their "positive changes in the aftermath of crisis" (1998) included applying the theory to broader experiences such as natural disaster and conflict. Further work (Calhoun and Tedeschi, 1992, 1999 and 2013) changed the focus to the validation of the theoretical PTG by clinical research (Shakespeare-Finch et al., 2014; Shakespeare-Finch, 2013) and applied further scholarship to the application of the theory to clinical practice. The latter always accompanied by prolific case studies illustrating strategies to facilitate PTG through inclinical settings. In "Facilitating posttraumatic growth- a clinician's guide" (1999), the authors provide an alternative to "burnout" and "vicarious trauma" responses in helping professionals, placing emphasis on the privilege and outcomes involved for "expert companions" rather than the perils of spending too much time professionally close to those suffering as a result of traumatic experience.

Morris (2015:252) in his chapter entitled "Growth" describes his first encounter with PTG theory, "Tedeschi's research has led him to a stunning conclusion: post-traumatic growth is far more common than post-traumatic stress disorder". This conclusion reached in the context of the continuing growth in the numbers of veterans and first responders (including police) who are being diagnosed with PTSD as a direct result of their experiences seems to fly in the face of contemporary popular media and clinical research. The cohort of Vietnam Veterans as well as those of the conflicts in Iraq and Afghanistan in the USA and elsewhere are now almost universally identified with PTSD (Bannink, 2014; Bistoen, 2016; Harms, 2015; Hinton & Good, 2015; Jones & Wessely, 2005; Joseph, 2012; Neocleous, 2012; Rogers, 2008; Seligman, 2012; Violanti, 2006; Young, 1997). The recent last minute cancellation by the Vietnamese Government of a ceremony to celebrate the 50th anniversary of the battle of Long Tan was likely to cause setbacks in the mental health of many Australian Vietnam veterans, according to the President of their Association, citing the group's well-recorded vulnerability to PTSD (ABC TV news: August 17, 2016). Morris goes on to express his initial reservations about "the idea that telling someone that trauma might actually be good for them seemed morally outrageous" (p. 259) and recalls that during his long treatment regime for PTSD within the US Veteran's Affairs programmes, "only a very few occasions where any sort of growth oriented thinking was encouraged", (p. 263) and wonders as a result "whether PTSD becomes a sort of self-fulfilling prophecy".[2]

The real possibilities of more positive trauma-related outcomes are revealed in a significant study by David Alexander, "Debriefing and body recovery: police in a civilian disaster" (in Raphael and Wilson, Eds. 2000) which is described in detail in Chapter 5 "Coping". This is a clear example of the effectiveness of appropriate debriefs and support for operational police under very challenging circumstances, which led to positive outcomes for those involved.

10.1 Post-traumatic Growth in the Interviews

Many of those interviewed recognised how their policing career had a positive impact on their lives. Pride in their vocation, a recognition of achievements and personal growth were often mentioned. Some whilst conducting their own well-being research found comfort in post-traumatic growth theory (Tedeschi & Calhoun, 1995). Attesting to such an experience of post-traumatic growth and the positive side of difficult police experiences one officer said, "When you have had bad experiences, hopefully you can learn from them. I should have been more affected than other coppers. My own experience of family tragedy helped me deal with victims".

A Senior Constable of almost 40 years of service was philosophical and forthright referring to the positives of his career said, "You're a policeman aren't you? I can only tell you this it's a magnificent career, a moral thing to do. It's such good fun!" It is difficult to reconcile the predictions of the damage done during a police career by exposure to trauma (McFarlane, 2011) with such enthusiasm particularly the reference to policing as "fun". This officer had nothing but enthusiasm for what he had achieved and experienced despite significant career-related experiences of tragedy, trauma, grotesque death and loss typical of most long police careers. This is resilience, optimism and post-traumatic growth writ large.

[2] See also Seligman (20122).

Making a contribution, making a difference and "giving something back", as well as the security of a well-deserved pension, all point to a positive view on the part of one of the officers interviewed. Said a retired Commissioned officer who served in Major Crime homicide investigations, "It's a very good career where you are able to give something back, I have been fortunate with my health and have a very good pension". This is in summary of a long career during which this officer moved out of major crime investigations because he recognised unwelcome impacts on his well-being into a less stressful role. Such a move was not the result of departmental intervention, but rather his own self-taught awareness of early signs of stress-related issues.

The successful outcome of investigations and the development of investigative competence as well as the process of reaching those outcomes, is also a potent protective factor for many. A Detective senior Sergeant put this aspect clearly, "In terms of the investigations, I want to find out why, I'm curious, I want to use my skill set, I want to be challenged. I am continually testing myself, it's all about our skills". This is a very positive view of policing from an officer involved in the investigation of sexual offences against children. Here the focus is clearly not on the hazards of such a career, rather on the challenges and positive outcomes. Again, clear indicators of growth, not disfunction.

Optimism not dwelling on negative experiences and a sense of career accomplishments were also identified as important indicators of good health, resilience and well-being among long-serving officers, "It has been everything I wanted and more, everything I expected… I dwell on the good things. If reincarnated I would do it all again. I love my job. I don't look forward to change but I don't think I have ever struggled in the job". A very long-serving female Senior Constable said, "I felt really good about what I had achieved after a while". The expression of her career in terms of her expectations around it being fulfilled, embracing the chance to do it all again and a strong sense of achievement are all present here. "Dwelling on the good things" is an almost textbook definition of resilience and optimism in the midst of significant and continual challenge (Schiraldi, 2011).

At the centre of post-traumatic growth theory, (Tedeschi and Calhoun, 2006, Chopko, 2010, Violanti, 2006, Padhy et al., 2015, Burke and Shakespeare-Finch, 2011, Burns et al, 2008, Middleton, 2016) is the capacity to view traumatic experiences positively, interpreting them as a contribution to learning and competence. An officer talked of such a relationship between building positively on sometimes negative experiences and outcomes, "you handled it, you got through it. You develop character through experience". Another was equally clear about the source of his personal and professional well-being, "Helping others helps me. I enjoy my life, friends and family". This being a clear indication of this officer's capacity to transfer positive aspects of policing into the personal sphere, "my life".

A Senior Constable in a training role had clearly thought about the personal benefits of her service, "I wouldn't be the person I am without all these challenges". Another reflecting on his 35 years of service was quite specific, "I see all this as post-traumatic growth". These two officers are clearly indicating what

Tedeschi and Calhoun (2005) and others have researched to confirm their post-traumatic growth theories. Recent research (Shakespeare-Finch & Lurie-Beck, 2014; Shakespeare-Finch et al., 2014) into the validity of the Post-traumatic Growth Inventory (Tedeschi & Calhoun, 1996) reflects comments similar to these from others who have experienced trauma and growth simultaneously.

Frequent references during my interviews to the importance of "camaraderie" to well-being and growth identify this as an important factor in growing through trauma. Many officers referred to the usually unspoken assurance that "Camaraderie is very important. We get to know each other well and that helps {cope with the stressors}". A Senior Constable, looking back on her long career and its challenges, said, "I have done some amazing things and enjoyed some fantastic camaraderie". A high ranking officer, referring to the most challenging experiences, added, "The troops rally around in difficult situations, comradeship comes out".

Four of the officers interviewed in my research were members of SAPOL's elite "Special Task and Rescue" group. STAR group is the frontline of policing in South Australia, being called upon in situations where armed offenders are posing a significant threat and where rescues and body retrieval are required. They are a very close knit group, and display a well-developed, informal peer support structure which becomes evident in challenging situations. Text messages of encouragement flow between on and off duty STAR group members after difficult taskings and informal debriefs are conducted. Said one officer, "You're into overtime, have a bit of a chill. We are all bonding. Off-loading without being judged". Another added, "We talk about things in a casual way after a big job". The intention within this group is to grow into the job and become more skilled, not to be damaged by it.

10.2 What Have We Learnt? Post-traumatic Growth and Policing

Post-traumatic growth theory and practice (Calhoun & Tedeschi, 2014) offers the possibility that trauma-related duties may have a positive effect on officer's well-being, enhancing "wellness" and resilience. The 50 interviews conducted with operational and retired officers, as well as those undertaken with psychiatrists and psychologists who had worked with them, confirmed that possibility. Despite the constant contact with death and societal mayhem, the majority of officers interviewed were well, enjoyed "the job", had a positive view of what they achieved and scored highly on the 1–10 scale of satisfaction. They were, however, aware of the scourge of PTSD and some felt threatened by the prospect of a sudden accumulated trauma response that might be beyond their control. The interviews shone a light on coping and resilience that revealed the importance of accumulating experience of confronting trauma in the context of a culture of support ("camaraderie") that is passed down from generation to generation of operational police. Put simply, officers either develop the capacity to cope, to distance themselves from horror, (referred to in the interviews as the "personal shield") or leave the job for less confronting alternatives.

Calhoun and Tedeschi (1996) cite Janoff-Bulman's (1989) concept of the importance of an "assumptive world" with regard to the consequences of individual experiences of traumatic events. Those who believe that the world is a safe place, that life is fair, that bad things only happen to other people who in some way deserve their fate, are often, according to Janoff-Bulmann likely to become anxious, depressed and traumatised by sudden, unexpected exposure to traumatic events. Police officer's assumptive worlds are not those of civilians. They have constant contact with death, violence and anti-social behaviour. They are trained to accept negative operational outcomes, their operational experience encourages hyper-vigilance (Gilmartin, 2002) and their confrontations with horror and trauma are usually expected by them as part of "the job". It is only the occasional operational event, for example, the death of a child or attendance at a fatal road crash involving a friend or family member that challenges their assumptions. In the context of post-traumatic growth and a duty related assumptive world, operational resilience may well be more predictable than a PTSD diagnosis. Police learn to expect bad things to happen and even over a 30-year operational career should be expected to develop resilience rather than PTSD. A typical SAPOL officer's assumptive world according to my interview data might be expressed thus:

> I expect to encounter death, violence and victimisation regularly. Most of the people I deal with on a daily basis are either criminal, non-functional, addicted, and self-destructive or victims of violence and oppression. I don't expect that most members of the public I deal with as a copper will respect me or the uniform. I can rely on my police colleagues (at my level) for support when I need it. SAPOL (the bosses) don't have my best interests at heart, don't trust my professionalism, have their own departmental and personal agendas and have forgotten what it's like to be operational. I expect bad things will happen to good people who don't deserve that fate. Sometimes I will encounter situations involving victims of violence, accident or other tragedies that will get through my protective shield. If I encounter such problems as a result of the job, I will need to find solutions myself. I need to take care of my own mental and physical health. I will be lucky if I get through my career without some trauma related issues. The people closest to me inside and outside "the job" are very important if I am to stay well. Despite all this, I love my job!

10.3 Future Research Possibilities

SAPOL, like many other Australian and International police organisations, is facing the challenge of maintaining the mental health of its officers like never before in its history. Reviews conducted by external authorities, (Cotton, 2016; Marin, 2012; Moss, 1999) independent research into policing and stress (Elntib & Armstrong, 2014; Flannery, 2015; Violanti & Paton, 2006; Woodberry, 1987) and the stories told by officers of their own isolated struggles with trauma (Henry, 2004; Horner, 2011; Mckay, 2005; Neil, 2014; Rogers, 1999; Sparkes, 2013) add up to a climate for change that is almost irresistible. Police Associations (unions) across Australia and elsewhere are adding to the clamour to dispense with the "tough it out" approach to policing and to listen to the voices of those at the centre of law enforcement. Early intervention, psycho-education, effective debriefs, peer support and easy access to counselling and support both internal and external are well and truly on the agenda. Changes in police recruitment and training to focus on resilience, optimism, physical and mental fitness are also prominent in this conversation. This is where the future of police health lies. Queensland Ambulance Service's "Priority One, Staff Support Services"(Wehr et al., 2017) provide a model for organisational reform in just this context.

I argue that police officers are not the hapless, slow-moving ignorant targets, of inevitable PTSD diagnosis, (McFarlane, 2011) but rather thoughtful, well-researched individuals whose sense of duty encourages them to adopt measures that contribute to their long-term well-being. Many are aware of the hazards of their profession and that leads to levels of anxiety that could be ameliorated with easy and encouraged departmental access to information and support as well as supervision that is provided by middle managers trained to detect early signs of trauma and access to resources to deal with them.

The typical "assumptive world" (Janoff-Bulman, 1989; Tedeschi & Calhoun, 1998) of a police officer encourages resilience in the face of trauma rather than PTSD. This should be at the centre of encouraging senior police management to embark upon the reforms outlined above in the interests of those they employ to keep society safe.

References

Bannink, F. (2014). *Post traumatic success: Positive psychology & solution-focused strategies to help clients survive & thrive.* WW Norton & Company.

Bistoen, G. (2016). *Trauma, ethics and the political beyond PTSD: The dislocations of the real*, Springer.

Brewin, C. (2003). *Posttraumatic stress disorder: Malady or myth?* Yale University Press.

Burke, K. J., & Shakespeare-Finch, J. (2011). Markers of resilience in new police officers: Appraisal of potentially traumatizing events. *Traumatology, 17*(4), 52–60.

Burns, C. M., et al. (2008). The emotional impact on and coping strategies employed by police teams investigating internet child exploitation. *Traumatology, 14*(2), 20.

Calhoun, L. G., & Tedeschi, R. G. (2014). *Handbook of posttraumatic growth: Research and practice.* Routledge.

Calhoun, L. G., et al. (1999). *Facilitating posttraumatic growth: A clinician's guide.* Routledge.

Caplan, G. (1964). Principles of preventive psychiatry.

Chopko, B. A., & Schwartz, R. C. (2013). The relation between mindfulness and posttraumatic stress symptoms among police officers. *Journal of Loss and Trauma, 18*(1), 1–9.

Cotton, P. (2016). Victoria Police Mental Health Review. An independent review into the mental health and well-being of Victoria Police employees. Australia.

Elntib, S., & Armstrong, T. (2014). Critical incidents' impact on front-line South African police personnel in light of the current briefing and debriefing strategies. *South African Journal of Psychology, 44*(4), 416–425.

Endersby, J. (2004). *Monsters in the dark.* Trafford Publishing.

Flannery, R. B. (2015). Treating psychological trauma in first responders: A multi-modal paradigm. *Psychiatric Quarterly, 86*(2), 261–267.
Frankl, V. E. (1968). *Man's search for meaning: An introduction to logotherapy*. Washington Squarer Press.
Gilmartin, K. M. (2002). Emotional survival for law enforcement. *ES Press, PMB, 233*, 2968.
Henry, V. E. (2004). *Death work: Police, trauma, and the psychology of survival*. Oxford University Press.
Hinton, D. E., & Good, B. J. (2015). *Culture and PTSD: Trauma in global and historical perspective*. University of Pennsylvania Press.
Horner, P. (2011). *Jack Knife: The crashing of a policeman- NSW police and PTSD*. Australia, Zeus Publications.
Huddleston, L. M., et al. (2006). Conceptualizing traumatic stress in police officers: Preemployment, critical incident, and organizational influences. *Traumatology, 12*(3), 170–177.
Janoff-Bulman, R. (1989). Assumptive worlds and the stress of traumatic events: Applications of the schema construct. *Social Cognition, 7*(2), 113–136.
Jones, E., & Wessely, S. (2005). *Shell shock to PTSD: Military psychiatry from 1900 to the Gulf War*. Psychology Press.
Joseph, S. (2012). *What doesn't kill us: A guide to overcoming adversity and moving forward*. Hachette UK.
Kates, A. (2008). *Copshock: Surviving Post Traumatic Stress Disorder (PTSD)*. Holbrook Street Press.
Marin, A. (2012). In the line of Duty. Ombudsman's report. Ontario, Canada.
McFarlane, A. C. (2011). *Many paths, one purpose. Expert forum*. Australian Centre for posttraumatic mental health.
Mckay, E. (2005). *Crime Scene-True stories from the life of a crime scene investigator*. Viking (Penguin) Australia.
Middleton, H. (2016). Flourishing and posttraumatic growth. An empirical take on ancient wisdoms. *Health Care Analysis, 24*(2), 133–147.
Morris, D. J. (2015). *The evil hours: A biography of post-traumatic stress disorder*. Health Affairs.
Moss, I. (1999). Officers under stress: A special report for Parliament under section 31 of the Ombudsman's Act. New South Wales, Australia.
Neil, B. (2014). *Under siege*. Australia: Harlequin Mira.
Neocleous, M. (2012). "Don't Be Scared, Be Prepared" Trauma-anxiety-resilience. *Alternatives, 37*(3), 188–198.
Padhy, M., et al. (2015). Optimism and psychological well-being of police officers with different work experiences. *SAGE Open, 5*(2), 2158244015580852.
Rees, B., & Smith, J. (2008). Breaking the silence: The traumatic circle of policing. *International Journal of Police Science & Management, 10*(3), 267–279.
Rivard, J. M., et al. (2002). Acute dissociative responses in law enforcement officers involved in critical shooting incidents: The clinical and forensic implications. *Journal of Forensic Science, 47*(5), 1–8.
Rogers, L. K. (1999). *PostTraumatic Stress Disorder: A police officer's report*. Proctor Publications.
Rowe, A., & Regehr, C. (2010). Whatever gets you through today: An examination of cynical humor among emergency service professionals. *Journal of Loss and Trauma, 15*(5), 448–464.
Schiraldi, G. R. (2011). *The complete guide to resilience: Why it matters how to build it and maintain it*. Resilience Training International.
Seligman, M. E. P. (2012). *Flourish: A visionary new understanding of happiness and well-being*. Simon and Schuster.
Shakespeare-Finch, J., & Lurie-Beck, J. (2014). A meta-analytic clarification of the relationship between posttraumatic growth and symptoms of posttraumatic distress disorder. *Journal of Anxiety Disorders, 28*(2), 223–229.
Shakespeare-Finch, J. E., et al. (2014). Promoting posttraumatic growth in police recruits: preliminary results of a randomised controlled resilience intervention trial. In *2014 Australian and New*

Zealand Disaster and Emergency Management Conference: Book of Proceedings-Peer Reviewed. Association for Sustainability in Business Inc.
Sparkes, A. (2013). *The cost of bravery*. Penguin Group, Australia.
Tedeschi, R. G., & Calhoun, L. G. (1995). *Trauma and transformation: Growing in the aftermath of suffering*. Sage Publications.
Tedeschi, R. G., & Calhoun, L. G. (1996). The posttraumatic growth inventory: Measuring the positive legacy of trauma. *Journal of Traumatic Stress, 9*(3), 455–471.
Tedeschi, R. G., & Calhoun, L. G. (1998). *Posttraumatic growth: Positive changes in the aftermath of crisis*. Routledge.
Tedeschi, R. G., & Calhoun, L. G. (2006). Expert companions: Posttraumatic growth in clinical practice. In *Handbook of posttraumatic growth: Research and practice* (pp. 291–310).
Violanti, J. M. (2006). The police: Perspectives on trauma and resiliency.
Violanti, J. M. (2014). *Dying for the job: Police work exposure and health*. Charles C Thomas Publisher.
Violanti, J. M., & Paton, D. (2006). *Who gets PTSD?: Issues of posttraumatic stress vulnerability*. Charles C Thomas.
Wastell, C. (2005). Understanding trauma and emotion: Dealing with trauma using an emotion-focused approach.
Wehr, T. E. M., Priority One, staff support services, Queensland Ambulance Service. (2017). *Priority One*. Queensland, Australia, Australian Society for Traumatic Stress Studies.
Woodberry, J. M. (1987). An examination of stress in the police force. South Australia.
Young, A. (1997). *The harmony of illusions: Inventing post-traumatic stress disorder*. Princeton University Press.

Chapter 11
Conclusions: Policing and Growth

This research sprang from a career-long interest in policing and a close professional association with police officers over a 35-year period. At the centre of my professional experience has been a focus on trauma, working with domestic violence survivors and perpetrators, homicide victim's families, victims of natural disaster and offenders in a prison setting. I shared this environment with police officers whose everyday tasks put them into situations of threat and danger as well as the necessity of confronting death, violence and societal mayhem. In the early 1980s, the first DSM was published, describing post-traumatic stress disorder as diagnosed in troops returning from the Vietnam War. At the time, I argued that it seemed unreasonable to diagnose this cohort, who had seen and been involved in a particularly ugly conflict, with a disorder upon their return. It appeared to me that their response was a "normal" reaction to a profoundly "abnormal" and traumatic experience. As my police-oriented career unfolded, I became interested in how my sworn colleagues dealt with their career challenges. I was and am fascinated by their apparent capacity to cope, to stay well, to "bounce back" and continue their duties and commitment to "the job" over many years, in the context of an organisation (SAPOL) that has at best a hands-off approach to their mental well-being.

I began my research by reviewing autobiographical accounts written by police officers who had retired "hurt on duty" from their careers after a PTSD diagnosis. Each account described their individual descents into high states of anxiety, sleep disturbance, depression, hyper-vigilance avoidance and other symptoms described in the Diagnostic Statistics Manuals (American Psychiatric Association, HYPERLINK "sps:refid::bib1|bib2") which in the 1980s focussed on military trauma but by the twenty-first century included "first responders" in the cohort of those who may be negatively impacted by the experiences central to their duties. The autobiographies had one common thread. In all cases, the police organisations who employed them showed no interest in their mental health, assuming that they would cope with the challenges of their occupation alone without support. This stems from the traditional masculine policing culture of "toughing it out" showing no emotion, simply dealing with the challenges of their careers.

A. Paterson, *Trauma and Resilience in Contemporary Australian Policing*,
https://doi.org/10.1007/978-981-16-4416-0_11

I chose therefore to research resilience and began the 50 officer interviews with the expectation that the career stories told would mirror those of the autobiographies. They did not. The aims of this research have been fulfilled with unique input from the 50 officers interviewed and the six clinicians who added their insights to the outcomes sought in my research. The data are rich and offer the opportunity for those involved to suggest changes that may encourage resilience rather than pathology as SAPOL members careers unfold.

11.1 The Significance of My Research

My professional history with SAPOL offered a rare opportunity to conduct qualitative police research examining in depth and detail how these officers have coped with the trauma-related challenges of their careers in the organisational context characterised by "command and control" management. I am familiar with police culture and with the organisation and am comfortable with the language and structures of policing. I am not an "outsider" and was not perceived by those interviewed as an academic. In line with Winlow's (2001) experience researching "Badfellas", I had access to police officers that very few (if any) academic researchers could have gained. I shared with Winlow "a detailed knowledge of the culture, my continued contacts within it, my age" (p. 12). From the outset, I had very strong support from the police union in South Australia (PASA) who showed little concern when SAPOL's Research and Survey Co-ordinating Committee denied approval for the conduct of the study. The questions that my interviews were intended to address (albeit indirectly) were "how has policing changed you?" and "How have you coped?"

11.2 How My Findings Connect with Earlier Work in Policing and Stress

The trauma literature traces the development of the PTSD diagnosis from "shell-shock" and "battle fatigue" of world wars one and two to the post-Vietnam period and beyond. The emphasis of much of the general research is on how the diagnosis has developed and been applied beyond war and conflict to other trauma related human experience such as that of police and first responders such as fire and ambulance officers. Much of the literature has a profoundly negative focus on the perils of trauma in such settings, much is predictive of the inevitable ill effects of such duties. Professor Alexander McFarlane puts this argument very clearly: "Even the healthiest individuals will become unwell when exposed to enough trauma" (McFarlane, 2011:1; Neil, 2014). What constitutes "enough trauma" is not defined but almost all of the 50 officers interviewed for this research were aware of the perils of PTSD and also described an awareness of the possible benefits of their chosen career (Morris,

2015; Seligman, 2012; Tedeschi & Calhoun, 1995; Young, 1997). Most were well and enjoyed their duties. Most had learned to distance themselves appropriately from scenes of death and carnage. Most recognised that their careers had changed them in positive ways, and most recognised positive outcomes, professional development and an overall sense of achievement. What would constitute a critical traumatic incident for civilians had little long-term impact on them. Their "assumptive world" (Janoff-Bulman, 1989) included an acceptance of the need to process other people's trauma as being external to them and allowed them to remain "well" even when exposed to "enough" trauma. This is post-traumatic growth, not disorder. These interviews, the literature review and discussion, is my original contribution to knowledge in the field of policing and posttraumatic growth.

The 50 in depth interviews and those with the six psychiatrists and psychologists provided a unique insight into the careers of the Police Officers and to the views of the clinicians who treat and assess them. Compared with the Faull and Loftus ethnographical approach (Faull, 2017; Loftus, 2009) which relied on conversations had while shadowing Police Officers on shift these were detailed, long conversations that ensured that SAPOL officer's voices were clearly heard in a context unique in South Australian policing.

11.3 The Limitations of My Research

Participants may have been "resilience enthusiasts" and not typical of SAPOL members who were attracted to the project to display and discuss their achievements in this area. It was decided not to ask officers interviewed to fill out either the short PTSD checklist (PCL) (Weathers et al., 2013) or its posttraumatic growth equivalent (Tedeschi & Calhoun, 1996), the PTG inventory, in the interests of maintaining a qualitative approach and maintaining the conversational tone of the interviews. Furthermore, interviews were not held with life partners of officers due to issues raised by Flinders SABS ethics committee.

The lack of approval for the project from the SAPOL RSCC may have limited input from SAPOL Executive management regarding innovations made in this area after my interviews with members concluded. Very few young officers (recent graduates from the academy) were interviewed.

11.4 Future Research

Partners of serving officers, if interviewed, would offer triangulation of—or dissonance to—their partners' resilience self-assessments. Interviews with executive-level SAPOL management and EAP psychologists and Social Workers could be conducted to further triangulate data. Emphasis on the value of Mitchell model CISD and its application in SAPOL review impact on those receiving debriefs and those who do not. Retirement is a significant issue for Police Officers, particularly after a long career in the front line. Research into their experience of such a significant change would be of great interest.

11.5 Resilience: The Themes that Emerged from the Interviews and Their Significance for Existing Theory

SAPOL's approach to organisational management and leadership was a frequent theme. Unlike much of the trauma and policing literature which focuses on duty-related stressors such as death, threat and violence, my interviewees revealed that the officers found SAPOL management approaches and the culture of management and leadership much more challenging. The psychologists and psychiatrists interviewed were even more forthright offering a unique insight into what one described as a "toxic psychological culture", characterised by managerialism, bullying a lack of trust and excessive management of risk. This is of great significance to the field of study, reinforcing those researcher's views (Paton, 2009; Shane, 2010; Stinchcomb, 2004) that a change of focus when assessing sources of stress in policing is timely.

The benefits and drawbacks of SAPOL culture were also a constant theme from my interviews. Policing culture is important to the operational resilience of individual officers in that they are aware that they are a "family", share and understand each other particularly when experiencing out of the ordinary operational experiences. Female officers in particular, rather than being more at risk of traumatic responses as some literature suggests, (Blok & Brown, 2005; Brough, 2016) are more likely to confide in each other and receive support when stressed, than their male colleagues, who a more constrained by macho expectations.

The history of women in SAPOL, how they entered the uniformed cohort in 1974 and how they overcame opposition from their male colleagues to fully engage in their duties and become part of the culture of "the job" is characterised by the profound impact of bullying and harassment and worse. The progress they have made in terms of their influence on organisational culture, the impact they have had on culture and practice testifies to their courage, tenacity and resilience. The female officers interviewed were clear that systemic discrimination, bullying and harassment had been a major challenge to their careers as police officers. This was also true of their perceptions of organisational responses to female parents in the organisation placing restrictions on opportunities for service and promotion. Some change is apparent, but this research and the voices of these female officers add urgency to the need for change.

The impact of death and bodies and other challenging tasks on individual officers revealed coping mechanisms that are not negative avoidance but rather learned and effectively enabling of resilience. This research reveals in detail the strategies officers use to create emotional distance between themselves and potentially distressing scenes of death, grotesque injury and the intense emotional responses of victims of crime or accident. Such mechanisms are often characterised as "avoidance" by some researchers, (Elntib & Armstrong, 2014; Flannery, 2015; Green, 2004; Kates, 2008; Kroes, 1976; Ménard & Arter, 2013; Moss, 1999; Nievas, 2015; Peters, 2009; Rees & Smith, 2008; Stone, 1999; Toch, 2002; Violanti, 2014) that at best offer only a temporary reprieve from the impact of trauma. My interview cohort, many with decades of experience, thought otherwise.

The interviews also revealed coping strategies that work for police in terms of their off duty lives. Many officers described in detail the strategies they have developed to create distance from their duties especially when they are off duty. It was important for many to undertake actions that symbolise and represent that distance, such as changing clothes when leaving for home, showering either before departing from work or immediately when arriving at home. Developing an off duty identity by volunteering at their children's school, at service and sporting organisations, not carrying a warrant card when off duty and cultivating and maintaining non-police friendships were prominent and contribute significantly to such strategies described by quantitative research in the field.

Asking for (seeking) help while operational, the critical importance of timely and early intervention when officers show signs of trauma, is often highlighted in policing literature but very rarely in the detail described by my interviewees. They described a reluctance to seek internal support from the SAPOL Employee Assistance Programme, largely because "it leaks" and could pose a threat that could be career ending. Many officers had arranged private resources outside of the organisation, at their own expense to meet such needs.

The importance of effective, regular and sustaining sleep was also a common theme expressed by officers interviewed. Many were aware that sleep disturbance is a significant symptom of PTSD and either described strategies they used to ensure sustaining sleep or to deal creatively with its absence. Some described temporary sleep disturbance after, e.g. a confronting homicide scene, which passed with time and reflection. Much research in this area focuses only on sleep disfunction or the negative impact on sleep patterns of long-term shift work.

Is PTSD a potential epidemic that threatens the careers and mental health of SAPOL members? Is a diagnosis or a "sub-threshold" response inevitable for long-serving police officers? All those interviewed displayed a significant knowledge of PTSD. Some had observed colleagues who had "broken" and wondered why, some had experienced periods when they were "near the edge" some had conducted their own research into symptoms, others through media and other conversations were anxious about the possibility of the build-up of stress from career experiences suddenly overwhelming them. Again, this level of detail goes beyond the data extracted from quantitative research, which often utilises inventories to obtain such information to a personal/professional expression of an anxiety, which has never been addressed by SAPOL. Simple psycho-education, embedded in routine training and information sessions would do so.

Post-traumatic growth is a completely different expectation! Many officers expressed high levels of satisfaction with the achievements of their careers in policing, as well as signs of personal growth, optimism and skill. Some described their career as "fun", many as "a moral thing to do" all in response to a "1–10" satisfaction question, scored highly. This was a profound contrast to much of the literature predicting dire and inevitable negative consequences of a career in policing. Optimism among officers interviewed was not uncommon as they described their careers as challenging but profoundly fulfilling. A common reason given for such an unexpected response was the importance of culture, camaraderie and the police family.

11.6 What is "Resilience" in Policing? Where Does It/Should It Come from?

Resilient police officers are able to turn up to undertake their shifts ready for whatever may occur. Many of the officers I interviewed expressed their enthusiasm for the unpredictability of their duty related experiences, and for the challenges around exercising their considerable power and discretion responsibly. Their "assumptive world" (Janoff-Bulman, 1989) is built as their experience of policing grows, as they build on their training and benefit from the wisdom passed down from their senior colleagues. Their resilience is developed as they encounter "out of the ordinary experiences" such as the death of a person they unexpectedly identify with or series of challenging events such a fatal motor vehicle accidents or sudden infant deaths that happen close together. Resilient officers develop the capacity to resist the temptation of cynicism about human nature and maintain an optimistic view of their duties and the world despite disappointing outcomes and their often negative experiences of leadership and management. Resilient officers recognise that SAPOL "won't take care of them" and therefore develop coping strategies of their own, often located outside of the organisation. Resilient officers have a clear perspective on the difference between their on and off duty lives and cultivate strategies to maintain that difference. They realise the importance of their families to their well-being unlike some of their colleagues who were in different times, "married to the job". They learn from negative experiences in relationships at work and at home. They recognise the importance of what they do and enjoy the professional culture that sustains it. Their levels of resilience largely come from within themselves and their close colleagues and not from the organisation's executive leadership and management. If SAPOL executive management was prepared to consider some basic, inexpensive innovations in dealing with duty and management-related trauma, through early intervention and prevention strategies, they would be able to simultaneously improve their image and relationship with those below them and save considerable expenditure on Workcover (work-related injury insurance) and mental health issues. I outline some strategies emerging from my research, below which may assist.

11.7 Recommendations: (Implications of My Findings for SAPOL and Other Police Organisations.)

1. The police academy/recruiting and training syllabus should develop an increased emphasis on self-care and resilience training. This should include a clear focus on the inevitable challenging experiences of a career in policing, and how to stay well.
2. Women should be encouraged to remain in the job by a practical focus on anti-discrimination and the prevention of harassment and bullying as recommended in recent reviews. Female officers who have children while serving should not be discriminated against as a result. PASA should ensure that the recent gender-related reviews of SAPOL should achieve permanent, identifiable and positive outcomes for women officers.
3. Sergeants should be trained to undertake early detection of mounting trauma reactions and offer peer support and training and critical incident debriefs to their teams. They should also be equipped to offer information to team members about confidential referrals to outside support agencies. This should ensure cultural change around asking for help penetrating deep into the organisation.
4. Support services external to SAPOL should be available in complete confidence to members as they are in other organisations. Confidential access to support services will greatly reduce the present reluctance among officers to seek timely help for trauma related issues.
5. Psycho-education and resilience training throughout the SAPOL career should become a priority as is IMOST for operational members. This will greatly reduce anxiety among members with regard to the perceived threat of a PTSD diagnosis. This should be compared with the recent distribution of the "Head Notes" booklet to SAPOL members, which predicted that they had a 25% chance of a PTSD diagnosis.
6. Resilience training for cadets and operational members should be delivered by peers as in the US Army (Seligman, 2012) and the Queensland Ambulance Service (Wehr et al., 2017).
7. Debriefs after carefully defined critical incidents "outside of the officer's ordinary experience" should be mandatory for all operational members and should be followed up appropriately over a following time span to ensure the resilience and well-being of those involved.
8. Although the distribution of self-help and mental health information such as "Head notes" and "A cop in the family" (Carroll, 2017, 2018) and the provision of "Emotional survival for law enforcement" lectures (Gilmartin, 2002) are well intentioned, they must not be seen as an alternative to departmental initiatives and policy that ensures access to meaningful support and resilience resources for SAPOL officers. Such responses continue to locate the responsibility for their mental with individual officers and ignore the necessity for radical change in police management and leadership, a major stressor for most police officers.

9. Executive management training in SAPOL, beyond the present "command and control" approach where the focus of management is ensuring compliance rather than people management (Chapin et al., 2008; Hanson & McKenna, 2011; Parsons et al., 2011; Pearson-Goff & Herrington, 2013) is critical to the well-being of police members. There is a clear necessity to increase person management skills through access to external management training for existing and aspiring SAPOL commissioned officers.
10. There is neither a PTSD epidemic in SAPOL nor the prospect of one. Police Officers in South Australia should enter and remain in the profession with the expectation that they will be supported by SAPOL to stay well, not that PTSD is an inevitable outcome of their career choice. Much of trauma and policing literature reviewed in my research encourages such an expectation that may contribute to the higher likelihood of a diagnosis. The recent "Head notes" (Carroll, 2017) distribution and the accompanying media response "Fight for our force: The black cloud that hangs over our police" (Kemp, 2017) were not helpful in this regard. What is required is an organisation and cultural response to these issues, not pamphlets and guest lectures.
11. Trauma information and psycho-education sessions for partners, wives and boy/girlfriends of SAPOL officers should be offered as an option to encourage "Family survival for law enforcement". As indicated above, effective support mechanisms are crucial to resilience and well-being, the family in whatever form is a crucial source of such support. Care, however, should be taken to ensure that family members are not drafted by SAPOL to become "whistle blowers" in terms of early symptoms but rather individuals who are better placed to offer effective support at critical points of their family member's career.
12. A significant number of the officers I interviewed for this research were retired from SAPOL, some recently. Most were coping with their transition as one put it from "a busy, highly experienced and competent Major Crime Detective Sergeant to a golfer!" At retirement, as the Police Journal describes it, the "last Shift" much more should be offered than the present physical examination. A competent career debrief, not unlike my interview format would be a very good start.
13. The role of the Police Association of South Australia (the Union) is crucial to change. They and their national police union colleagues are very aware of resilience issues as indicated by their support of my research in the context of SAPOL's refusal to grant permission for the research to proceed. The potential impact of PASA, for example, on the cultural reluctance of officers to seek timely support and regular mental health "checkups" is immense as is their opportunity to counsel SAPOL executive management to change the focus of their present "command and control" management to what Cotton (2016) calls "people oriented leadership". With the addition of contemporary management theory into its training arsenal, SAPOL could achieve such a change in the next decade.

Police organisations across the globe are notoriously resistant to change and challenge (Scraton, 1985; Sparrow, 2016) particularly when it involves a significant rethink of long held cultural beliefs and practices. The officers interviewed for this research were crystal clear about the need for radical change in the way they are supported, managed and lead. They take good care of themselves but realise that thus far SAPOL takes little care of them. These are not a disgruntled minority, most have a very strong commitment to "the job" and enjoy being police officers. Their well-being and resilience up until now have been their responsibility, particularly the women who were interviewed have had their resilience tested by decades of bullying, harassment, disadvantage and worse. Recent reports and research (Jenkins, 2015; Paterson, 2014; Vincent, 2016) make a similar future impossible. Police leaders must act on all these issues to ensure that their members are supported and encouraged by competent, well-trained people-focussed mangers, peers such as their Sergeants who are trained to offer them debrief and early intervention to ensure their resilience. The 13 recommendations above are not the result of academic thought bubbles but represent the voices of the officers who gave their time and career experience to this project. Here is an opportunity for SAPOL to avoid a potential crisis and to take the lead into a new era of policing where resilience and growth are more common than disorder and anxiety.

References

American Psychiatric Association. (1980). *Diagnostic statistics manual of mental disorders*. USA: American Psychiatric Pub.

American Psychiatric Association. (2013). *Diagnostic and statistical manual of mental disorders (DSM-5®)*. American Psychiatric Pub.

Blok, D., & Brown, J. (2005). *The gendered nature of policing among uniformed operational police officers in England and Wales*. Department of Psychology: School of Human Sciences, University of Surrey, November.

Brough, P. (2016). Women in policing: Exploring challenges associated with career progression and related health and well-being impacts. South Australia, Police Health.

Carroll, M. (2017). "Head notes" A social and emotional well- being/mental health initiative for South Australian police officers. Police Association of South Australia. Adelaide: SA Government and SAPOL.

Carroll, M. (2018). "A cop in the family" Police Association of South Australia. Adelaide: SA Government and SAPOL.

Cotton, P. (2016). Victoria Police Mental Health Review. An independent review into the mental health and well-being of Victoria Police employees. Australia.

Chapin, M., et al. (2008). Training police leadership to recognize and address operational stress. *Police Quarterly, 11*(3), 338–352.

Elntib, S., & Armstrong, T. (2014). Critical incidents' impact on front-line South African police personnel in light of the current briefing and debriefing strategies. *South African Journal of Psychology, 44*(4), 416–425.

Faull, A. (2017). *Police work and identity: A South African ethnography*. Routledge.

Flannery, R. B. (2015). Treating psychological trauma in first responders: A multi-modal paradigm. *Psychiatric Quarterly, 86*(2), 261–267.

Gilmartin, K. M. (2002). Emotional survival for law enforcement. *ES Press, PMB, 233*, 2968.

Green, B. (2004). Post-traumatic stress disorder in UK police officers. *Current Medical Research and Opinion, 20*(1), 101–105.

Hanson, R., & McKenna, P. F. (2011). Respectful leadership: The emergence of upward nobility as a way of life in policing. *Policing, 5*(4), 287–299.

Janoff-Bulman, R. (1989). Assumptive worlds and the stress of traumatic events: Applications of the schema construct. *Social cognition, 7*(2), 113–136.

Jenkins, K. (2015). Independent review into sex discrimination and sexual harassment, including predatory behaviour in Victoria Police. Victoria, Australia: Victorian equal opportunity and human rights commission.

Kates, A. (2008). *Copshock: Surviving Post Traumatic Stress Disorder (PTSD).* USA: Holbrook Street Press.

Kemp, M. (2017). Fight for our force: The black cloud that hangs over our police. The Advertiser. Adelaide: South Australia.

Kroes, W. H. (1976). *Society's victim, the policeman: An analysis of job stress in policing.* IL: Thomas Springfield.

Loftus, B. (2009). *Police Culture in a changing world.* UK: Clarendon Studies in Criminology.

McFarlane, A. C. (2011). *Many paths, one purpose. Expert forum.* Australian Centre for posttraumatic mental health.

Ménard, K. S., & Arter, M. L. (2013). Police officer alcohol use and trauma symptoms: Associations with critical incidents, coping, and social stressors. *International Journal of Stress Management, 20*(1), 37.

Morris, D. J. (2015). *The evil hours: A biography of post-traumatic stress disorder.* Health Affairs.

Moss, I. (1999). Officers under stress: A special report for Parliament under section 31 of the Ombudsman's Act. New South Wales, Australia.

Neil, B. (2014). *Under siege.* Australia: Harlequin Mira.

Nievas, V. (2015). Posttraumatic stress disorder and police officers. *Australian Police Journal, 69*(4).

Parsons, A., et al. (2011). Effective policing: Management influence and the commitment of senior police personnel. *Policing & Society, 21*(1), 1–26.

Paterson, K. (2014). Modern, motivated, progressive and professional? Flexible work practices and the retention of female members in SAPOL. *Australasian Policing, 6*(1), 21.

Paton, D. (2009). *Traumatic stress in police officers: A career-length assessment from recruitment to retirement.* Charles C Thomas Publisher.

Pearson-Goff, M., & Herrington, V. (2013). Police leadership: A systematic review of the literature. *Policing* pat027.

Peters, R. F. (2009). *Police under pressure (A donkey on the edge).* HEAS Publications

Rees, B., & Smith, J. (2008). Breaking the silence: the traumatic circle of policing. *International Journal of Police Science & Management, 10*(3), 267–279.

Scraton, P. (1985) *The State of the police.* Pluto Pr.

Seligman, M. E. P. (2012). *Flourish: A visionary new understanding of happiness and well-being.* Simon and Schuster.

Shane, J. M. (2010). Organizational stressors and police performance. *Journal of Criminal Justice, 38*(4), 807–818.

Sparrow, M. (2016). *Handcuffed: What holds policing back, and the keys to reform.* Brookings Institution Press.

Stinchcomb, J. B. (2004). Searching for stress in all the wrong places: Combating chronic organizational stressors in policing. *Police Practice and Research, 5*(3), 259–277.

Stone, V. (1999). *Cops don't cry: A book of help and hope for police families.* Creative Bound.

Tedeschi, R. G., & Calhoun, L. G. (1995). *Trauma and transformation: Growing in the aftermath of suffering.* Sage Publications.

Tedeschi, R. G., & Calhoun, L. G. (1996). The Posttraumatic growth inventory: Measuring the positive legacy of trauma. *Journal of Traumatic Stress, 9*(3), 455–471.

Toch, H. (2002). Stress in policing. *American Psychological Association Journal.*

Vincent, N. (2016). Sex discrimination, sexual harassment and predatory behaviour in South Australia Police. Independent review. South Australia: Equal Opportunity Commission.

Violanti, J. M. (2014). *Dying for the job: Police work exposure and health.* Charles C Thomas Publisher.

Weathers, F., et al. (2013). *The PTSD checklist for DSM 5 (PCL-5).* National Centre for PTSD.

Wehr, T. E. M., Priority One, staff support services, Queensland Ambulance Service. (2017). *Priority one, staff support services.* Australian Society for Traumatic Stress Studies.

Winlow, S. (2001). *Badfellas: Crime, tradition and new masculinities.* Bloomsbury Academic.

Young, A. (1997). *The harmony of illusions: Inventing post-traumatic stress disorder*. Princeton University Press.

Appendix A
Information Sheet for Police Participants

Professor Fiona Verity.

School of Social and Policy Studies.

Flinders University.

GPO Box 2100.

Adelaide SA 5001.

Fiona.verity@flinders.edu.au.

"Resilience in policing".
Information sheet for Police participants

Academic Supervisors:

Professor Fiona Verity and Professor Willem De Lint, Flinders University.

Researcher: Mr Andrew Paterson, PhD Candidate, Flinders University.

Dear Sir or Madam,

I write to invite you to participate in a research project where Police members will be interviewed by Andrew Paterson, a PhD student from the School of Social and Policy Studies at Flinders University. This study is being supervised by me, Professor Fiona Verity, and Professor Willem De Lint, Flinders University.

A. Paterson, *Trauma and Resilience in Contemporary Australian Policing*,
https://doi.org/10.1007/978-981-16-4416-0

The project:

The purpose of the research is exploring "resilience" among Police Officers:—how they have dealt with the challenges of policing. Retired members will also be interviewed.

In particular, Andrew is researching how exposure to the trauma encountered in the day to day events of Policing is handled by members and the organisation and how members might stay healthy on the job.

The interviews will be relaxed and completely confidential in a location either at the Police Association offices, Flinders University or a place of your choice. The Police Association is very supportive of this project.

Participation in the research will be confidential.

Your role in this:

In an interview with Andrew that may last up to 1 hour, tell the story of your police service with regard to your experiences around traumatic and potentially stressful incidents encountered on the job. Andrew may ask clarifying questions as you speak with him. No questionnaires will be involved. You are, of course, entirely free to discontinue your participation at any time or to decline to answer particular questions.

\\userOP\P\PATE0010\prefs\Desktop\Info sheet for Policing research January 2015.doc

Updated 28 June 2006

The consent process.

Andrew will ask you to fill in a consent form once he has explained the process to you prior to the interview.

Are there any risks or discomforts if I am involved?

Telling your career story may bring back memories of experiences you found difficult and confronting. If these memories are a problem, the interview will be terminated and arrangements made, if you require them, for you to receive independent support from a qualified professional. Lifeline can be contacted on 13 11 14 and beyond Blue on 1300 22 4636. Both services are free.

Contact details

Andrew can be contacted on (Mob.) 0434187249 or email: Andrew.paterson@flinders.edu.au.

Privacy and confidentiality:

The notes taken by Andrew during the interview will be sent to you for your approval of their accuracy before they are used in the research thesis. The thesis itself will not identify participants in any way. Your participation in the interviews will not be disclosed to SAPOL management or your colleagues. Notes of the interviews will not include your name. The electronic records of interview notes will be password protected. No voice recordings will be taken.

How the conclusions and recommendations will be published:

The final PhD thesis will, after examination, be available on the University website. Electronic copies will be available to participants on request. Hard copies will be provided to SAPOL management.

Possible benefits to Policing in South Australia:

This research is focused on understanding the stresses of the job, and how they are dealt with, from the perspective of Police Officers. This study will examine ways that you and your colleagues can be encouraged to stay healthy based on your experience, and that of police organisations in Australia and overseas. Management's role in that process will also be examined. Andrew is basing his research on post-traumatic growth theory, which unlike PTSD places the focus on how confronting trauma might also contribute to growth as a professional law enforcement officer, as well as growth in other areas of life. Police organisations and associations in Australia are aware of issues like these. This study may well encourage change where it is needed.

Any enquiries you may have concerning this project should be directed to me at the address given above or by telephone on (08) 82013437 or e-mail fiona.verity@flinders.edu.au

Thank you for your attention and assistance. Yours sincerely

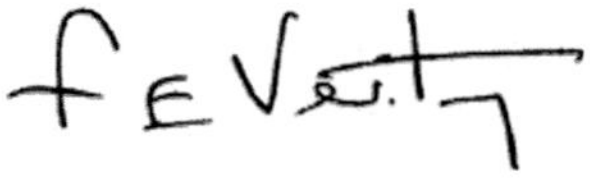

Professor Fiona Verity

Appendix B
PASA Support Letter

POLICE ASSOCIATION OF SOUTH AUSTRALIA

27 Carrington Street
Adelaide SA

PO Box 6032
Halifax Street
SA 5000

T (08) 8212 3055
F (08) 8212 2002
www.pasa.asn.au

MC:ah 7101/12

18 August 2015

Associate Professor Lorna Hallahan
Chair
Social & Behavioural Sciences Research Ethics Committee
Flinders University
GPO Box 2100
ADELAIDE SA 5001

Dear Associate Professor

I write in respect of Phd. Candidate Andrew Paterson's research dealing with resilience among police in Australia.

The Police Association of South Australia (PASA) is an organization that represents the professional and industrial interest of its members, drawn exclusively from sworn members of all ranks of the South Australia Police. Membership is voluntary and currently we represent some 99.3% of sworn members of SA Police.

PASA is registered pursuant to the *Fair Work Act* as a trade union. By its own rules, PASA is a non-sectarian and apolitical organization.

The primary purpose of PASA is to promote the interests of the members of the police service by all means consistent with the rules.

The welfare of our members is a primary concern.

Having considered Andrew's higher degree research proposal, the association is pleased to support Andrew in his endeavours. To that end, we will inform our members of the research and encourage their participation.

The *Police Journal* – our flagship publication – will publish a letter from Andrew inviting contact by our members and we will write a 'news story' for publication on our member only website to promote Andrew's research.

Yours sincerely

MARK CARROLL
PRESIDENT

ABN 73 802 822 770

A. Paterson, *Trauma and Resilience in Contemporary Australian Policing*,
https://doi.org/10.1007/978-981-16-4416-0

Appendix C
SAPOL Research and Survey Committee Letter

29 June 2015

Mr. Andrew Paterson,
9 Belvedere Court
Aberfoyle Park SA 5159.

Dear Mr. Pateron,

Subject: Resilience among police in Australia: Cops aren't authorised* to *be traumatised!

Thank you for your request to the South Australia Police Research and Survey Coordination Committee (RSCC) regarding the above matter. I wish to advise that your request was considered by the RSCC at its meeting on 11 June 2015.
After careful consideration of your proposal, I regret to inform you that the RSCC is unable to approve your application. The proposed field of work has already being considered internally to be undertaken within the organisation.

While we cannot assist you on this occasion, the Committee wishes you well in future post- graduate research endeavours. Should you have a new proposal for research, you are welcome to supply it for new consideration.

Yours sincerely,

Phil Hoff
Superintendent
Officer in Charge
Strategy, Policy
and Programs
Section.

A. Paterson, *Trauma and Resilience in Contemporary Australian Policing*,
https://doi.org/10.1007/978-981-16-4416-0

Appendix D
Information Sheet for Psychiatrists and Psychologists

School of Social and Policy Studies.
Flinders University.

GPO Box 2100.

Adelaide SA 5001.
Fax: + 61 8 xxxx xxxx.

Fiona.verity@flinders.edu.au.
CRICOS Provider No. 00114A.

Information Sheet for Psychiatrists and Psychologists.
"Resilience in Policing" Research Project.

Academic Supervisors: Professor Fiona Verity and Professor Willem De Lint, Flinders University.
Researcher: Mr Andrew Paterson, PhD student, Flinders University.

Dear Sir or Madam,

I write to invite you to participate in a research project where Police members will be interviewed by Andrew Paterson, a PhD student from the School of Social and Policy Studies at Flinders University. This study is being supervised by me, Professor Fiona Verity and Professor Willem De Lint, Flinders University.

A. Paterson, *Trauma and Resilience in Contemporary Australian Policing*,
https://doi.org/10.1007/978-981-16-4416-0

Description of the study:

You are invited to participate in a research project focusing on "resilience" among Police Officers:—how they have dealt with the challenges of Policing. This study is being conducted by Andrew Paterson, a PhD student from Flinders University..

Purpose of the study:

The study is exploring how exposure to the trauma encountered in the day to day events of Policing is handled by members and the organisation, and how members might stay healthy on the job. In particular, the project seeks to explore the utility of employing Post-Traumatic Growth in Police organisations as a means to respond to stress and trauma.

What will I be asked to do?

You will be asked to take part in an interview that will last no more than an hour. Andrew is particularly interested in the nature of any professional contact you might have had with serving or retired Police Officers. This will be completely confidential in a location either at Flinders University, or a place of your choice.

What benefit will I gain from being involved in this study?

The sharing of your experiences will contribute to knowledge about future responses to trauma and stress experienced through the course of police work, and how resilience can be enhanced.

Will I be identifiable by being involved in this study?

We do not need your name and you will be anonymous. Once the interview has been typed-up and saved as a file, the notes will then be destroyed. Any identifying information will be removed and the typed-up file stored on a password-protected computer that only the researcher (Mr Andrew Paterson) will have access to. Your comments will not be linked directly to you.

Are there any risks or discomforts if I am involved?

The investigator anticipates few risks from your involvement in this study. If you have any concerns regarding anticipated or actual risks or discomforts, please raise them with the investigator.

How do I agree to participate?

Participation is voluntary. You may answer "no comment" or refuse to answer any questions and you are free to withdraw from the interview at any time without effect or consequences. A consent form accompanies this information sheet. If you agree to participate please read and sign the form and send it back to the researcher at Andrew.Paterson @flinders.edu.au.

How will I receive feedback?

The notes from your interview will be summarised and given to you by the investigator if you would like to see them and check them for accuracy.

Any enquiries you may have concerning this project should be directed to me at the address given above or by telephone on (08) 82013437or e-mail fiona.verity@flinders.edu.au.

Thank you for your attention and assistance.

Yours sincerely.

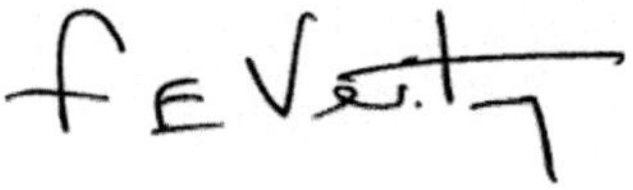

Professor Fiona Verity

This research project has been approved by the Flinders University Social and Behavioural Research Ethics Committee (Project number 6684). For more information regarding ethical approval of the project, the Executive Officer of the Committee can be contacted by telephone on 8201 3116, by fax on 8201 2035 or by email human.researchethics@flinders.edu.au